SUBSTANCE ABUSE PREVENTION

A Multicultural Perspective

Edited by
Snehendu B. Kar

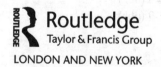

Routledge
Taylor & Francis Group

LONDON AND NEW YORK

First published 1999 by Baywood Publishing Company, Inc.

2 Park Square, Milton Park, Abingdon, Oxfordshire OX14 4RN
52 Vanderbilt Avenue, New York, NY 10017

Routledge is an imprint of the Taylor & Francis Group, an informa business

First issued in paperback 2018

Library of Congress Catalog Number: 98-47889

Library of Congress Cataloging-in-Publication Data

Substance abuse prevention : a multicultural perspective / edited by
  Snehendu B. Kar.
      p.   cm.
   Includes bibliographical references (p.   ) and index.
   ISBN 0-89503-194-9 (cloth)
     1. Substance abuse - - United States - - Prevention.   2. Children of
  minorities - - Substance use - - United States.   3. Minorities - - Substance
use - - United States.   I. Kar, Snehendu B.
HV4999.2.S795   1999
362.29'17'0973 - - dc21   98-47889
                                                                                     CIP

ISBN 13: 978-0-89503-194-5 (hbk)
ISBN 13: 978-0-415-78471-9 (pbk)

"When races come together, as in the present age, it should not be merely the gathering of a crowd; there must be a bond of relations, or they will collide with each other."

Rabindranath Tagore, in "On Education,"
Talks in China (Visva Bharati), 1925

Nearly seventy years later, the 1992 Los Angeles civil unrest once again proved how prophetic Tagore was. This book is dedicated to those who are committed to promoting our understanding and quality of life of multicultural societies.

SBK
Los Angeles, 1998

Foreword

I am delighted to be a participant and a supporter of the initiative that led to this volume. Three recent trends underscore the significance of this timely review. First, substance abuse prevention has emerged as a national priority with the recognition that cigarette smoking and alcohol consumption are major contributors to the three leading causes of death and disability among Americans: cancer, heart disease, and stroke (McGinnis and Foege, 1993). It is estimated that alcohol and other drug abuse costs American taxpayers about seventy billion dollars each year in preventable health care costs, law enforcement, auto accidents, crimes, and lost productivity (USDHHS, 1997).

Second, as the field of public health matured, a new paradigm of public health emerged in response to our changing patterns of death and disability and the need for population-based prevention interventions in partnership with the community (Afifi and Breslow, 1994). Improved standards of living, along with successful public health campaigns of the past decades that applied innovations in medicine, have eradicated or effectively controlled many infectious diseases that were leading causes of death and disability in the earlier part of this century. We now face new sets of threats to our lives against which we do not have medically effective preventive measures such as vaccines or antibiotics. Aspects of our lifestyles, including the use of tobacco, alcohol, and other drugs, are now among our real leading causes of death and disability. These risk behaviors occur within the larger socio-cultural context of our communities; we need effective population-based strategies to prevent these risk factors. The core of the new public health paradigm consists of three key functions: *assessment* of risks and determinants, *policy development*, and *assurance* of conditions and services necessary for optimal health. This new paradigm of public health, with its focus on population-based disease prevention and health promotion (DPHP) strategies, is a most appropriate modality for substance abuse prevention as well.

Third, communities are becoming increasingly multicultural; in many large metropolitan areas, no single ethnic majority exists. This trend will continue and will lead us to a truly multicultural society. The role of culture on health status, risks, and quality of life has been well documented. But we have yet to fully understand the dynamics of multi-ethnic communities that affect health risks and effective prevention strategies.

For these reasons, we must develop a sound understanding of the determinants of substance abuse prevention in multicultural communities from a public health perspective. Our school of public health is delighted to take a first step in this direction. Our Public Health Practice Office, under the leadership of Professor Snehendu B. Kar, has accepted the challenge of this State-of-the-Art-Review by established researchers and academicians from the disciplines of substance abuse, public health, and related fields, along with community leaders dedicated to substance abuse prevention. As we approach the twenty-first century, our school is committed to remaining at the leading edge of research, teaching, and professional services that are more responsive to the needs of our communities and profession. The lessons learned from this review will be an important force in that endeavor. I am also convinced that this volume would be an important resource to other schools of public health and allied fields, the substance abuse prevention community, policy planners, and the community at large.

Finally, I wish to congratulate and thank the authors of this volume and the participants in this State-of-the-Art-Review process for their dedication and pioneering contributions. We owe our gratitude to the Bureau of Health Professions, Health Resources Service Administration (HRSA) for a Grant that made this project possible; special thanks are due to Mr. Ron Merrill, Captain Berry Stern, and Ms. Anne Kahl of that Bureau for their unqualified support. Last but not least, I wish to acknowledge Professor Kar for providing the leadership for this important project and thank his staff at the Office of Public Health Practice, Ms. Kirstin Chickering, Ms. Felicia Sze, Ms. Shana Alex, and Ms. Darcy Richards, for their dedicated professional support.

Abdelmonem Afifi, Ph.D.
Dean, School of Public Health
UCLA
August 20, 1998

REFERENCES

Afifi, A. and Breslow, L. (1994). The maturing paradigm of public health. *Annual Review of Public Health,* 15:223-235.
McGinnis, J. M. and Foege, W. H. (1993). Actual causes of death in the United States. *Journal of the American Medical Association,* 270(18):2207-2212.
USDHHS: U.S. Department of Health and Human Services (1997). *Substance Abuse— A National Challenge, Prevention Treatment and Research at HHS.* Fact Sheet, December 20.

Acknowledgments

I would first like to thank all the authors who contributed to this work, as well as the other participants of the State-of-the-Art-Review (STAR) Conference on Substance Abuse Prevention, held in September of 1997 at the UCLA Campus. Without their contributions, the issues and ideas that are presented in this volume would not have come so sharply into the public focus. We are thankful also to the Health Resources and Services Administration, Bureau of Health Professions, for making this project possible through a grant from that office. In particular, special thanks to Ron Merrill, Branch Chief, Barry Stern, Program Officer, and the late Anne Kahl, Program Officer; without their support, this project would not have been possible. And we wish to thank Dean Abdelmonem Afifi and Associate Dean Gale Winting for their continuous support of the Office of Public Health Practice and its work within the UCLA School of Public Health.

The UCLA Office of Public Health Practice staff also made invaluable contributions to this work. Special thanks to Felicia Sze, who not only coordinated the entire STAR Conference, but also involved herself heavily in compiling each chapter into the final work. Without her tireless efforts on behalf of this project, it would have been impossible to create this volume. Additionally, thanks to Shana Alex for her editorial assistance during the final phase of preparing the book. Finally, thanks to Kirstin Chickering, Jasmeet Gill, and Cathy Pascual for their contributions to the research and compilation of data for my own chapters.

Last but not least I am deeply indebted to my family, especially to Sanji Kar, for graciously sacrificing countless hours and trips we could have enjoyed together, while I carved out time for this project and to Robin Kar JD, for many stimulating debates which sharpened my own thoughts about equity and ethical imperatives for public health.

This volume represents the first major published book to come out of the UCLA Office of Public Health Practice. We are pleased to have the opportunity to contribute to both the fields of substance abuse prevention and of public health practice in multicultural communities; this work also has implications for the field of empowerment and participatory research. We hope that this book will enrich researchers and practitioners alike.

Contents

PART I
Conceptual and Methodological Issues
in Substance Abuse Prevention

INTRODUCTION

Substance Abuse Prevention State-of-the-Art-Review Project

Snehendu B. Kar and Felicia Sze

Substance Abuse Prevention: A Multicultural Perspective is the outcome of a State-of-the-Art-Review (STAR) project, directed by Professor Snehendu B. Kar at the Office of Public Health Practice of the University of California, Los Angeles School of Public Health. Funding for the commission of these chapters was provided from a grant by the Health Resources and Services Administration (HRSA). The objective of the Substance Abuse Prevention State of the Art Review (STAR) was to carefully review and evaluate available literature and professional expertise in community-based alcohol, tobacco, and other drug (ATOD) prevention in multicultural communities and to draw implications for public health policy, research, teaching, and practice. The emphasis of this project focused on multicultural communities where diverse cultures come into contact and interact to form a new culture, both dynamic and different from each of its parts.

With many works being published in the area of substance abuse prevention, the question may be posed, "Why produce another volume discussing substance abuse prevention?" We consider the following as important books in our field; they are related to our interest but they do not duplicate the scope of this volume:

1. Botvin, G., Schinke, S. and Orlandi, M. (1995). *Drug Abuse Prevention with Multiethnic Youth.* Ságe: Thousand Oaks, CA.
2. De La Rosa, M. and Adrados, J.L.R. (1993). *Drug Abuse among Minority Youth: Advances in Research and Methodology.* National Institutes of Health Publication No. 93-3479.

1

3. Langton, P., Epstein, L. and Orlandi, M. (1995). *The Challenge of Participatory Research: Preventing Alcohol-Related Problems in Ethnic Communities.* Department of Health and Human Services Publication No. (SMA) 95-3042.
4. Sussman, S. and Johnson, C.A. (1996). Drug abuse prevention: Programming and research recommendations. *American Behavioral Scientist,* 39(7).

However, this new volume addresses contemporary issues that are not addressed in these works: (1) this volume concentrates on a public health paradigm with an emphasis on primary prevention rather than treatment or secondary prevention, (2) many of these books focus on individual ethnic groups, with little focus on the unique, multicultural interaction that occurs when diverse ethnic or cultural groups reside together, (3) in addition to the discussions focusing on ethnic issues, the proposed volume on substance abuse prevention has special sections dedicated to specific issues focusing on substance abuse among women and prevention programs targeting women and substance abuse in religious communities, broadening the definition of culture away from just ethnic/racial identities, (4) these works are also mostly dated (before 1995), and (5) this new volume, with the inclusion of recommendations from the workshop, introduces the current issue of community partnership in substance abuse prevention programs, research, and policy.

The STAR initiative is part of the agenda of the Office of Public Health Practice, which is concerned with prevention efforts in multicultural and high-risk communities. The Office of Public Health Practice provides leadership and coordination of activities to make the UCLA School of Public Health more responsive to the needs of our community and profession by establishing practice linkages with health agencies and health departments to fulfill teaching, service, and research functions. In line with the objectives of the Office of Public Health Practice, an alternative focus of the STAR that developed with the workshop in September 1997, was the development of bridges between research, teaching, and community-based entities to form community partnerships to coordinate and track community empowering research projects.

The authors of the chapters were selected in consultation with the Substance Abuse Prevention STAR Advisory Committee for their demonstrated expertise in substance abuse and public health issues and presented their work at the *Substance Abuse Prevention in Multicultural Communities: A Public Health Perspective* workshop at UCLA in September 1997. Representatives from academic and research institutions, community based organizations, and government agencies attended this workshop and contributed to the critique of these chapters. Final recommendations from this workshop on top-ranking priorities in the areas of teaching, research, programs, and policy were developed through consensus in small, breakout sessions. These recommendations were prioritized into the final recommendations from the workshop.

Among the results of the workshop were recommendations for new chapters to fill perceived gaps in the topics covered by the volume. The first additional chapter covered issues from a community perspective and was written by a group of professionals working in substance abuse oriented community based organizations in Los Angeles. The second additional chapter addresses policy issues in regards to substance abuse prevention and is authored by Dr. Ruth Roemer, a former president of the American Public Health Association and an expert in public health law.

This volume is divided into three sections. Section one consists of five chapters that deal with conceptual and methodological issues related to substance abuse research and prevention. The second section consists of four chapters dealing with cultural issues in substance abuse research and prevention within specific ethnic/cultural groups. The third section consists of four chapters; three of these focus on policy and pragmatic issues, while the last chapter presents a summary of key issues and recommendations, including a proposed conceptual model for substance abuse research and intervention in multicultural communities.

The first chapter, authored by Snehendu Kar and Shana Alex, gives an introduction to trends affecting substance abuse and prevention in multicultural communities and to the importance of the new public health paradigm as a major strategy for community based risk prevention and reduction. With a substance abuse problem that affects all communities and the changing demographics of the United States population, the nation is charged with the development and accurate evaluation of well-planned substance abuse prevention programs from a multicultural perspective that emphasize the development of the relationship between research institutions and the community. This chapter outlines some general issues that affect the development of substance abuse prevention efforts in these multicultural communities, including the nature of the health care system, the communication revolution and emergence of media as a risk factor, the importance of community participation and empowerment, and specific areas of concern when working within the public health paradigm in multicultural communities. Kar and Alex discuss a community health improvement model from the Institute of Medicine and its implications for substance abuse prevention, along with the use of participatory research, empowerment, and evaluation in the development of effective prevention programs.

The second chapter, authored by Mary Ann Pentz, et al., provides a conceptual framework for substance abuse prevention work in multicultural communities through the discussion of general and specific issues in planning prevention research in multi-ethnic communities, research methods and conduct, ethnic/racial community considerations, and contraindications to general models of community organization. Conditions are discussed under which the definition of prevention, theoretical assumptions about behavior change, program readiness and planning, role of the researcher, and type of evaluation may differ according to the ethnic status of the community. Studies are summarized for their attention to these conditions. The authors recommend extensive formative evaluation for drug abuse prevention planning, as well as careful attention to the development of appropriate research hypotheses, designs, measures, and analyses.

The third chapter, authored by Gauri Bhattacharya, expands on the role of women and mothers in community-organizing for empowerment and addresses how the empowerment of women can be utilized to prevent substance abuse. This chapter examines the characteristics of cultures that support parents' desires to nurture their children and then to extend these characteristics into the context of community organizing for use as an effective approach to preventing children and adolescents from abusing drugs. The partnership between parents and the community is viewed as instrumental in reducing the demand for (an individual-level factor) and the supply of (a community-level factor) drugs. The author reviews examples of community organizing efforts initiated by women that are based on cultural strengths that honor the values of parental caring and commitment. She develops a conceptual framework by which parents' concerns about drug abuse can be translated into collective actions via the community organizing process. Guided by the cultural competence perspective, this framework is grounded on the relevant research of drug abuse. The author emphasizes that although women are associated with the provision of care, society as a whole should accept and operationalize those values in the context of drug abuse prevention among children and adolescents.

In the fourth chapter, Phyllis Ellickson focuses on school-based substance abuse prevention programs where she describes the prevalence of substance abuse among adolescents, gender and racial/ethnic differences, psychosocial factors contributing to drug use, and the effectiveness of well-known prevention programs, such as the DARE program. This chapter seeks to provide information on what works in drug prevention and how our efforts might be improved. The author also assesses the degree to which drug use, risk factors, and program effectiveness vary across different ethnic/racial groups.

The fifth chapter, authored by Christopher Ringwalt, et al., explores a model of ethnic identity in African-American adolescents and discusses the utilization of the development of ethnic identity as a protective factor in substance abuse prevention programs. With steady increases in the prevalence and severity of adolescent risk behaviors, policy makers and practitioners are more often tailoring prevention programs to the needs of specific populations. In response, Rites of Passage and other ethnic identity development programs that target minority adolescents are proliferating nationally. In this chapter, a conceptual framework by which ethnic identity may be considered a key domain that protects against risk factors is introduced. Also, findings of studies that have investigated the empirical link between ethnic identity, adolescent risk behaviors, and the various risk and protective factors believed to mediate or moderate these behaviors are summarized.

The sixth chapter, authored by Melvin Delgado, deals with cultural issues and addresses substance abuse in the Latino community. This chapter discusses the extent of substance use in the Latino community and provides several examples of prevention strategies that have been used in this community in the past. The chapter consists of five sections that overview approaches toward substance abuse prevention, challenges in defining the problem in the Latino community, substance abuse prevalence data for the Latino community, innovative intervention strategies, and principles for organizing and prevention.

The seventh chapter, authored by Lawrence Brown and Stanley John, discusses the prevalence of substance abuse in the African-American communities, its consequences on the communities, cultural issues, and a brief evaluation of existing prevention efforts. This chapter elaborates on the challenges and theoretical basis for current HIV prevention efforts and looks at the interface between HIV prevention and substance abuse prevention. Brown and John focus on the diverse spectrum of African-American issues pertaining to substance abuse and the social, economic, and medical consequences of substance abuse in these communities.

The eighth chapter, co-authored by Saskia Subramanian and David Takeuchi, addresses the complexity of substance abuse issues in a population as diverse as the Asian/Pacific Islander community and the challenges that present to us for prevention research and practice in these communities. This chapter reviews the past and current research on substance use and abuse among immigrants with a special focus on Asian Americans. Initial findings of this review indicate that this problem is a far more complex issue than previously conceptualized and the authors recommend more systematic work in linking social science theories with methods with program interventions.

Chapter nine, drafted by Kathy Sanders-Phillips, focuses on substance abuse issues among Black and Latina women: the prevalence of abuse in these communities, psychosocial factors that contribute to this abuse, and how these psychosocial factors can be integrated into prevention programs targeting these communities. Existing data indicate that drug use in women is significantly influenced by psychosocial factors including levels of depression, anger, alienation, and powerlessness, as well as social experiences such as exposure to community violence, perceptions of stress, and levels of social support. The author recommends that successful drug prevention programs for women must acknowledge and address psychosocial factors such as experiences of racism, oppression, and ethnic identity that may promote drug use in women, particularly among low-income Black or Latina women.

C. Anderson Johnson authors the chapter that reviews evidence supporting specific ingredients necessary for program effectiveness and discusses the implications for standards for prevention programs. The author reviews tobacco, alcohol, and other drug abuse prevention programs for empirically validated effectiveness, mechanisms of mediation, and implications for public policy. The chapter delineates characteristics of various successful programs, including social influences-based school programs and "comprehensive" community programs. Systematic problems that contribute to poor dissemination and maintenance of STAR prevention programming are discussed and steps for resolution are suggested.

Chapter eleven, by Ruth Roemer, focuses on the policy issues surrounding the issues of tobacco and alcohol abuse prevention. The central theme of this chapter is that effective prevention strategies depend upon a well-coordinated campaign that includes legislation, public health education, and social action for prevention. Drawing the lessons learned from successful alcohol and tobacco prevention initiatives, this chapter analyzes key legislative and social action strategies for reducing both the demand for and the supply of tobacco, alcohol, and other drugs in the community.

Chapter twelve, written by Earl Massey, Raquel Ortiz, and Shana Alex, describes the problems from the perspective of community based organizations (CBOs) working in the field of substance abuse. They discuss the goals of a CBO working within a multicultural community, as well as the methods used to achieve these aims. The authors also review, from their insider's perspectives, the obstacles that prevent substance abuse prevention practitioners to fully fulfill their potential within the community. They conclude with a discussion of how researchers and CBOs can better work together in the future.

The closing chapter, by Snehendu Kar, Kirstin Chickering, and Felicia Sze summarizes overlying themes that are prevalent throughout the different chapters, including diversity in multicultural communities, lack of data/research, generalizability of models and programs developed for one community to other communities or multicultural communities, ethnicity as a proxy for other factors, and policy implications. We refer back to the conference proceedings for recommendations for policy, programs, research, and professional education in the field and discuss the follow-up programs that have grown out of the STAR project. The chapter presents a proposed model for substance abuse prevention that focuses on proximal and distal determinants of abuse and prevention. Additionally, implications for further research, programs, and policies are delineated.

We expect that the unique topics covered in this volume will add to the body of knowledge concentrating on substance abuse prevention in multicultural communities, but we would also like to acknowledge that the findings here have implications beyond simply substance abuse programs. The underlying models and ideologies defined in this volume are translatable into a myriad of different issues facing multicultural communities; as the American population becomes increasingly diverse, these issues will have corresponding increasing importance. We would like to point out that most of these studies have concentrated on school-based programs and may have implications for community-based programs. Because the emphasis of the public health paradigm concentrates largely on early, primary prevention, many public substance abuse prevention programs focus on youths, but this should not preclude us from continuing prevention efforts into adulthood. Additionally, we have touched on issues of gender and religion, but feel that both these realms within multiculturalism need to be further explored.

We are at a critical junction in the formation of an age of a multicultural nation with a unique interface of diverse cultures, giving the United States the exciting opportunity to step forward and take this challenge to make our nation stronger and healthier. With a public health perspective, focusing on primary prevention, we hope that communities and researchers can utilize the information we have compiled in this volume in order to work together to provide for a substance-free future.

PART I

Conceptual and Methodological Issues in Substance Abuse Prevention

CHAPTER 1

Public Health Approaches to Substance Abuse Prevention: A Multicultural Perspective

Snehendu B. Kar and Shana Alex

This chapter has two aims: first, to review the major socio-cultural trends that constitute the ecological environment that affects community based substance abuse prevention interventions, and second, to review the contemporary public health paradigm which provides a framework for effective community based substance abuse prevention policy and interventions. Specifically, the chapter reviews the following trends as they relate to substance abuse prevention: (1) substance abuse as a public health threat, (2) changing health needs and the health care system, (3) demographic imperatives and multiculturalism, (4) communication revolution and risks, and (5) the new public health paradigm: risk-reduction from a multicultural perspective. Implications of these trends for substance abuse prevention are discussed.[1] The subsequent chapters in this volume address specific research and intervention issues as they related to various domains of substance abuse prevention.

SUBSTANCE ABUSE AS A PUBLIC HEALTH THREAT

Substance abuse (alcohol, tobacco, and other illicit drug abuse) is a major threat to public health as it causes significant adverse effects on health and

---

[1] Due to space limitation we do not discuss several important trends and events which may affect health of populations, but do not directly affect substance abuse; these include environmental hazards, political and economic turmoil, global warming, natural disasters, and war and famine.

quality of life of Americans. According to a recent study, substance abuse kills over fourteen thousand Americans annually (DHHS, 1997a). In 1995, there were 142,164 cocaine-related emergency room episodes alone (National Center for Health Statistics, 1997). Cigarette smoking and other tobacco uses are also major contributors to the three leading causes of deaths among Americans: heart disease, cancer, and stroke (McGinnis and Foege, 1993; National Center of Health Statistics, 1996). The latest data indicate that, for the total population, drug-related deaths increased 23 percent from 3.8 to 4.7 per 100,000, from 1987 to 1996 (DHHS, 1998c). Since 1990, this rate has actually increased 40 percent among Hispanics and 21 percent among African Americans (DHHS, 1998c). It is estimated that alcohol and other drug abuse costs American taxpayers about seventy billion dollars each year in preventable health care costs, law enforcement, auto accidents, crimes, and lost productivity (DHHS, 1997a).

During the last two decades, there has been a decline in the overall use of illicit drugs (see Table 1). In 1996, an estimated thirteen million Americans (or 6.1% of those age 12 years and above) were current drug users; this was about one half of the 1979 peak of 25.4 million current drug users. While the overall rate of drug abuse in the United States has fallen by one-half in the last fifteen years, this positive development is overshadowed by an increase in drug abuse—notably among the youth. Most recent data contained in *Health, United States 1998* (DHHS 1998b, Table 65, pp. 277-278) show increased use of tobacco, marijuana, cocaine, alcohol, and inhalants among adolescents. Among high school seniors,

Table 1. Trends in Selected Drug Use Indicators, 1979-1996
(in Millions of Users)

Selected Drug Abuse Indicators	1979	1982	1985	1988	1990	1991	1992	1993	1994	1995	1996
Any illicit drug use	25.4	N/A	23.3	15.2	13.5	13.4	12.0	12.3	12.6	12.6	13.0
Past month (current) cocaine use	4.7	4.5	5.7	3.1	1.7	2.0	1.4	1.4	1.4	1.5	1.7
Occasional cocaine use	N/A	N/A	7.1	5.1	3.7	3.8	3.0	2.7	2.4	2.5	2.6
Current marijuana use	23.6	21.5	18.6	12.4	10.9	10.4	9.7	9.6	10.1	9.8	10.1
Lifetime heroin use	2.3	1.8	1.8	1.8	1.5	2.4	1.7	2.1	2.1	2.5	2.4
Any adolescent illicit drug use	4.1	2.8	3.2	1.9	1.6	1.4	1.3	1.4	1.8	2.4	2.0

Source: National Household Survey on Drug Abuse, National Institute on Drug Abuse (1979-91), and Substance Abuse and Mental Health Services Administration (1992-1996).

cigarette smoking increased from 27.8 percent in 1992 to 36.5 percent in 1997. Similarly, marijuana smoking in this group has doubled from 11.9 percent in 1992 to 23.7 in 1997. While alcohol use remained steady for five years (51.3% and 52.7% respectively) heavy alcohol use, defined as five or more drinks in a row at least once in two weeks, increased among seniors from 27.9 percent in 1992 to 31.3 percent in 1997. Use of cocaine nearly doubled from 1.3 percent in 1992 to 2.3 percent in 1997. The rates of increase in cigarette smoking, alcohol, and marijuana among female high school seniors were greater than the rates among the males (DHHS, 1998b, Table 65, pp. 277-278). Finally, in the recent year, fewer high school seniors perceived parental and peer disapproval of marijuana, heavy drinking, experimental use of cocaine, and smoking (DHHS, 1998c).

In 1997, 39 percent of high school seniors had reportedly smoked marijuana in the past year (MTFS, 1997). Lifetime use of marijuana among tenth and twelfth graders increased between 1996-1997. Among the twelfth graders, lifetime use of marijuana rose from 44.9 percent in 1996 to 49.6 percent in 1997 (MTFS, 1997). A recent study also reported a significant increase in cocaine use and availability among tenth graders. Tobacco usage also remains a constant problem among American adolescents. In 1996, an estimated 29 percent of Americans, including 4.1 million adolescents between 12-17 years old, were current smokers (MTFS, 1997). Between 1996-1997, cigarette smoking during the past month among twelfth graders (use during past 30 days of interview) also increased from 34 to 36.5 percent. Daily cigarette smoking among the seniors increased to 24.6 percent, the highest level since 1979. It is also disturbing to note that, among the youth, perception of availability of drugs has increased while at the same time perception of harmful effects of drugs has decreased (MTFS, 1997).

Table 2 presents the available data on substance use among adults and students by selected ethnic groups. Available data show significant differences in tobacco use by ethnicity and gender. The differences in alcohol and marijuana use among the students are less pronounced across the three ethnic groups. Against the common ethnic stereotype, African-American students show a significantly lower reported rate of tobacco and marijuana use as compared to the other ethnic groups. Adult African Americans, however, have a rate of overall tobacco use that is slightly higher than Whites, both of which are significantly higher than both Latinos and Asian/Pacific Islander rates of usage. The rates of alcohol usage also show differences among the ethnic groups, with what data is available. While only 43 percent of Hispanics report having at least one drink in the past month, as opposed to the White response rate of 54 percent and Black of 42 percent, Hispanics have a higher rate of binge and heavy drinking than both of the other ethnic groups.

The figures for marijuana usage reveal an important pattern consistent in all the ethnic groups for which data exists; the increase in the rate of usage between eighth to tenth grade far surpassed the change in the rates from tenth to twelfth grade. For White students, marijuana usage jumped 17.5 percent from eighth to

Table 2. Substance Abuse by Ethnicity and Other Subgroups

Categories	Total (%)	White (%)	Black (%)	Hispanic (%)	Asian/Pacific Islander (%)
TOBACCO:					
Use in the last 30 days—					
8th grade[a]	19.4	22.8	10.9	19.1	N/A
10th grade[a]	29.8	34.4	12.8	23.0	N/A
12th grade[a]	36.5	40.7	14.3	25.9	N/A
Use by adult men[b]	N/A	27.6	31.4	27.6	25.1
Use by adult women[b]	N/A	24.4	22.7	15.1	5.8
Overall use by adults[b]	N/A	25.9	26.5	18.9	15.3
ALCOHOL:					
At least one drink in the past month for people age 12+[c]	51	54	42	43	N/A
Five or more drinks on the same occasion in the past month for people age 12+[c]	15.5	16.1	13.1	16.7	N/A
Five or more drinks on the same occasion at least five different times in the past month for people age 12+[c]	5.4	5.5	5.3	6.2	N/A
Used in the past month—					
Men[c]	58.9	61.2	52.3	54.8	N/A
Women[c]	43.6	47.7	33.5	31.1	N/A
OTHER DRUGS:					
Marijuana:					
Use in the last 12 months					
8th grade[a]	17.7	17.8	15.3	21.8	N/A
10th grade[a]	34.8	35.3	28.4	36.8	N/A
12th grade[a]	38.5	38.7	30.4	36.4	N/A
Any illicit drug use:					
Ever used					
Men[c]	40.0	41.6	40.1	32.2	N/A
Women[c]	29.9	32.6	27.0	19.6	N/A

[a]Monitoring the Future Study (1997)
[b]DHHS (1998a)
[c]Substance Abuse and Mental Health Services Administration (1996)

tenth grade, as opposed to a 3.4 percent increase from tenth to twelfth grade. Younger Black students had an increase of 13.1 percent, as compared to a 2 percent increase between the older age groups. While the rate of marijuana usage for Hispanic students rose 15 percent from eighth to tenth grade, it actually dropped .4 percent between tenth and twelfth grade. This overarching pattern does not apply to either the tobacco use data in Table 2 or the data (not shown, since it is not broken down by ethnicity) regarding overall alcohol use, both of which show more constant and slow growth in their usage as the age of the subject increases.

Within a particular ethnic group, significant differences exist between genders and generations. Table 2 shows substance use differences by ethnicity and gender for smoking. Whites have less gender difference in the rate of smoking than other groups, while Asian/Pacific Islanders have a 19.7 percentage point difference in smoking rates between genders. Hispanics and Blacks also show significant gender difference in the rate of smoking, 12.5 percent and 8.7 percent, respectively. Data has also shown that gender differences in regards to alcohol and drug use are significant (see Table 2). Overall, men use both alcohol and illicit drugs at a much higher rate than women. For alcohol, in particular, the ethnic differences emerge across gender divisions. The difference between the rate of usage for White men and women is only 13.5 percentage points, but the difference between Black men and women is 18.8 percentage points. For Hispanics, the disparity grows; the difference between men's and women's alcohol usage in the past thirty days of the interview is a huge 23.7 percentage points. Clearly, while substance abuse is a problem for both genders, in general, men of all ethnicities have this problem more than their female counterparts.

In recognition of these problems, substance abuse prevention has emerged as an important national priority and as a major challenge to those concerned with health and well-being of Americans. The Clinton administration has declared substance abuse prevention a top priority. Under the direction of General Barry McCaffrey, the national Drug Control Policy includes a range of strategies including interdiction, law enforcement, prevention, treatment, research, and public education for substance abuse prevention. According to McCaffrey, "We know that the heart and soul of the nation's counterdrug strategy is to keep our young people from using illegal drugs—particularly marijuana—as well as drinking alcohol and smoking cigarettes" (DHHS, 1997b).

Often substance abuse occurs concurrently with other health and behavioral problems known as the Problem Behavior Syndrome (Jessor and Jessor, 1977). Risk-taking behaviors interact with one another and accentuate their overall adverse effects; frequently one problem may affect other problems (e.g., effects of drunk driving on auto accidents, adolescent substance abuse on problems at school or with law enforcement authorities). Consequently, substance abuse prevention cannot be examined or addressed as an isolated problem. The complex relationships among several problems which occur along with substance abuse present a major threat as well as an opportunity to design and test new paradigms of prevention. While substance abuse seldom occurs in isolation, research and interventions often deal with substance abuse as a separate problem. There is a need for a systems approach which integrates substance abuse within the ecological context in which it occurs.

We need to explore new prevention strategies that are based upon the lessons learned from three distinct but interrelated fields: (1) substance abuse prevention research, (2) the new public health paradigm which focuses on community based comprehensive health risk reduction, and (3) related human service programs, especially education and social welfare.

CHANGING HEALTH NEEDS AND THE HEALTH CARE SYSTEM

Our health risks and health care needs have undergone significant changes as the leading causes of death have shifted from infectious diseases to chronic diseases during the twentieth century. The current ten leading causes of death in the United States are, in the following order: heart diseases, cancer, stroke, chronic obstructive pulmonary diseases, accidents, pneumonia/influenza, diabetes, HIV/AIDS, suicide, and chronic liver diseases including cirrhosis (National Center for Health Statistics, 1996). This list of leading causes of death illustrates two important points. First, almost all of the infectious diseases, which were among the leading causes of death in 1900, are absent on this list. There are still some infectious diseases on this list including a new infectious disease HIV/AIDS, but deaths are now predominantly due to chronic diseases and injuries. Second, while there were effective clinical and medical preventive measures against the old infectious diseases (e.g., vaccinations, antibiotics), this is not true in the case of the current leading causes of death. For instance, there are no vaccinations, antibiotics, or drug that can prevent cancer, cardiovascular diseases, injuries, accidents, and HIV/AIDS. Effective prevention of these leading causes of death can only be achieved through changing personal health risk-taking behavior and social conditions which promote health risks and behavior.

Nearly one-half of current deaths are due to behavior rooted in culturally influenced lifestyles. Two careful analyses of relative affects of four categories of determinants of deaths revealed that about 50 percent of the premature mortality is due to behavior and lifestyles; 20 percent of premature deaths are attributable to genetic factors, another 20 percent to environmental factors, and 10 percent to inadequacies of health care (DHHS, 1980; McGinnis and Foege, 1993). Major lifestyle related risk behaviors that affect premature mortality are tobacco use, unsafe sex, eating habits, sedentary lifestyles, use of alcohol and other drugs, violent and abusive behavior, and risk-taking behavior leading to injury (Lee and Paxman, 1997). A recent analysis of "real causes of deaths" (McGinnis and Foege, 1993) shows that health-risk behavior including tobacco, alcohol, and drug abuse

Table 3. Real Causes of Death, 1990

Cause of Death	Percentage of Total Deaths	Number of People in U.S. that Died
Tobacco	19	400,000
Diet/activity patterns	14	300,000
Alcohol	5	100,000
Microbial agents	4	90,000
Toxic agents	3	60,000
Firearms	2	35,000
Sexual behavior	1	30,000
Motor vehicles	1	25,000
Drug use	<1	20,000

Source: McGinnis and Foege, 1993

are among the "Real Causes of Death" (see Table 3). Thus, it is clear that effective prevention will depend upon our better understanding of behavioral determinants of risks deeply rooted in socio-cultural domain. These lifestyle behaviors are rooted in our culture and occur in socio-cultural contexts; prevention of these risks would have to deal with socio-cultural factors and forces beyond the individuals.

Studies also show that interventions that focus on individuals using a clinical paradigm are grossly inadequate to alter risk-taking behavior. An example is the MRFIT project, perhaps the most expensive intervention ever designed, to modify behavior among high-risk subjects to reduce cardiovascular risks. The MRFIT project, which lasted ten years and at a cost of 180 million dollars, was unsuccessful in producing sustained behavioral changes among a population of patients at high cardiovascular risk (Syme, 1997).

On the other hand, community based campaigns that combined robust communication and health education, along with increased services and social action, have produced significant impacts. Examples include the North Karelia heart disease prevention program in Finland (National Public Health Laboratory of Finland, 1981), child survival program in rural India (Bang, et al., 1990), family planning campaigns in third world nations (Piotrow, et al., 1997; Rogers, 1973), and tobacco control initiatives supported by Proposition 99 in California. This new reality places a sobering challenge on social and behavioral scientists to generate adequate knowledge base for community based prevention intervention.

Our health care system has also undergone a major transformation. The two dominant characteristics of our current health care system are its emphasis on: (1) provision of clinic based personal health services at the expense of community based prevention, and (2) cost containment to protect profit for the medical service providers at the expense of community based preventive care for all. Medical innovations and increased medical services do not necessarily have commensurate impact on health status of population at large. For instance, the United States has the highest per capita expenditure for health care in the world; yet, the health status of Americans as a whole ranks below the European nations and several nations in Asia (DHHS, 1998b). This anomaly is largely due to two reasons: (1) heavy investment on expensive clinical and personal health services at the expense of primary prevention, and (2) inadequate access to health care among high-risk populations including the poor and ethnic minorities (Kar, 1990; Lee and Paxman, 1997). However, the practice of medicine continues to become increasingly specialized, and continues to emphasize clinical and high-tech interventions to treat illness and trauma at the expense of prevention of health-risk behavior (e.g., substance abuse) and changing social conditions that enhance health risks (e.g., accessibility of illicit drugs). Curative care consumed the lion's share of health case costs; primary prevention received frequent lip service but inadequate funding from the legislators and health care organizations alike. For instance, in 1996, of the total of $1,035.1 billion in national health expenditures, only 3.4 percent (or $35.5 billion) was spent on government sponsored public health activities which included community based prevention strategies and 3 percent for research and construction activities. In contrast, 87.6 percent or $907.2 billion was spent for personal health care services (DHHS, 1998b, p. 346). During this phase, health interventions in the United States increasingly focused on individual lifestyle changes to combat the leading health risks (e.g., smoking cessation and prevention, exercise and dieting, seat-belt use, use of condoms/safe sex).

The private sector, especially large employers who are concerned with increasing health care costs, act as the driving force behind the current emphasis on health care cost containment. Strategies used by employers to cut health care costs include shifting costs to employees, eliminating dependents' coverage, and an emphasis on managed care (Lee and Paxman, 1997). The primary goal of managed care, the dominant paradigm of our current medical care, is to save costs by eliminating services which the providers consider unnecessary. This system affects the public in two important ways. First, the decisions about what services are included or excluded are usually made by managed care staff who are interested in cost savings rather than by the physicians who are more interested in patient care. Second, managed care is limited to personal health services and does not support community based disease prevention interventions. Furthermore, the high cost of health insurance leaves a large segment of population, the poor and large proportion of minorities, without access to health care. Nationally, about 15 percent of people are without any health insurance (Lee and Paxman, 1997); the percentage of uninsured is significantly higher among the minority and poor. For instance, in Los Angeles county where no single ethnic group is in the majority, as much as 32 percent of the population is not covered by health insurance; among Latinos, as high as 40 percent are uninsured (Table 4).

Our current health care delivery system is not responsive to primary prevention including substance abuse prevention. Public health, on the other hand, is

Table 4. Ethnicity, Health, and Quality of Life by Selected Indicators
Los Angeles County, California, United States

	Los Angeles	African American	Asian American	Latinos	Whites
Population:					
1990 census	8,863,164	10.6	10.3	37.8	40.8
1997 estimate	9,771,386	9.6	13.3	42.5	34.2
Families below poverty 1990	18.9	30.9	14.1	26.3	12.8
Birth rate 1992 per 1000 people	22.3	22.3	18.8	36.7	10.1
Infant death rate per 1000 live births	7.2	16.2	4.6	6.3	6.9
Student % 1993	100.0	12.1	11.0	54.2	22.5
Public school 1990	100.0	10.6	10.3	37.8	40.8
Graduation: 1992 %	60.0	53.0	88.0	50.0	71.0
High school dropout %	20.4	30.9	14.1	26.3	12.8
Uninsured 1992 %	31.0	20.0	19.0	39.0	15.0
Deaths per 100,000— all causes	509.3	789.6	318.3	420.6	508.6
Heart disease per 100,000	149.7	239.2	97.0	113.6	151.8
Suicides per 100,000	10.3	7.5	5.8	6.0	14.7
Accidents per 100,000	25.2	31.3	14.1	27.4	25.0
AIDS cases in 1992 per 100,000	Males: 101 Females: 6	201 19	23 1	83 7	111 4
AIDS deaths per 100,000	23.6	39.2	3.0	17.9	29.0
Alcohol/drug overdose death— % of drug deaths by ethnicity	100	19.5	N/A	20.6	57.8

Source: United Way of Greater Los Angeles, 1994.

deeply concerned with population based prevention, including substance abuse prevention (see definition of public health mission and the list of ten "Essential Public Health Services" proposed by the Public Health Functions Committee and adopted by all major public health associations and organizations in the nation. Source: Public Health Foundation (1995)). The new public health paradigm advocates in favor of a population based empowerment and prevention strategy in partnership with the public. Consequently, there is a pressing need for the two fields, public health and substance abuse prevention, to join forces for common concerns.

DEMOGRAPHIC IMPERATIVES AND MULTICULTURALISM

According to the 1990 census, Whites comprise 83.9 percent of the national population. When only non-Hispanic Whites are counted, however, that figure drops to 75.9 percent, meaning minorities make up almost one-quarter of the population of the United States; that number will only become larger as the dual effects of increased minority immigration and higher minority fertility ripple through society. In 1995, the Hispanic fertility rate of 2.9 children per woman was considerably higher than the White and Asian/Pacific Islander rate of 1.9 children per woman. Black women also have a lower fertility rate than Hispanics at 2.4 children per woman, but this is still significantly higher than the rate for Whites. At this point, 31 percent of the nation's children belong to a minority group, which illustrates the future capacity for minorities to become a larger proportion of the total population than at present (American Demographics, 1991).

This trend will result in an unprecedented situation in this country, in which intergenerational conflict will cross ethnic lines as the overall elderly population becomes much less diverse than the younger population. Not only was the original population cohort, now the elderly, less diverse to begin with, but as people age, the mortality rate is higher for non-Whites than for Whites. For example, overall life expectancy for Whites is 76.8 years, but only 70.2 years for Blacks (DHHS, 1998b), meaning that the elderly population over seventy will be disproportionately White.

From the historical high of 89.5 percent in 1950, the percentage of non-Hispanic Whites in the population will slip by the year 2050 to comprising only 52.8 percent of the population, according to estimates by the Census Bureau. At that point, Hispanics *alone* will become 25 percent of the total population of the United States, surpassing the percentage of any other minority group (U.S. Census, 1996). Along with this, however, the percentage of Asian-Americans is growing at the fastest rate (U.S. Census, 1990). Although their fertility levels equal that of Whites, their immigration levels will cause Asian/Pacific Islanders to rise from 3 percent of the population in 1990 to a projected 9 percent in 2050 (U.S. Census, 1990), tripling their percentage but actually growing at an even faster rate when looking at raw numbers. Over the last part of the twentieth century, the annual number of Asian/Pacific Islander immigrants has more than quadrupled from less than 50,000 people in 1965 to over 200,000 in 1994 (National Academy of Sciences, 1997).

To the dismay of the "assimilationists," who insist that all Americans should melt into one dominant culture and embrace a unified identity, evidence reviewed above show that our society is becoming increasingly multicultural. By 1990, in 186 counties, including 15 of the largest metropolitan statistical areas in the nation, Whites were minorities; non-White minorities comprised a majority of the population. The number of multicultural communities will continue to increase (American Demographics, 1991). Indeed, the 2000 Census format is considering expanding the number of ethnic sub-categories to around fifty-two.

According to multiculturalists, "assimilation" has become a term associated with giving up a person's original ethnic identity in favor of some amorphous idea of "Americanism" (Glazer, 1997). In other words, to assimilate is to lose one's identity with original culture and heritage, which has in turn spawned the notion of keeping different cultures intact within the overarching society of the United States. Many ethnic minorities reconcile their dilemma of retaining original ethnic identity on one hand and of becoming "American" on the other by accepting a dual or hyphenated identity (e.g., Asian-American, Hispanic-American). A recent study reports that ethnic minorities often live a dual life; while they agree that in the public domain the "American" culture and English language must prevail, within their homes and in personal domains they prefer to retain their original culture (Taylor and Lambert, 1996). Increasing rates of mixed marriages further compounds the problem of ethnic identity; for instance, a bicultural identity may not be adequate for the children when both parents have separate bicultural identities (e.g., children of Hispanic-American and African-American parents). For these and other reasons, the meaning and measures of multiculturalism and personal identity remain as unresolved issues and pose significant challenges to multicultural research and policy. At the aggregate level, however, increasingly larger proportions of the population identify themselves as members of different ethnicities. Indeed, in a recent volume, Nathan Glazer, an eminent sociologist and a leading advocate of the assimilationists, conceded that multiculturalists have won the national debate, and that: "We are all multiculturalists now" (Glazer, 1997). The crucial implication of this pervasive social trend is that social policies and programs, including substance abuse prevention, must be based upon a multicultural perspective for two reasons: (1) the deantological imperative, and (2) the utilitarian imperative.

The "deantological" or moral imperative derives from the essential values in our Bill of Rights; all citizens, regardless of their race or origin, have certain inalienable rights, which include the right of equal protection against threats to their lives. Substance abuse threatens the lives of individuals and the safety of communities. Therefore, the nation is morally bound to provide all people access to this basic right of prevention and protection from death and disability, regardless of ethnicity and national origin. A truly multicultural strategy should base its health programs commensurate with the needs of the population, which entails designing prevention information and services in a form acceptable to the different cultures. Interventions would have to be specially designed to provide "equal protection" to all ethnic groups in a multicultural community; this means that in some cases special efforts would have to be made to meet the criteria of equal protection for all. An example would be culturally appropriate special programs for non-English speaking ethnic minorities or high-risk populations.

In more practical terms, the "utilitarian" imperative states that a risk-reduction intervention should be so designed as to maximize its objective at the least cost and effort. From a utilitarian standpoint, a multicultural perspective in substance abuse prevention is essential for two reasons. First, an effective intervention should protect all ethnic groups because if it fails in one the entire community suffers from the consequences of that failure. There is strong evidence that in a multi-ethnic community, cultural groups may have different priorities regarding health, economic, and social issues that influence its members (DHHS, 1998b; Kar, et al., 1996; United Way, 1994). Second, some ethnic groups demonstrate culturally rooted protective factors (resilience) against certain risks; for instance, lower rates of substance abuse exist among several Asian-American and Latino groups (as was discussed earlier in this chapter with Table 2). Available data shows that in Los Angeles, Latinos have the lowest level of health insurance coverage (a proxy measure of access to health care) and yet infant mortality rate among the Latinos is lower than that among the Whites and nearly two and one-half times lower than the African Americans (Table 4). An understanding of these and other cultural buffers will help develop interventions that may benefit other groups and the entire society. A better understanding of factors in substance abuse prevention that are common to all ethnic groups and unique to each will help us design interventions that are more effective and hence will maximize the benefit to all.

Regrettably, reliable data on tobacco and substance abuse by all major ethnic groups is not readily available; when available, the statistics tend to combine all Hispanics/Latinos into one group and all Asian-American subgroups into a single group. These two ethnic groups consist of descendents of extremely diverse cultural/national origins. Often intra-group variations are so extreme that combining these disparate cultures into a single group defeats the very purpose of ethnic comparison. For instance, placing the fifth-generation Japanese and Chinese Americans or the high achieving Asian Indians with the extremely different recent Asian immigrants, such as Hmongs, Laotians, and Cambodians into a single group of Asian Americans raises the question: what meaningful purpose is served by using such an ethnic classification? Lack of knowledge about the levels of substance abuse and their determinants by important ethnic groups, especially among recent immigrants, is a major research need.

Significant differences among ethnic groups appear in their health and quality of life indicators. In order to provide a snapshot of a multicultural community, Table 4 enumerates eighteen indicators by ethnicity for Los Angeles County, one of the most multicultural regions in the world. According to the 1990 Census, no one ethnic group held the majority position within this area, with non-Hispanic Whites accounting for only 40.8 percent of the population. Estimates for 1997 make non-Hispanic Whites a minority, with only 34.2 percent of the population, as compared to Latinos at 42.5 percent, African Americans at 9.6 percent, and Asian Americans at 13.3 percent. The data on Table 4 points to deeper problems related to health and substance abuse risks across four ethnic groups.

For example, African Americans have the highest percentage of families living below the poverty level, the highest infant death rate, the highest high school drop-out rate, the highest rate of death per 100,000, the highest rate of heart disease, the highest homicide rate, the highest rate of accidents, and the highest rate of AIDS related deaths. Many of these risks have been linked to increased substance abuse. Interestingly, however, non-Hispanic Whites have the highest rate of suicides and alcohol/drug overdose-related deaths in the county, despite having the lowest rate of families below the poverty level and the lowest high school drop-out rate, two factors that are often linked with self-destructive behavior. The data in Table 4 suggest complex relationships among socio-cultural factors and health risks. The causes of substance abuse cannot be understood by a simple linear model; both quality of life indicators and cultural factors seem to be intermingling to form a more complex picture.

Intergenerational Conflict

Intergenerational conflict affects all ethnic groups; often youth and their parents do not view the same values and norms of life in the same manner, creating dissonance that may lead to deviant behavior including substance abuse. When this tension is exacerbated by acculturation stress, the results can be serious discord within the family unit. In general, intergeneration conflict and stressful parent-child relationships have been implicated in deviant behavior, including substance abuse among the youth (Bhattacharya, 1998; Félix-Ortiz, et al., 1998; Leland and Samuels, 1997). Conversely, positive parent-child bonding, modeling, and parental supervision is believed to serve as protective mechanisms against substance abuse by adolescents. Intergeneration conflict can vary significantly by ethnicity and acculturation experience.

Family structure, dynamics, and acculturation experience may vary significantly by ethnicity. In some cultures (e.g., Asian American), respect for the elderly and for parental authority play a more important role in shaping intergenerational relationships than in other cultures. Male authority and "machismo" are believed to exert relatively greater influence on family dynamics among Latinos and many Asian-American groups than among African-American and

White families. In addition, some ethnic groups have significantly greater proportions of single-parent families headed by women, with African Americans having the highest proportion.

Finally, intergeneration conflict and clash of values has always been most pronounced between first-generation immigrants and their children born in the United States (Kar, et al., 1998; Smart and Smart, 1994). The parents are socialized with the norms of their culture of origin, tending to hold on to many of these values related to their children's behavior, particularly when dealing with children's autonomy, dating, marriage, and career choice issues. A dual standard also exists between dealing with male and female children. For these and other reasons concerning culturally influenced family dynamics, children from different ethnicities experience very different socialization processes and parent-child relationships. These and other trends, including increasing divorce rates, have significant impact on the quality of parent-child relationships. This means that when we study a sample of students in a school in a multicultural community, we are by no means dealing with a homogenous population. Yet most surveys tend to study groups of students by grades/age and gender cohorts; they do not further examine ethnic differences. Such studies may give us rates or averages for population as a whole but conceal the very processes of risk taking behavior that we need to understand for effective interventions in multicultural communities.

Research on intergenerational conflict among immigrants has shown that even when the children in a family are also first-generation immigrants along with their parents, the adolescents tend to acclimatize more quickly to their new country, causing friction with the older members of the family (Baptiste, 1993). Our exploratory study of Japanese Americans and Indo-Americans revealed that first the Indo-Americans, who are overwhelmingly first generation immigrants, reported significantly greater levels of intergenerational conflicts than the Japanese Americans who were all descendents of immigrants for several generations (Kar, et al., 1998).

We do not have well-designed studies across major ethnic groups to assess the levels of substance abuse and to understand the determinants which are common to major groups and those unique to each. For instance, the literature suggests that acculturation stress and intergeneration conflicts can enhance deviant behavior including substance abuse. Furthermore, intergeneration and inter-gender conflicts tend to be most serious between the first and second generation immigrants; with acculturation process, the subsequent generations increasingly converge toward the national trends. And yet we have no national study of substance abuse levels and their determinants by several major ethnic groups and recent immigrants. For instance, Asian Americans are the fastest growing minority in the nation. But our literature search failed to identify more than a handful of published papers that examined and compared substance abuse among Asian Americans and Latinos, two of which were published extremely recently by authors from this volume.

Our own exploratory study on acculturation and quality of life compared the Indo-Americans (Asian-Indian) who are mostly foreign-born and Japanese Americans who are almost always born in the United States (Kar, et al., 1998). We hypothesized that Indo-Americans will have higher acculturation stress than the Japanese Americans. As expected, acculturation stress, intergeneration and inter-gender conflicts were more pronounced among the Indo-Americans than among the Japanese Americans. At the same time, the reported level of current cigarette smokers among the Indo-American is significantly lower than that among the Japanese Americans (5.7% and 23.8% respectively). More significantly, less than 1 percent of Indo-American women were current smokers, compared to 20.5 percent Japanese-American women (Kar, et al., 1998). Both groups had reportedly lower levels of cigarette smoking than the national averages. The Indo-Americans reported higher level of alcohol use (at least 1 drink past thirty days of interview month) than the Japanese Americans: 54.7 percent and 48.1 percent respectively. The national average of alcohol use in 1996 was 51 percent for the entire population age twelve and older, and 54 percent among Whites (SAMHSA, 1996). It is important to point out that our sample included subjects twenty-one years and older (not 12 years and older) and that the difference (between 54.7, 54, and 51 percents) may not be statistically significant. Illicit drug use was reported by less than 3 percent Indo-American respondents. These results do not speak about the protective factors operating against cigarette smoking and substance abuse among the Indo-Americans. Perhaps Indo-Americans find other ways to cope with their acculturation stress and inter-generation conflicts. A relatively higher alcohol use by the Indo-American men suggests such a possibility. We do not have systematic knowledge about substance abuse among Asian Americans and Latinos, especially among the recent immigrants (first and second generations). It appears that these cultures have buffers that contribute to lower rates of substance abuse. We need more multicultural comparative research in order to better understand the nature of these buffers and use this knowledge for the benefit of others.

COMMUNICATION REVOLUTION AND RISKS

We present here our analysis of the communication media as they affect our contemporary society in general and substance abuse prevention in particular. Modern communication systems can have important positive and negative influences, especially on impressionable children, and consequently it is important to review media influences on substance abuse and prevention from a multicultural perspective. Historically, organized communication and health education have been an integral part of every successful public health movement. There are several useful volumes that review the processes and effects of communication for public health and risk reduction. The purpose of this chapter is not to summarize the expanding field of health communication, but rather to review key issues, which may determine the effectiveness of communication for substance abuse prevention in our increasingly multicultural communities. These issues require further attention by researchers and substance abuse prevention professionals alike.

We first draw attention to a sample of notable volumes on health communication to assist the readers in the event they are interested in studying these in greater depth. These include a valuable volume, which reviews theories and practice of public health communication campaigns by Rice and Atkin (1989). This volume examines the role of mass communication including social marketing in various health promotion campaigns. A volume by Backer, Rogers, and Sopory (1992) focuses on how to design effective communication campaigns based upon their review of which methods effectively achieve their goals. This volume presents ten principles that work; these are: (1) use multiple media, (2) use a combined media and interpersonal strategy, (3) use audience segmentation approach, (4) use celebrities and entertainment programs to attract and sustain attention, (5) use simple and clear message, (6) emphasize positive behavior not negative consequences, (7) emphasize current rewards not distant consequences, (8) involve power figures and organization, (9) take advantage of timing, and (10) use formative evaluation (Backer, et al., 1992, p. 12). This volume contains twenty-seven generalizations about health communication and seven additional generalizations specific to substance abuse and high-risk behavior in youth. According to these authors, substance abuse campaigns for high risk youth should: start when children are age eleven or twelve, increase awareness of broader context affecting substance abuse, include messages to parents of high risk youths, deal with major themes in the development of adolescent identity, use peer models instead of adult celebrities, promote positive images and lifestyles, and use the radio to promote the desired message (Backer, et al., 1992, pp. 33-34).

Another volume, edited by Piotrow, et al. (1997), focuses on the lessons learned from the worldwide family planning and reproductive health movement during the past decades, along with its implications for health communication in the United States. A volume edited by Harris deals with the role of new media and technologies in transformation of personal and public health (Harris, 1995). This volume is based upon the tenets of chaos theory of complexity which holds the "rule of first forces" paramount; the first intervening events and influences have disproportionately greater influence on outcomes. According to this rule of first forces, modern and emerging media have an overwhelming influence on health-related outcomes and on the public itself. Specifically, this volume examines the role of the national information infrastructure and its role in enhancing accessibility of health information through modern media systems. Another noteworthy volume is a special issue of the American Behavioral Scientist edited by Ratzan (1994). This volume focuses on the challenges of health communication for the twenty-first century with special emphasis on the needs, technologies, and constraints of health communication. All of the above volumes make important contributions to our understanding of the complex issues involved in health communication in our contemporary society.

These and other volumes in their genre focus on communication process from an assimilationist perspective; they examine the process and impact of communication media on the American culture and public as a whole. They do not address communication issues and challenges unique to multicultural communities. For instance, while the importance of cultural sensitivity is sporadically mentioned, there is no serious discussion of how relative values and norms of different ethnic groups, ethnic communication networks, and inter-ethnic dynamics or conflicts in a multicultural community affect health communication. Works by Gudykunst (1988), Kim and Gudykunst (1988), and Kreps and Kunimoto (1994) have appropriately raised important conceptual and methodological issues in intercultural communication processes. The latter volume specifically deals with multicultural communication in health care settings, but the focus here is on health care professionals and organizations not on multicultural communities. We discuss here those issues, which can affect population based substance abuse prevention in multicultural settings.

Culture, Communication, and Health Behavior

Cultural/ethnic differences in quality of life and achievements (Sowell, 1996), health status, and substance abuse risks have been discussed by several authors (Cazeres and Beatty, 1994; Cruickshank and Beevers, 1989; DHHS, 1998a, 1998b; Harwood 1981; Howard, 1995; Langton, 1995; Orlandi, 1992; Penn, et al., 1995; Sussman and Johnson, 1996). It is important to recognize that communication and media from outside sources (or induced communication) do not bypass or neutralize socio-cultural factors, which determine health related behavior and outcomes. Induced communication must interact with culturally conditioned health related beliefs, values, knowledge, attitudes, and practices (BVKAP); these forces in combination with planned communication interventions can affect health behavior of people (Kar, et al., 1998). A significant lesson we have learned from earlier communication studies is that effective communication programs should not be based upon the old "hypodermic model" of communication, which held that messages injected by powerful media into a community will be a sufficient cause for changing people's behavior independent of social and cultural influence. This model conceptualized the public as passive, captive subjects manipulated by externally induced powerful communication intervention. The concepts validated by behavioral science and communication research, including cultural relativity, selective perception, selective retention, interpersonal influence, group pressure, and value maximizing behavior, to name a few, are sufficient to reject the old hypodermic model of communication. It is therefore important for us to conceptualize health communication as a sub-system of the total system that affects health related risks and behavior.

We conceptualize one such system to look at important forces, which, along with effective communication, influences health related behavior of individuals in traditional and modern cultures (see Chapter 13 for details). The basic tenet is that culturally conditioned BVKAP influence the health related behavior of its members through five dimensions/processes: belief about disease etiology, preferred modality of treatment, locus of decision/responsibility, communication and social relations, and accessibility of services. These forces influence not only how and which sources of health related information will be taken seriously, but also how personal health decisions are made. The cultural beliefs and norms about smoking, drinking, substance abuse, and their consequences can either reinforce or negate the effects of communication on these matters from outside sources. Substance abuse prevention and intervention should therefore strive to understand those cultural factors and utilize them to create effective programs.

Interestingly, in most cases, the traditional societies do not completely reject the methods of modern societies, but rather prefer to focus on other means as the primary forms of health care and keep the modern methods as supplementary. Within minority groups, however, a diversity of practices exist; for instance, a recent Asian immigrant raised with Eastern medicinal practices may follow those original customs in his or her new country more strongly than a fourth-generation Asian American will. Therefore, attention must be paid to the communication networks and sources that are believed to be most credible by the members of certain ethnic groups, so that meaningful and relevant partnerships are built, empowering communities for prevention efforts.

Media Explosion and Fragmentation

During the last four decades there has been an unprecedented media explosion, consisting of two facets. First, there has been a rapid expansion in the total volume of media access to a population in a given area. Second, there has been a rapid diversification in media designed to serve a wide range of population segments, including many ethnic media. More TV programs, newspapers, and communication materials are now produced and distributed to serve an increasingly diverse audience, both globally and locally.

During the last four decades, television has replaced the earlier domination of radio to the extent that it is now impossible to avoid the ubiquitous presence of TV sets. As of mid-1998, there were estimated ninety-eight million television-containing households in the United States (Nielsen, 1998a). Multiple TV set families have emerged in response to diverse interests within the same family. Satellite and cable networks have made it possible for news and other programs to travel instantaneously across the globe. One can watch live events across the globe as they shape our lives. Poor, half-clad villagers in India can witness bikini clad youths on Baywatch or Beverly Hills 90210, which shapes their (mis)perceptions of American culture and lifestyles. Violence and other risk-taking behaviors that are glamorized in the media, including alcohol use and smoking, are accepted as signs of the good life and of the emancipation of youth and women. The world has now shrunk into what Marshall MacLuhan had once termed as a Global Village. And yet, underlying this obvious growth of television, there are profound changes in the ways television reaches people, or rather, how people use television. Only recently, television broadcasts were the monopoly of three TV networks (ABC, CBS, and NBC); today most major metropolitan areas have access to over one hundred channels. The question is: why?

It has become apparent that the media must diversify itself to be responsive to the needs of the diverse segments of our population. The major broadcast network channels are no longer appealing to all audiences; for example, network TV viewership has significantly declined from 90 percent in 1970 to only 60 percent in the 1990s (UCLA Center for Communication Policy, 1997), as more people are patronizing alternative channels and sources of news and entertainment. New commercial products are being developed and marketed to diverse population segments through a wider range of channels. A major impetus for this diversification is due to the increasing diversity among the audience by age, gender, ethnicity, and special interests. There are now separate channels exclusively dedicated to news, sports and physical fitness, cooking, religious services, movies, and ethnic interests.

There are significant differences in TV viewership by ethnicity. For instance, Neilsen ratings for primetime viewing during the 1998-99 season (Nielsen, 1998a) show that nine of the top ten programs seen by Americans as a whole were broadcast by NBC. However, the ten top ranked programs for African-American viewers during the same time period were broadcast by FOX, ABC, and NBC (Nielsen, 1998b), showing that this group watches a greater variety of networks, and can be reached by other cable stations with equal or better impact. Interestingly, while the general population watches CBS, NBC, and ABC (in that order), Blacks watch mostly UPN, FOX, and WB (Nielsen, 1998b). Hispanics also have markedly different viewing patterns than the general population. For example, fully 16 percent of Hispanic households watched "Maria La Del Barrio" on Univision during the 1996-97 season, making it the single highest rated television show among all networks for Hispanic viewers during that time period (Nielsen, 1998c). This show does not even appear in the top 100 programs for the general population for the same time period. Unfortunately, we do not have data on TV viewership by Asian-American preferences. The trend then is both expansion and diversification of TV viewers. The same trend holds true for newspapers and other printed media. For instance, one incomplete list included seventy-two ethnic newspapers in English and other languages serving the Los Angeles community alone (Pearlstone, 1990).

In a multicultural community, media and communication seeking behavior may vary significantly by different ethnic groups. A recent study in Los Angeles confirms this phenomenon (Table 5), showing the differences in sources of the health related information obtained by four ethnic groups. While at the aggregate

Table 5. Sources of Health Related Information in Los Angeles (Percent)

Source	Total (n = 2054)	Non-Hispanic White (n = 924)	Hispanic (n = 679)	African American (n = 200)	Asian American (n = 251)
Television	33.7	27.5	44.3	28.5	32.1
Doctors	31.5	37.3	24.9	42.5	19.1
Newspapers	31.4	33.5	28.3	20.5	40.6
Printed materials (books, magazines, pamphlets, etc.)	31.0	31.5	29.8	37.8	26.7
Family	12.3	12.6	14.1	6.0	11.6
Friends	12.2	10.2	16.1	7.5	12.7
Radio	5.6	4.4	7.7	5.0	7.1
Hotlines	1.7	2.1	1.3	1.0	1.6
Other	7.3	7.5	9.0	3.5	5.2

Source: Los Angeles County Department of Health Services, 1994.

level, television appears as the most common source, it is not the most frequent source of health information across all groups. TV is the most common source among the Latinos only; the fourth important source among the Whites, third most important source among African Americans, and the second most important source among the Asian Americans. Among the Whites the three most common sources are in this order: doctors, newspaper, and other printed materials. Among the African Americans the ranking sources are: doctors, printed materials, and television. Among the Asian Americans the ranking sources are: newspaper, TV, and printed materials. Finally, among Hispanics, the most common sources are: TV, printed materials, and newspapers. Interestingly, there has been much interest in special hotlines, but they are used by less than 2 percent of the survey respondents. It should be noted, however, that those who use hotlines may be in a current crisis situation and need help during specific times, rather than requiring general health information.

If the results above reflect the reality of a multicultural community, it raises a major question as to how effective are the mainstream media, including network television stations and printed media, for communicating prevention information across major ethnic groups and how can we best reach these groups. We must go beyond the naïve assumption that because TV is believed to influence various behaviors including violence and substance abuse, we can use major network stations as our primary communication media for substance abuse prevention for at least two reasons. First, the cost of purchasing TV time is prohibitively high; often a thirty-second spot on a primetime program may cost up to one half-million dollars. Communication research tells us that a message to be effective must be simple and frequently repeated. Most local health departments or substance abuse programs do not have sufficient budgets to sponsor such expensive media campaigns. Second, even if we have budget to broadcast ten spots (at an estimated cost of 5 million dollars), with so many channel choices it remains difficult to pinpoint which station will be most effective in reaching the targeted communities.

Media as a Risk Factor

Notwithstanding the potential for the positive role of communication, both conventional (TV, printed media, etc.) and emerging (Internet, Web sites, and online service, etc.), media has actually become a risk factor, especially among the children, for two reasons: (1) the cumulative effects of repeated depiction and glamorizing of sex, substance abuse, and violence in the news and entertainment media, and (2) the use of media by alcohol and tobacco industries targeted to reach high-risk population segments, including children and minorities. The extent to which media depiction of violence and sex affect antisocial behavior has been an area of lively debate; several Presidential Commissions on pornography and violence examined extensive evidence to answer this question. Experts often disagree on the degree of media effects on the public in general. There is, however, a consensus that depictions of drugs, sex, and violence can have significant effects on young and impressionable children. It is this conviction that led tobacco and alcohol industries to target their products to children and people of color by utilizing mass media.

Television viewing is a major domain of our lives. According to the Center for Media Education (CME), most children watch three to four hours of TV per day; they spend approximately 1500 hours in front of TV compared to 900 hours in classrooms per year. On average, a child sees over 20,000 commercials each year and, by age twenty-one, a viewer will be exposed to over a million commercials on TV. A teen will have seen 100,000 alcohol commercials before he/she reaches drinking age. Children who watch TV excessively are more likely to be obese, use alcohol and drugs, and engage in sexual activities earlier (CME, 1998a). Industries also compete to increase "brand loyalty" among viewers by engaging in aggressive marketing campaigns and commercials, including sponsorships of sports and entertainment events, free giveaways, and awards. Media is also used to target minorities and women in particular. For instance, there is a greater concentration of tobacco billboards in predominantly African-American communities; women's magazines also glamorize cigarette smoking as indicators of emancipation and independence. The agenda is to saturate the market with a steady flow of messages to create an image of reality in which smoking, drinking, and sexual adventure are integral parts of a happy, independent, and successful lifestyle.

Emerging media is expanding at a phenomenal pace; this includes online services, Web sites, VCS, and interactive media. According to one estimate, nearly five million children age seventeen and below used the Internet in 1996 (Jupiter Communications, 1998). The CME study referred to above reports that alcohol and tobacco companies are using online media to promote their brands through sophisticated marketing techniques. There were more than thirty-five brands of alcohol products promoted via the Internet by major alcohol companies during the scope of the study. There are also indicators that tobacco companies are increasing their online advertisements. For instance, in 1997 Brown and Williams began Lucky Strike brand ads in the San Francisco bay area, and some tobacco companies have set up Web sites targeted to youth in other countries, but these are also easily accessible to children in the United States (CME, 1998b).

We agree with the assessment that: "We are moving from the Age of Mass Communication to the Age of Interactive Communication, in which many of the old communication models will be insufficient or redundant" (Chamberlain, 1996, p. 43). According to one estimate in 1996, 35 percent of homes in the United States had home computers. Between 1994 and 1995, the number of home computers has doubled (The Economist, 1995). With the rapid decline in computer costs and a competitive market, the number of home computers and online subscribers is likely to increase rapidly. The emerging media offer literally countless sources from which a viewer can, at his/her will, access and personalize a search of information. In 1996, there were seven million subscribers of online services in the United States. A minor can easily join chat rooms (and purchase commodities online) without necessarily having to provide proof of age. Aggressive use of emerging media promoting sexually explicit materials, advertisements of cigarettes and alcohol promotions have become so prevalent that the conventional and new media have emerged as a risk factor for our children.

The question is: how do we deal with the role of media as a risk factor? Substance abuse programs will never have sufficient resources to match tobacco and alcohol industries in a media war, as was briefly mentioned in the previous section. Nor will commercial media help us by launching educational campaigns. Consequently, we must increasingly mobilize community-based resources and alternative strategies to combat the avalanche of risk promotion and reinforcement messages in the media. These include: (1) legislative measures and activism, (2) public education for normative change, (3) targeted education for those at risk, (4) community empowerment and organization, and (4) coalitions for health promotion and risk reduction. Several authors in this volume have reviewed strategies and factors that seem effective; but much work needs to be done in the area of media use and effects in multicultural communities.

THE NEW PUBLIC HEALTH PARADIGM: RISK REDUCTION FROM A MULTICULTURAL PERSPECTIVE

The field of public health has undergone a recent paradigm shift; the emerging framework offers an important foundation on which to develop community-based, comprehensive risk reduction and health promotion interventions, including substance abuse prevention. The mission of the new public health paradigm is to promote physical and mental health, and prevent disease, injury, and disability. The three functions of public health are *assessment* of health status, needs, and determinants, *policy development* to meet health needs of populations, and *assurance* of services and conditions necessary for people to be healthy (Institute of Medicine, 1989). In order to meet its mission and functions, the Public Health Functions Steering Committee has defined ten "Essential Public Health Services" which were adopted by all major public health associations and organizations in the nation. These essential services are: (1) monitor health status, (2) diagnose health problems and hazards, (3) inform, educate, and empower people about health issues, (4) mobilize community partnership to identify and solve health problems, (5) develop policies and plans that support individual and community health efforts, (6) enforce laws and regulations that protect health and ensure safety, (7) link people to needed personal health services, (8) assure competent public health workforce, (9) evaluate effectiveness, accessibility, and quality of public health services, and (10) research for new insight and innovative solutions (Public Health Foundation, 1995). The seminal idea of this new public health paradigm is that disease prevention and health promotion requires both individual and societal actions and that such a strategy must have the active partnership of the public or community. Public health differs from a clinical discipline, such as medicine, in three distinct ways: (1) its goal is prevention, not treatment, of disease, (2) its level of intervention is the community or public, not individual patients, and (3) its *modus operandi* is population based prevention through participation of the public as active partners. Its scope includes all preventable health risks including substance abuse. By nature, public health is essentially an interdisciplinary and applied field. Operationally, it must work closely with state and community organizations that deal with health and human services.

History of Public Health

Historically, public health has gone through three overlapping phases: (1) control of communicable diseases, (2) dual-epidemic control, and (3) community-based public health practice. The first phase began in mid-1800s, when public health emerged as an organized social action to control communicable diseases (Afifi and Breslow, 1994; Lee and Paxman, 1997; Turnock and Handler, 1997). During this first phase, public health focused on better application of modern scientific innovations. Improved sanitation and robust public health interventions through applications of innovations in medicine and in microbiology, including development of vaccinations and antibiotics, helped control or eradicate major infectious diseases of that time (e.g., smallpox, plague, cholera, typhoid, polio, tetanus, diphtheria, malaria, tuberculosis). Organized public health actions worked along with improved maternal and child health care, rapid industrialization, and improved standard of living to accomplish their goals. The immediate effects were rapid reductions in infant mortality and the extension of life expectation. This was the golden age of public health, as the field was generally credited with playing a major role in the dramatic reduction of mortality rates due to epidemics of preventable communicable diseases.

The success in the control of communicable diseases ushered in the phase of dual-epidemics. During this second phase, which began between early- and mid-twentieth century, while some of the old communicable diseases still persisted at a significantly lower level, chronic diseases, injury, and new infectious diseases (e.g., HIV/AIDS) emerged as the leading causes of death in the United States. Consequently, public health was challenged to deal with a dual set of leading causes of death and illness, both chronic and infectious, simultaneously.

The third and current phase of public health has evolved from the widely shared recognition that a radical paradigm shift is needed to achieve the health objectives of our nations and to meet the mission of public health as a profession as well. Three influential developments served as the impetus for the new public health paradigm: the *Alma Ata Declaration* on Primary Health Care (WHO/UNICEF, 1978), *Healthy People 2000: National Health Promotion and Disease Prevention Objectives* (DHHS, 1991), and *The Future of Public Health* by the Institute of Medicine (IOM, 1989). The first document, endorsed by over 165 nations, underscored that basic health care is a fundamental human right and that governments/nations should develop a primary health care (PHC) strategy to provide accessible, affordable, and culturally acceptable preventive and clinical services to all. The second document focuses on the health needs of the general public in the United States. In the late 1970s, under the leadership of the Department for Health and Human Services of the United States, massive efforts were invested to define health objectives for the nation as we approach the twenty-first century. This landmark document attempted to define the health needs of our nation and identified over 300 health objectives, including several dealing with substance abuse (DHHS, 1991). Since then, these objectives have significantly influenced our federal, state, and local health initiatives as well as those funded by private foundations involved in health. This development has significantly refocused our national attention on public health approaches for disease prevention and health promotion.

Finally, in the late 1980s, the influential Institute of Medicine of the National Academy of Sciences undertook an in-depth review of the field of public health. Its landmark report titled *The Future of Public Health* (IOM, 1989) concluded that the United States had lost sight of its public health goals and had neglected the necessary public health activities needed for a healthy population (IOM, 1989). The report defined public health as ". . . what we, as a society, do collectively do to assure the conditions in which people can be healthy." It identified the three core functions of public health as: assessment, policy development, and assurance of services and conditions necessary for good health. Finally, the IOM concluded that public health schools/programs at universities in the United States had become more like academic teaching and research units; it admonished both the public health schools and the profession at large to join forces and to become more engaged in communities to achieve the mission of public health and health objectives of our nation (IOM, 1989).

Community Participation and Empowerment for Risk Prevention

The new public health paradigm, which focuses on population based prevention in partnership with the public, has significant implications for substance abuse research and interventions. First, tobacco and substance abuse prevention is a major item on the public health agenda. Recent progress made in controlling tobacco abuse, especially among the adult population, and HIV/AIDS transmission rates further support the importance of community based prevention interventions using a public health paradigm. Second, the history of public health contains dramatic success stories when massive community based preventive interventions helped eradicate or control major epidemics; these include smallpox, polio, tuberculosis, and malaria to name a few. The lessons learned from these and other effective population-based public health programs would be valuable for substance abuse prevention. The synergy generated through a combined effort by specialists in substance abuse, public health, and the community is perhaps the only sensible way to deal with the daunting challenge of substance abuse by our communities, especially by our younger generation.

In recognition of the importance of a collaborative relationship between researchers and the community as equal partners for public health, the Division of Health Promotion and Disease Prevention of the Institute of Medicine strongly advocates a Community Health Improvement Process (CHIP) model (IOM, 1997, p. 7). Like other areas of health-risk prevention research, this model (Figure 1) would complement conventional and basic research related to substance abuse and would significantly enrich substance abuse prevention strategies in communities. The central tenet of the IOM's proposed participatory research model is that: ". . . a wide array of factors influence community's health, and many entities in the community share the responsibility of maintaining and improving health. Responsibility shared among many entities, however, can easily become responsibility ignored or abandoned" (IOM, 1997, p. 5). The report furthermore claims that: "a community health improvement process (CHIP), that includes performance monitoring, as outlined in this report, can be an effective tool for developing a shared vision and supporting a planned and integrated approach to improve community health" (IOM, 1997, p. 5). Finally, "The committee concluded, however, that individual communities will have to determine the specific allocation of responsibility and accountability" (IOM, 1997, pp. 5-6). It requires a partnership between researchers and the community concerned at each step. The Community Health Improvement Process (CHIP) model proposed by the Institute of Medicine (IOM) includes two principal interacting cycles: (1) the problem identification and prioritization cycle, and (2) analysis and implementation cycle (see Figure 1).

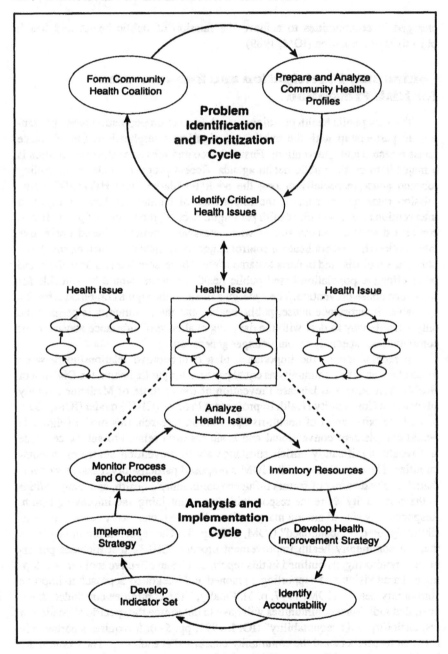

Figure 1. The community health improvement process (CHIP).
Source: IOM, 1997

The problem identification and prioritization cycle includes formation of a community health coalition, which plays critical roles in identification and ranking of problems as perceived by the community. In the second cycle, the community participates as an equal partner to "devise, implement, and evaluate the impact of health improvement strategies to address the problems" (IOM, 1997, p. 6). Through a pre-established performance monitoring system, the community together with the researchers controls the entire health improvement process. We believe that such a participatory model is more appropriate, and perhaps the only sensible approach, for prevention research and intervention among multicultural communities where the cultural and linguistic difference between the researchers and the ethnic subgroups could pose insurmountable barriers.

Finally, the importance of performance measurement and development of appropriate indicators for monitoring program progress cannot be over emphasized. Public health has been concerned with and involved in development of health promotion indicators for decades (Kar, 1989). Strategies included extensive use of consensus methods (e.g., Delphi Technique) for identifying contextually and culturally appropriate indicators at both the individual and community levels (Kar, 1989). Recently, in recognition of the importance of process evaluation, the Office of National Drug Control Policy has taken the lead in developing a guideline for *Performance Measures of Effectiveness: A System for Assessing the Performance of the National Drug Control Strategy* (McCaffrey, 1997). This guide presents targets of impact in three domains: supply of drugs, demand for drugs, and drug-related consequences (McCaffrey, 1997, pp. 17-18). It is important to note that these global impact targets would have to be calibrated to suit the conditions of multicultural communities and specific ethnic groups. Furthermore, it is important to identify "targets" and performance indicators that are relevant for measuring community norms related to substance abuse and prevention readiness in major ethnic groups. This is still an uncharted area and will require creative applications of participatory research and evaluation methods to complement standard quantitative methods.

Because of the pervasive nature of substance abuse and the changing demographical nature of our society, future prevention and intervention research must have a multicultural and participatory focus. Future programs must also take into account the various cultural and communication differences among ethnicities, tailoring their message and methods specifically for the targeted group. However, without further research on the nature of substance abuse and its prevention within different ethnic groups, practitioners will often be working without a hard scientific base to support their programmatic decisions.

The serious gaps in our current knowledge related to substance abuse prevention in multicultural communities are: (1) what are the relative risks by major ethnic groups, (2) what are the socio-cultural and behavioral determinants common to major ethnic groups and unique to each, (3) whether past interventions which are effective among White Americans will be effective across other major ethnic groups, (4) how to mobilize community resources, especially the cultural capitals or positive attributes that serve as protective mechanisms against substance abuse, and (5) what are the effective methods for organizing and empowering diverse communities (with distinctly different language, cultures, and acculturation levels) for collective action for substance abuse prevention. Lack of knowledge in these critical areas and inadequate use of available research due to the lack of communication among researchers, policy planners, practitioners, and community remain the serious barriers to effective prevention.

REFERENCES

Afifi, A. and Breslow, L. (1994). The maturing paradigm of public health. *Annual Review of Public Health*, 15:223-235.

American Demographics (1991). *American Diversity, Desk Reference Series, #1*. Ithaca, NY: American Demographics Magazine.

Backer, T. E., Rogers, E. M. and Sopory, P. (1992). *Designing Health Communication Campaigns: What Works?* Sage Publications: Newbury Park, CA.

Bang, A., Bang, R., Tale, O., Sontakke, P., Solanki, J., Wargantiwar, R. and Kelzarkar, P. (1990). Reduction in pneumonia mortality and total childhood mortality by means of community-based intervention trial in Gadchiroli, India. *The Lancet*, 336:201-206.

Baptiste, D., Jr. (1993). Immigrant families, adolescents, and acculturation: insights for therapists. *Marriage & Family Review*, 19(3-4):341-364.

Bhattacharya, G. (1998). Drug use among Asian-Indian adolescents: Identifying protective/risk factors. *Adolescence*, 33(129):169-184.

Cazeres, A. and Beatty, L. A., Eds. (1994). *Scientific Methods for Prevention Intervention Research*, NIDA Research Monograph 139, NIH Publication No. 94-3631.

Chamberlain, M. A. (1996). Health communication: Making the most of new media technologies—An international overview. *Journal of Health Communication*, 1:43-50.

CME (1998a). *Frequently Asked Questions*, Center for Media Education Website: Washington, D.C.

CME (1998b). *Alcohol and Tobacco on the Web: New Threats to Youth (Executive Summary)*. Center for Media Education Website: Washington, D.C.

Cruickshank, J. K. and Beevers, D. G. (1989). *Ethnic Factors in Health and Disease*. Butterworth-Heinemann: Oxford.

DHHS: U.S. Department of Health and Human Services (1980). *Ten Leading Causes of Death in the United States in 1977*. Public Health Service, Centers for Disease Control: Atlanta, GA.

DHHS: U.S. Department of Health and Human Services (1991). *Healthy People 2000: National Health Promotion and Disease Prevention Objectives*. U.S. Dept. of Health and Human Services, Public Health Service: Washington, D.C.

DHHS: U.S. Department of Health and Human Services (1997a). *Substance Abuse—A National Challenge, Prevention Treatment and Research at HHS*. Fact Sheet, December 20th.

DHHS: U.S. Department of Health and Human Services (1997b). *Drug Use Survey Shows Mixed Results for Nation's Youth, Use Among Younger Adolescents Appears to be Slowing.* Press Release, December 20th.

DHHS: U.S. Department of Health and Human Services (1998a). *Tobacco Use Among U.S. Racial/Ethnic Groups—African Americans, American Indian and Alaska Natives, Asian Americans and Pacific Islanders, and Hispanics: A Report of the Surgeon General.* Atlanta, Centers for Disease Control and Prevention.

DHHS: U.S. Department of Health and Human Services (1998b). *Health, United States, 1998.* DHHS Pub. No. 98-1232, Center for Disease Control and Prevention, National Center for Health Statistics: Hyattsville, MD.

DHHS: U.S. Department of Health and Human Services (1998c). Healthy people 2000 progress review: Substance abuse—alcohol and other drugs. *Prevention Report,* 13(2):11-12.

The Economist, (1995). The Internet society. *The Economist,* 336(7921):S5.

Félix-Ortiz, M., Fernandez, A. and Newcomb, M. (1998). The role of intergenerational discrepancy of cultural orientation in drug use among Latina adolescents. *Substance Abuse & Misuse,* 33(4):967-994.

Glazer, N. (1997). *We are All Multiculturalists Now.* Harvard University Press: Cambridge, MA

Gudykunst, W. B. (1988). Uncertainty and anxiety. In Y. Y. Kim, and W. B. Gudykunst (Eds.), *Theories in Intercultural Communication,* Sage Publications: Newbury Park, CA.

Harris, L. M., Ed. (1995). *Health and the New Media.* Lawrence Erlbaum Associates: Mahwah, NJ.

Harwood, A., Ed. (1981). *Ethnicity and Medical Care.* Harvard University Press: Cambridge, Massachusetts and London, England.

Howard, J. M. (1995). Alcohol prevention research in ethnic/racial communities: framing the research agenda. In P. A. Langton (Ed.), *The Challenge of Participatory Research: Preventing Alcohol-Related Problems in Ethnic Communities,* SAMSHA, DHHS Publication No. (SMA) 3042:3441.

Institute of Medicine (1989). *The Future of Public Health.* National Academy Press: Washington, D.C.

Institute of Medicine (1997). *Improving Health In The Community: A Role of Performance Monitoring.* Institute of Medicine, National Academy of Sciences, National Academy Press: Washington, D.C.

Jessor, R. and Jessor, S. (1977). *Problem Behavior and Psychosocial Development: A Logitudinal Study of Youth.* Academic Press: New York, San Francisco, London.

Jupiter Communications (1998). In CME, *Frequently Asked Questions,* Center for Media Education Website: Washington, D.C.

Kar, S. B., Ed. (1989). *Health Promotion Indicators and Action.* Springer Publications: New York.

Kar, S. B. (1990). Primary health care: Implications for the medical education. *Academic Medicine,* 65(5):301-306.

Kar, S. B., Chickering, K. and Pascual, C. (1996). *Public Health Practice in a Multicultural and Underserved Los Angeles Community: A Case Study* (Monograph). Bureau of Health Professionals/Public Health Service: Washington, D.C.

Kar, S., Jimenez, A., Campbell, K. and Sze, F. (1998). Acculturation and quality of life: A comparative study of Japanese-Americans and Indo-Americans. *Amerasia Journal*, 24(1):129-142.

Kim, Y. Y. and Gudykunst, W. B., Eds. (1988). *Theories in Intercultural Communication*, Sage Publications: Newbury Park, CA.

Kreps, G. L. and Kunimoto, E. N. (1994). *Effective Communication in Multicultural Health Care Settings*, Sage Publications: Thousand Oaks, CA.

Langton, P. A. Ed., (1995). *The Challenge of Participatory Research: Preventing Alcohol-Related Problems in Ethnic Communities*. SAMSHA:DHHS Publication No. (SMA) 3042.

Lee, P. and Paxman, D. (1997). Reinventing Public Health. *Annual Review of Public Health*, 18:1-35.

Leland, J. and Samuels, A. (1997). The new generation gap (Black families). *Newsweek*, 129(11):52-58.

Los Angeles County Department of Health Services (1994). *LA County Annual Health Risk Assessment*. Information from data on CD-ROM.

McCaffrey, B. R. (1997). *Performance Measures of Effectiveness (PME): A System for Assessing the Performance of the National Drug Control Strategy*, Office of National Drug Control Policy, Washington, D.C.

McGinnis, J. M and Foege, W. H. (1993). Actual causes of death in the United States. *Journal of the American Medical Association*, 270(18):2207-2212.

MTFS (1997). *Monitoring the Future Study, 1997*. Institute for Social Research, Survey Research Center: University of Michigan.

National Academy of Sciences (1997). Immigration: Who wins, who loses. *Issues in Science and Technology*, 14(1):87-89.

National Center for Health Statistics (1996). Fastats A-Z. From the *Monthly Vital Statistics Report*, 46(1 Supplement).

National Center for Health Statistics (1997). *Health, United States, 1996-7*. U.S. Department of Health and Human Services.

National Public Health Laboratory of Finland (1981). *Community Control of Cardiovascular Diseases*. WHO, Regional Office for Europe: Copenhagen.

Nielsen Media Research (1998a). *Household Network Primetime Report for the Week of 7/6/98-7/12/98*. From the Nielsen Media Research Website.

Nielsen Media Research (1998b). *African American Household Viewership*. Presentation given to The Summit on November 3, 1998: New York.

Nielsen Media Research (1998c). *1998 Report on Television*. Nielsen Media Research: New York.

Orlandi, M. O., Ed. (1992). *Cultural Competence for Evaluators, A Guide for Alcohol and Other Drug Prevention Practitioners Working with Ethnic/racial Communities*, DHHS Publication No. (ADM) 92-1884.

Pearlstone, Z. (1990). *Ethnic LA* (pp. 151-153). Hillcrest Press: Beverly Hills, CA.

Penn, N. E., Kar, S. B., Kramer, J., Skinner, J. and Zambrana, R. (1995). Ethnic minorities, health care systems, and behavior. *Health Psychology*, 14(7):641-646.

Piotrow, P. T., Kincard, D. L. and Rinehart, W. (1997). *Health Communication: Lessons from Family Planning and Reproductive Health*. Praeger Publishing Group: Westport, CT.

Ratzan, S. C., Ed. (1994). Special Issue: Health communication: Challenges for the 21st century. *American Behavioral Scientist*, 38(2).

Rice, R. E. and Atkin, C. K., Eds. (1989). *Public Communication Campaigns*. Sage Publications: Thousand Oaks, CA.

Rogers E. M. (1973). *Communication Strategies for Family Planning*. Free Press: New York.

Smart, J. and Smart, D. (1994). The rehabilitation of Hispanics experiencing acculturative stress: Implications for practice. *Journal of Rehabilitation*, 60(4):8-14.

Sowell, T. (1996). *Migrations and Cultures: A World View*. Basic Books: New York.

Substance Abuse and Mental Health Services Administration (1996). *National Household Survey on Drug Abuse* (Part 6). Department of Health and Human Services.

Sussman, S. and Johnson, C. A., Eds. (1996). Special Issue: Drug abuse prevention: Programming and research recommendations. *American Behavioral Scientist*, 39(7).

Syme, S. L. (1997). Community participation, empowerment, and health: Development of a wellness guide for California. *1997 Wellness Lectures*, The California Wellness Foundation and the University of California:147-167.

Taylor, D. and Lambert, W. (1996). The meaning of multiculturalism in a culturally diverse urban American area. *The Journal of Social Psychology*, 136(6):727-740.

Turnock, B. and Handler, A. (1997). From measuring to improving public health practice. *Annual Review of Public Health*, 18:261-282.

UCLA Center for Communication Policy (1997). *The UCLA Television Violence Report 1997*. University of California, Los Angeles, CA.

United Way of Greater Los Angeles (1994). *State of the County Databook: Los Angeles 1996-97*. United Way: Los Angeles, CA.

U.S. Census Bureau (1990). *1990 Census*. Department of Commerce, US Census Bureau Website.

U.S. Census Bureau (1996). *Estimate for 1996 US Population*. Department of Commerce, US Census Bureau Website.

WHO/UNICEF (1978). *ALMA-ATA 1978 Primary Health Care: Report of the International Conference on Primary Health Care*. WHO: Geneva, Switzerland.

CHAPTER 2

Multi-Ethnic Considerations in Community-Based Drug Abuse Prevention Research

Mary Ann Pentz, Sadina Rothspan,
Gencie Turner, Silvana Skara,
and Serineh Voskanian

Community-based approaches to drug abuse prevention have received increasing attention in recent years. The rationale for using the entire community to plan and implement a drug prevention strategy is that such a strategy is likely to include more channels for program delivery, program exposure, and opportunities for repetition and diffusion of prevention messages and changing the social norm for drug use than are available from single channel programs such as school or parent programs (Pentz, 1993). As this chapter will discuss, most of the community-based drug abuse prevention research conducted thus far has focused on communities that are either primarily white, with smaller ethnic groups represented within the larger white community, or communities that represent primarily one ethnic group. Few community-based prevention efforts have deliberately focused on multi-ethnic communities, defined as communities that represent multiple, sizeable ethnic populations within a circumscribed community, region, or neighborhood. Federal research agencies are currently exploring whether drug abuse and other chronic disease risk behaviors require specialized prevention interventions for multi-ethnic communities, particularly whether unique interventions are required for each type of community or whether certain principles of community-based prevention research might be universal or generalizable across communities regardless of ethnic status. The remainder of this chapter addresses this question.

ISSUES IN PLANNING PREVENTION RESEARCH IN MULTI-ETHNIC COMMUNITIES

General Issues

Several general issues should be considered first in planning prevention research in multi-ethnic communities, among them: (1) the stereotype of equating ethnicity with risk; (2) cultural themes of health, disease, and prevention; and (3) acculturation stress.

Equating Ethnicity with Risk

Two disturbing assumptions surround prevention with minority populations: preventive interventions that have already been developed on white populations will not generalize to different ethnic groups; and minority (ethnic) groups are at higher risk for drug use and other diseases than whites.

Results of epidemiological and prevention studies do not support these assumptions. Rather, results suggest that minority/ethnicity as a risk factor may be a proxy for socioeconomic status (e.g., Johnson, et al., 1990; Murray, et al., 1988). Ironically, minority interest groups may note the lack of available preventive services and fiscal resources as an argument for needing increased or different resources than other populations. An increase in drug abuse risk resulting from a lack of preventive services, again, is an economic rather than an ethnic issue. The same economic argument can be applied to predicting poor implementation and diffusion of prevention programs, which in turn are related to continued drug use problems in communities (see the ethnic validity model, Javier, 1992).

Cultural Themes of Health, Disease, and Prevention

Results of anthropologic research, using primarily ethnographic methods of observation, have yielded several cultural themes pertinent to the conduct of prevention research in multi-ethnic communities. Health is regarded in some cultures as a slow process of environmental and personal accommodation and a sense of well-being, self-esteem, and personal wholeness vs. a set of observable physical indicators (Landrine and Klonoff, 1992). Disease is perceived as a lack of accommodation and wholeness, with symptoms in some cultures described in terms of good vs. bad blood or hot vs. cold, rather than prevalence rates of drug use or other disease risk behavior (Landrine and Klonoff, 1992). In the specific case of drug use, quantitative indices of abuse are not as meaningful as indices of cultural rejection (Caetano and Medina-Mora, 1988; Legge and Sherlock, 1990-91). Principles of prevention may not be as meaningful as slow evolution of well-being and healing. Western societal preventive intervention tools of education, social support-seeking, resources, and independence may not be relevant or may require reinterpretation in terms of self-value and growth, confidante and family support, and interdependency (Fisher, Auslander, Sussman, Owens, and Jackson-Thompson, 1992). Skills-related prevention concepts of verbal communication, peer group, and group peer pressure situations may not be as important as non-verbal communication or identification of what constitutes a peer group, depending on what is normative and valued by the community (Schilling, Schinke, Nichols, and Botvin, 1989). Identifying a population or community as at risk, based on an epidemiologically defined set of risk criteria, may not be as meaningful or as motivating as redefining risk in terms of a general population or community "anomie" (Landrine and Klonoff, 1992; Hawkins, Catalano, and Miller, 1992).

Acculturation Stress

Communities populated by one dominant minority group or mixed minority groups, or which are experiencing a rapid in-migration of one or more minority groups, may be subject to several stressors on their capacity to organize effectively for prevention. The stressors may include attributions of helplessness and difficulty of acculturation to majority social norms for behavior (Landrine and Klonoff, 1992; Pentz, 1994). Attempting to accommodate to majority norms, minority communities may show an unusually high tolerance for conditions that would be considered unacceptable to other communities. Thus, by the time a critical incident or initiating event to community organization for drug abuse prevention does occur, it may serve as a flash point for aggressive or destructive behavior before positive organization can be realized (Oetting and Beauvais, 1991; Pentz, 1994). The prevention researcher should anticipate that a multi-ethnic community undergoing acculturation stress is likely to react quickly, and often negatively, to proposals for prevention research that have few, or delayed timelines for tangible products.

Specific Issues

In addition to general issues of conducting research with different ethnic groups, four specific issues are relevant to conducting prevention research in multi-ethnic communities. The *universality of prevention* relates to whether multi-ethnic communities require different prevention strategies from single ethnic or primarily white communities. The issue of *theory* relates to whether theories that have been developed from research on white populations may not be applicable to multi-ethnic communities, and/or whether only theories developed from anthropological or ethnographic research specific to ethnic groups are applicable. *Organization* relates to whether multi-ethnic communities should be prepared and organized for community-based drug abuse prevention differently from other communities, including whether the unit that defines community and readiness for prevention may differ across ethnic populations. Finally, the methodological issue of the *conduct of research* encompasses the role of the researcher at each stage of research and community organization development, emphasis on formative vs. summative evaluation research, and the role of ethnographic measures and designs compared to typical methodologies used in prevention outcome research.

To determine whether and how these issues have been addressed in research, a selective review of the drug abuse prevention literature was conducted. The review was constrained to a Medline search of published studies since 1990 that used a community-based approach to drug abuse prevention for or including youth, included one or more ethnic groups, and evaluated ethnicity for its relationship to process, implementation, and/or outcome. The review yielded twenty studies. Where particular themes emerged, results of this review are used to illustrate or support a conclusion about each issue.

Universality of Primary Prevention vs. Need for Tailored Prevention

Most drug abuse prevention programs that have been evaluated and shown to have significant effects on youth drug use are universal in the sense that the assumptions about behavior change and the methods used to induce behavior change are intended to be applicable across youth, regardless of ethnicity. Most programs have been school-based (Hansen, 1992). Among the few utilizing a community-based approach to drug abuse prevention, assumptions about the universality of prevention for different ethnic groups are less clear. For example, some studies of community-based drug abuse prevention have purposely applied the same prevention programs or strategies across the community, regardless of ethnic make-up of the community population, or applied programs previously developed on white populations to different ethnic groups (e.g., Butterfoss, Goodman, and Wandersman, 1996; Galbraith, et al., 1996; Schinke, Orlandi, and Cole, 1992; Schinke, Jansen, Kennedy, and Shi, 1994; St. Pierre, Kaltreider, Mark, and Aiken, 1992; Shea, Basch, Wechsler, and Lantigua, 1996). However, more than half of the reviewed studies have assumed that each ethnic group and community is different, thereby requiring development of intervention "from scratch" (e.g., Schorling, et al., 1997; Baldwin, et al., 1996; Delgado, 1996; Hernandez and Lucero, 1996; Vorheees, et al., 1996; Amodeo, Wilson, and Cox, 1995; Cheadle, et al., 1995; Ellis, et al., 1995; Kaufman, Jason, Sawlski, and Halpert, 1994; Groth-Marnat, Leslie, and Renneker, 1996; Walton, Ackiss, and Smith, 1991). It is not known whether assumption of automatic differences between ethnic groups is a function of source or criteria for research funding, a real possibility since several recent federal research announcements have been tied to developing or testing prevention strategies specifically designed or tailored to different ethnic groups (e.g., CSAP community partnership and high risk youth research announcements).

Research indicates that preventive interventions aimed at changing social influences on drug use have shown the most significant effects on delaying the onset of tobacco, alcohol, and marijuana use in adolescents. An underlying assumption of these programs is that the cognitive-behavior change principles of skills modeling, rehearsal, feedback, and practice are adaptable to any ethnic population or culture because participants generate their own skills situations (Bandura, 1977). Based on these principles, social influences programs appear to be effective, whether they teach counteractive skills specific to drug use or broader social skills that can be applied to counteracting drug use influences (Botvin and Botvin, 1992; Hansen, 1992; Tobler, 1992).

Limitations in research designs have prohibited determining whether the magnitude of prevention program effects is the same for different ethnic groups, including African-American, Hispanic, and American-Indian youth (e.g., see Botvin, et al., 1989; Johnson, et al., 1990; Oetting and Beauvais, 1991; Schilling, Schinke, Nichols, and Botvin, 1989), however, results thus far suggest that social influences approaches to prevention are effective with, as well as adaptable to, multi-ethnic groups. These results are consistent with epidemiological studies, which have shown similar patterns of social influences as risk factors for drug use among white and several different ethnic groups of adolescents (e.g., Bachman, Johnston, and O'Malley, 1991; Johnson, et al., 1990). It is logical to assume that social influences approaches should also apply to broader, community-based drug prevention efforts developed in multi-ethnic communities.

Theoretical vs. Atheoretical Approach to Behavior Change

Also referred to as the distinction between theory-based and action research, this issue is two-pronged: whether any existing theory is applicable to different ethnic groups, and/or if a theory is applicable, whether it should be a theory that is specifically derived from anthropological or ethnographic research on ethnic groups. Ten of the reviewed studies were based on theories that are assumed to fit all populations and communities, regardless of ethnicity; prominent among these theories are social learning and other theories of social influence, which focus on individual or intra-personal level modeling and previous behavior as behavior change influences, as well as situational or interpersonal level setting and social normative influences (e.g., Johnson, et al., 1990; Kaufman, et al., 1994; Schinke, et al., 1992, 1994; St. Pierre, et al., 1992; Shea, et al., 1996; Weiner, Pritchard, Frauenhoffer, et al., 1993). Three studies utilized social action theories or models that presume tailoring of a prevention program for a specific population, particularly based on social group influences like community leader networking (Baldwin, et al., 1996; Butterfoss, et al., 1996; Ellis, Reed, and Scheider, 1995). The remaining seven studies were considered atheoretical, based on either lack of use or lack of reference to any theory in the development and testing of a prevention program (Amodeo, et al., 1995; Cheadle, et al., 1995; Groth-Marnat, 1996; Schorling, 1997; Yin and Kaftarian, 1997). Thus, the majority of the studies reviewed presume use of a theory-based prevention strategy, using theory that can be applied across or with different ethnic groups with various degrees of tailoring. Where theory was employed, behavior change influences were limited primarily to either person or situation/group level factors. From a research perspective, use of theory was also related to use and explanation of a protocol for community organization and process, experimental control, and reporting of outcomes.

The relative advantage of using theory in planning community drug abuse prevention programs, and the typical situations in which theory is used, are shown in Table 1 (Pentz, 1995a). Lack of theory may be most associated with community drug abuse prevention efforts that are community-driven, that is, initiated and planned by the community with little or no impetus from research. Typically, these efforts take the form of a search for drug abuse prevention or treatment services, a response to a drug abuse crisis, a recognized gap in service delivery, and/or a funding opportunity. In contrast, theory is associated with research-driven prevention efforts which derive from funded research or a specific research

Table 1. Implications of Community- and Research-Driven
Prevention Programs

	Community-Driven	Community Research Partnership	Research-Driven
Theory	Atheoretical	Integrated p × s × e theory, with attention to acculturation	Integrated
Model	None	Structural + Process	Structural + Process
Organization	Grassroots, bottom-up	Interdependent top-down, bottom-up	Top-down
Process	Iterative	Flexible sequential	Fixed Sequential
Accountability	Anecdotal information, no. served, or none	Anecdotal + no. served + program evaluation	Research
Experimental Control	None	Moderate	High
Projected Effects	Unknown	High	Weak-Moderate
Generalizability	None	High, with cultural adaptation	Low, no cultural adaptation

Reprinted with permission from M. A. Pentz, "Prevention research in multi-ethnic communities: Developing community support and collaboration, and adapting research methods," in Botvin, G.J., Schinke, S. and Orlandi, M. (Eds.), *Drug Abuse Prevention with Multi-ethnic Youth*, California: Sage, 1995.

question that can be addressed by testing the effectiveness of a specific prevention approach. Community prevention efforts which entail the active partnership between community constituents, leaders, and researchers, may rely on the use of a more integrated theoretical perspective that includes environmental influences rather than on a single theory or a set of individual theories.

From a theoretical perspective, community based prevention can be expressed as the interaction of person × situation × environment level factors (see Figure 1). Person level factors are intra-individual variables that predict which community leaders will organize for drug abuse prevention and how actively they will participate. Variables include non-smoking status and previous civic service involvement of community leaders (see Pentz, 1986; Pentz and Montgomery, unpublished manuscript). Situation level factors involve inter-individual variables including regular communication among leaders of different community agencies and centrality of communications (Freeman, 1978; Galaskiewicz, 1979; Valente and Pentz, 1990). Finally, environment level factors involve existing system level variables that support community organization for prevention, including active representation of businesses, re-allocating existing resources, and concise, well disseminated prevention-oriented policies (Green, Kreuter, Deeds, and Partridge, 1980; Pentz, 1989; Pentz and Trebow, 1997).

Several researchers have proposed adaptations of the p × s × e perspective to multi-ethnic communities. Some, like Fisher, et al. (1992) and Baranowski (1992), propose that a traditional behavior change model can be applied, with ethnic and community-specific applications of modeling, natural contingencies, cues, self-attribution, and self-efficacy as p level factors; skills and social support as s factors; and empowerment as an e factor. For example, social support for adolescents in a multi-ethnic community would be interpreted as the use of a confidante and high density, informal social networks vs. a trusted, credible adult or professional. Empowerment would be sought through locality or neighborhood development, volunteer partnerships, and use of an initial lead or host agency vs. large-scale community organization for drug abuse prevention, professional partnerships, and initial establishment of an independent community organization. Sussman, among others, proposes that the p × s × e perspective be tailored further to the multi-ethnic community by including perceptions of the majority culture or other communities, and attention to physical space, crime, and housing at the neighborhood level (Sussman, 1992). This perspective requires that community organization would necessarily address deficits in basic care and the physical environment as a major, and perhaps first, component of a prevention strategy (Fisher, et al., 1992).

Organizing the Community

Organizing a community for drug abuse prevention involves consideration of at least four factors: (1) identifying the unit of "community" for intervention;

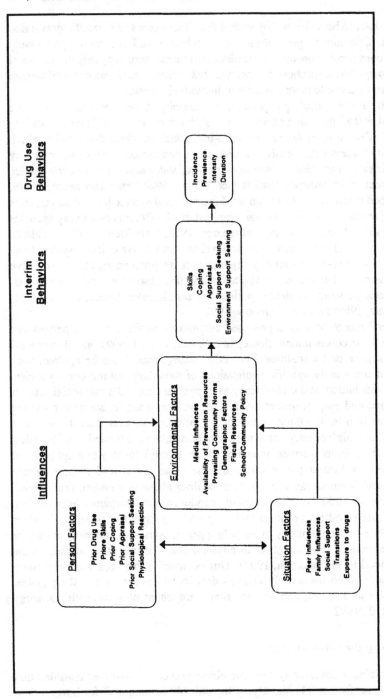

Figure 1. Person × situation × environment influences on drug use behavior in the community (General MPP Model). Reprinted with permission from Pentz, M.A. Primary prevention of adolescent drug abuse. In: *Applied Developmental Psychology*, (C.B. Fisher, R.M. Lerner (Eds.) pp. 435–474). New York: McGraw-Hill, 1993.

(2) assessing and preparing the community for readiness for prevention; (3) determining a structure by which individuals or groups responsible for prevention will be organized to plan and implement intervention; and (4) agreement of responsible parties to a process by which the intervention will be planned, implemented, and monitored.

Unit of Community—There are several complexities involved in applying prevention research to multi-ethnic communities. The first is identifying what constitutes a "community." Sarason and others have emphasized that a community can be identified on the basis of geographic, social/sociocultural, and psychological boundaries; all three boundaries should be considered in developing and tailoring of preventive interventions to the specific needs and resources of the community (Sarason, 1974).

Community Readiness—Research from education, mass communications, school and community psychology, and social work suggest several indicators of community readiness for prevention (Boruch and Shadish, 1983; Brown, 1993; Chavis and Wandersman, 1990; Fisher, et al., 1992; Goodman and Steckler, 1990; Pentz, 1986; Pentz and Valente, 1993; Perkins, Florin, Rich, Wandersman, and Chavis, 1990; Pretsby and Wandersman, 1985; Sarason, 1974; Wandersman and Giamartino, 1980; Zimmerman and Rappaport, 1988). These are organized in sequence in Figure 2. Community self-recognition or identity presupposes all other criteria for readiness, followed by perceived awareness and importance of the prevention problem and the need for prevention research, and perceived opportunity for intervention, which will vary according to whether the community's typical *modus operandi* is passive, active, or reactive to related community problems.

Regardless of demographic characteristics, communities are expected to vary in their readiness to organize for comprehensive drug abuse prevention. They are also expected to vary in terms of specific types of existing agencies to include in a community organization for drug abuse prevention, the focus of the community organization on prevention, early intervention and/or treatment, and the timing of local government involvement. Identifying community readiness and tailoring organizational strategies to fit community needs may be expressed roughly as a function of community type. Based on community psychology and organization development literature, a typology of communities is proposed based on three criteria: (1) whether a community is defined as a recognizable geographic, social, and psychological unit (Pentz, 1986; Sarason, 1983); (2) whether the perceived empowerment of community and government leaders to effect drug prevention is high or low (Wallerstein and Bernstein, 1988); and (3) whether formal groups or agencies for drug prevention exist prior to the development of an integrated community organization for drug abuse prevention (Pentz, 1986; Wandersman, 1981). Crossing the three criteria yields eight categories or types of communities (see Table 2). In general, communities that are well defined, with empowered

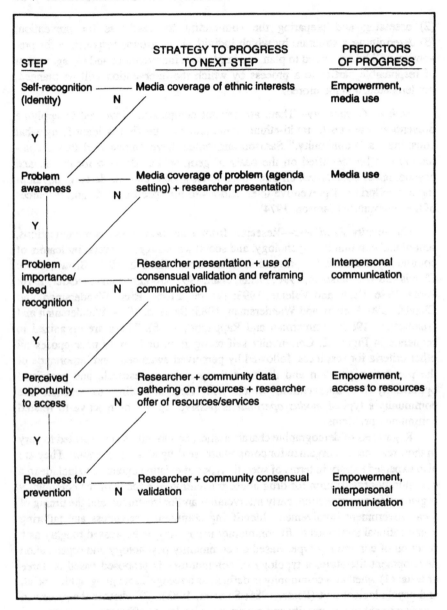

Figure 2. Model of community readiness.
Reprinted with permission from Pentz, M.A., "Prevention research in multi-ethnic communities: Developing community support and collaboration and adapting research methods," *Drug Abuse Prevention with Multi-Ethnic Youth,* Botvin, Schinke, Orlandi (Eds.), California: Sage, 1995a.

Table 2. Community Readiness and Empowerment

	Community Type			Organizational Strategies			
Defined Unit	Level of Empowerment	Formal Organizations for Drug Prevention	Length of Time to Organize	Types of Agencies to Include	Focus of New Community Organization	Timing of Local Government Involvement
1. Yes	Mod-High	Present	2-6 mos.	Business, media, school, parent, youth groups, youth service, health/medical	Primary Intervention + Early Intervention + Treatment	Late
2. Yes	Mod-High	Absent	6 mos.-1.5 yrs.	Business, media, school, parent	Primary Intervention + Early Intervention[b]	Mid
3. Yes	None-Low	Present	2+ yrs.	Media, school, parent, youth group, youth service	Early Intervention + Treatment	Early-Mid
4. Yes	None-Low	Absent	2+ yrs.	School, youth group	Early Intervention[b]	Early
5. No	Mod-High	Present[a]	1-1.5 yrs.	School, health/medical	Early Intervention + Treatment	Mid-Late
6. No	Mod-High	Absent	2+ yrs.	School, parent	Early Intervention[b]	Early[c]
7. No	None-Low	Present[a]	2+ yrs.	School, youth group, youth service, health	Treatment	Early-Mid[c]
8. No	None-Low	Absent	—	School	N/A	Late or Not at all[c]

[a]County-level organizations
[b]Early intervention limited to schools, e.g., SAP and peer counseling groups
[c]County-level government

Reprinted with permission from M.A. Pentz, A comprehensive strategy to prevent the abuse of alcohol and other drugs: Theory and methods. In Coombs, Ziedonis (Eds.), Handbook on Drug Abuse Prevention, Allyn and Bacon, 1995b.

leaders and existing structures for drug prevention, could be expected to organize most quickly, incorporate more types of agencies with less threat of territoriality, focus on primary prevention as a major objective but have sufficient resources to include early intervention and treatment, and manage without local government involvement until later phases of intervention focus on policy change.

The typology has not been evaluated experimentally; thus, typing criteria, time periods, and organizational strategies should be considered approximate. As the relationships between community characteristics and organizational capacities are evaluated systematically in future research, the typology can be expected to shift and expand. Also, changes in secular trends in drug use and acceptance of drug abuse prevention strategies nationally can be expected to contribute to changes in conceptualizing the typology.

Organizational Structure—Several overviews of prevention research suggest a bi-polar tendency of communities to organize for prevention, either as a result of grassroots, bottom-up pressure in response to a critical negative event or chronic condition; or as part of a researcher/expert, top-down plan prompted by an organization or funding opportunity (e.g., Giachello, 1992; Goodman et al., 1996; Pentz, Alexander, Cormack, and Light, 1990; Pentz, et al., 1986; Rothman, 1979). The published literature suggests that ethnic and multi-ethnic communities tend to organize at the grassroots level, or, if initially prompted by research, may reject what is perceived as white or majority tenets of research (cf. Chavis and Wandersman, 1990; Oetting and Beauvais, 1991; Pentz, 1994). Little is known about whether rejection of research-driven community organization by multi- ethnic communities is due to lack of access to prevention researchers, distrust of researchers, or failure of researchers to recognize and "package" prevention in terms of the community's perceived needs, norms, and solutions (Pentz, et al., 1986).

The most effective strategy for organizing communities for prevention may be a combined top-down/bottom-up, community/research partnership (Altman, 1986; Pentz, 1994). Characteristics of and research predictions about prevention based on a balanced community/research partnership, are shown in Figure 1. However, little is known about whether top-down or bottom-up approaches to community organization for drug abuse prevention are more or less effective for integrating new groups with any existing community agency and local government initiatives and groups. A third issue is maintaining the function of local government as providing environmental support for a non-drug use social norm in the community. Since local government oversees the use of law enforcement in the service of drug abuse prevention, it may be difficult to inhibit the development or perceived development of local government as a community "watchdog" of drug abuse, a function which could engender resentment rather than cooperation from community residents and agencies.

Organizational Process—Once the unit of community intervention has been determined and the community is ready for prevention and a structure for decisions about planning and implementation of programs is determined, then the process by which research and programming are implemented, refined, and maintained must be specified. Butterfoss, et al. (1996), in applying a process model to community partnership sites funded by the Center for Substance Abuse Prevention, pays particular attention to the process by which community leaders achieve and recognize their empowerment to make change. For example, community leaders must first move toward readiness for prevention (see Figure 2) before agreeing upon specific prevention objectives to complete for their community; completion of each objective is acknowledged by the group and plans for future objectives are initiated. In another example, community leaders and researchers agree to move through ten planning steps, with achievement of each step (e.g., needs assessment of the community) completed before the next step is attempted (Pentz, 1986). These planning models require that community leaders be systematic in their decisions and show long-term commitment to the organizational process. In multi-ethnic communities with fractured support, divisiveness of leaders, or leader turn-over, such a systematic long-term process may not be achievable.

Among the reviewed studies, fourteen of the twenty included a planning period. While only five of these could be determined to have followed a systematic, established protocol for planning (Butterfoss, et al., 1996; Ellis, et al., 1995; Johnson, et al., 1990; Shea, et al., 1996; Yin, et al., 1997), the finding that fourteen used a planning period to successfully develop program or research materials suggests that use of an organizational process model in multi-ethnic communities is feasible. Furthermore, twelve of the twenty studies reported developing or tailoring program and research materials for their communities, a finding which suggests that most researchers and community leaders expect to modify programs for use with different ethnic groups.

A GENERAL MODEL OF COMMUNITY PREVENTION RESEARCH

A model of community prevention research should specify the structure, process, implementation, maintenance, and outcomes of community organization. The expanded model presented here in Figure 3 allows for flexible choices at each step to accommodate the special needs of ethnic/racial communities.

Baseline Community Characteristics

Baseline community characteristics are represented by the same physical/demographic, social, and psychological constructs used to define boundaries of communities, as suggested by Sarason (1974) and others (Wandersman and Giamartino, 1980). Physical characteristics include the physical condition of the

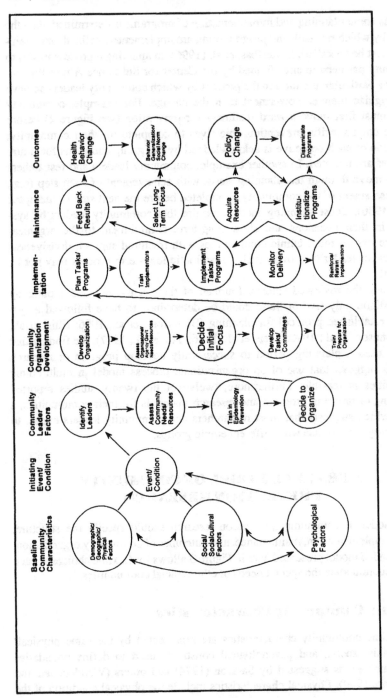

Figure 3. A general model of community organization.

Reprinted with permission from Pentz, M.A. Alternative models of community prevention research. Langton, Eptstein, Orlandi (Eds.), Challenge of Participatory Res. CSAP cultural competence series 3: Rockville, MD, 1996.

community, size, residential stability, racial/ethnic make-up, income, home/ business ownership, urbanicity, and population density; as well as the physical resource plant represented by the number and size of financial, informational, and support networks among existing organizations within the community (Galaskiewicz, 1979; Perkins, et al., 1990). Social characteristics include the centrality of communications among existing organizations; the level of support or conflict between organizations, schools, mass media, and local government; positive community acceptance (versus passive tolerance) of new and existing minority groups; acculturation of minority groups to the community (versus general societal acculturation); and sense of affiliation among minority groups. Psychological factors include the perceived and actual empowerment of the community, existing organizations within the community, and individuals to effect health behavior change; the perceived and actual readiness of the community to participate in such change; and the level of community upset or intolerance for existing conditions.

Initiating Events or Conditions

Initiating event(s) or conditions serve as catalysts to community organization. Event(s) can represent negative or positive community life events to which a community reacts by initiating the process of community organization around the event topic. An acute negative community life event, such as a tragic drunk-driving death of an adolescent on the night of graduation, increases community awareness of youth alcohol problems and can escalate to the level of a perceived community crisis if all population groups in the community have directly experienced a similar type of event or have been mobilized by the local mass media to empathize with the affected group. An example is drunk-driving deaths as a catalyst to the organization of Mothers Against Drunk Driving (MADD) groups in communities across the United States.

Chronic adverse conditions in a community may also serve as a catalyst to community organization. In this case, no particular event triggers organization; rather, community residents and leaders have already had preliminary discussions about community needs; the discussions evolve into community organization. Perkins and Associates (1990) have evaluated a model of participation in community block associations that showed an association between chronically poor physical conditions in a neighborhood and subsequent participation among residents who expressed an affiliation with the neighborhood. Chronic acculturation stress may also serve as a catalyst for change (Landrine and Klonoff, 1992).

Community Leader Identification and Preparation

Leaders undergo a process to prepare for formal community organization. Leaders may be leaders of existing formal organizations in the community, for example, directors of local health agencies, youth agencies, churches, parent groups, schools. If the community has had a prior history of failure with formal organizations, however, residents may decide to nominate grassroots leaders from the resident population who are known and respected by residents but who have served in no formal leadership capacity prior to organization.

Leaders prepare for formal organization in three steps: (1) an informal consensual assessment of the condition and readiness of the community for organization (initial needs/resources assessment); (2) arranging and participating in initial training in the etiology, epidemiology, prevention, and treatment of the community problem that fostered the initiating event or condition for organizing; and (3) meeting to formally agree to organize. Agreement to organize may be impeded if mass media coverage is negative, and/or if community leaders do not believe that they are empowered by residents, local government, or other existing organizations to address the community problem (Florin and Wandersman, 1990). In two studies of neighborhood block organizations in racially mixed metropolitan areas, the Neighborhood Participation Project in Nashville and the Block Booster Project in New York City, Florin and Wandersman concluded that blocks receiving professionally provided training in organization development and materials for suggested programs were significantly less likely to decline in participation after ten-month follow-up.

Community Organization Development

Katz and Kahn (1978) have noted that organizing communities effectively to address a particular problem or goal requires initial resources, a structure recognized by leaders and residents, specific production activities, and outputs or outcomes. Prestby and Wandersman (1985) added factors that contribute to organization maintenance as well as development, including the acquisition of other resources, monitoring of implementation, and feedback to the community.

Initial community organization will vary as a function of individual community differences in baseline characteristics, initiating events or conditions, and community leader factors, particularly community readiness and community and leader perceptions of empowerment. In addition to these individual differences, the particular form of organization will vary systematically according to several parameters: resource networks, incentive systems, problem acuteness, problem generalization, and problem approach.

Resource networks include but are not limited to financial support, information/communication, and physical and social support and transportation (Galaskiewicz, 1979; Florin and Wandersman, 1990). Leaders will tend to centralize their communications and new organizational efforts around the sources of these networks.

For example, in a disaffected, isolated minority community with no indigenous business leaders and a distrust of local government run by whites, new community organization might mobilize around neighbors who represent an active communication or transportation network. Organization would be from the grassroots level, or bottom up; local government would be excluded or delayed in involvement until such time as the community organization as a group felt empowered to demand local policy change regarding the community problem.

Incentive systems include material, solidary [sic], and purposive (Clark and Wilson, 1961). The incentives drive initial and maintained interest of community leaders in participating in community organization, as well as the general objectives and goals of the organization. For example, if community leaders and residents perceive a lack of goods, services, and facilities as the major means to improve the community and eliminate the presenting problem, then the organization will be structured to acquire and reinforce participants with materials as an initial focus, with tasks and work committees oriented toward the acquisition of specific types of materials.

Other parameters involve the initiating event or condition. If a community's problem is acute *and* little is known about its community-specific etiology and epidemiology, community leaders may decide to organize an initial task force to investigate the problem's size and origins before deciding on a course of intervention. A task force is usually mobilized quickly, gives rapid feedback to community leaders and residents about the scope of the problem, and then is disbanded and/or replaced with other, more permanent structures to plan, deliver, and monitor interventions to address the problem. If the problem is acute *and* specific, the community may organize as a coalition of community leaders or as a formal community organization that is independent of but includes representatives of other existing organizations. A coalition is structured to represent a formal "united front" against the presenting community problem which includes local government representatives as part of its membership and has local policy change as an explicit or implicit goal.

If the community problem is chronic, pervasive, indicative of general adverse conditions in the community, *and* likely to generalize to other problems and events, community leaders may opt for general community development rather than development of a specific task force, coalition, or community organization.

The development of an effective community organization effort requires operationalizing goals as a series of tasks with definite timelines for achievement, delegation of tasks to specific individuals or committees which serve as substructures to the larger community organization, and training or preparing individuals or committees in methods to accomplish these tasks. The tasks, and thus substructures, vary according to either the content of the community problem or the end health behavior change target.

Thus far, the steps from assessing baseline characteristics through community organization development represent a planning period. Among the studies selectively reviewed for this article, thirteen out of twenty, or more than half, reported a planning period that included one or more of the phases described in the community organization model. Length of planning varied, from several months, to three years, the latter in the case of the CSAP community partnerships (Yin and Kaftarian, 1997). The remaining studies involved generalizing an existing community organization model to different ethnic groups or communities.

Implementation

Actual implementation of the community organization's work, or "production input," involves at least five measurable steps: (1) outlining specific tasks or programs to be implemented, with required resources, delegated personnel, and timelines; (2) identifying and training implementors, whether they are indigenous to the community or a combination of indigenous personnel and outside experts; (3) implementing tasks or programs according to a standardized protocol used for training and agreed upon by the community organization; (4) formal monitoring, evaluation, and feedback about the quality of implementation, ideally by individuals who are independent of training and implementation and thus are assumed to be more objective; and (5) provision for regular reinforcement and retraining of implementors, to maintain their motivation to continue implementation, and to cope with personnel turnover in communities. Consistently, research and program evaluation studies have shown that effects of preventive interventions on health behavior are highly dependent on the quality of implementation *as designed* (Pentz, 1995b).

Maintenance

While program monitoring during the implementation phase involves giving at least periodic feedback to program implementors, use of regular feedback of results of community organization and intervention is critical during the maintenance phase. Depending on the initiating event and initial focus of organization in the community, potential long-term foci include prevention of problems that have been shown to be co-morbid with the initial community problem, for example, a long-term AIDS prevention focus that is linked to initial alcohol and drug abuse prevention; prevention of chronic diseases linked to the initial problem, for example, a long-term focus on cancer prevention that is linked to early smoking prevention; or general health promotion that expands an initial focus on nutrition. Maintenance will also depend on the acquisition of new physical, financial, and social resources to carry out programs that represent the long-term focus of the organization (Prestby and Wandersman, 1985).

Outcome

Measurable outcomes of community organization include changes in prevalence rates of the target health behavior. For example, two-thirds of the studies reviewed reported drug-use or drug-use-related outcomes. Other outcomes include generalization of organizational and prevention program effects to other related health behaviors; changes in community acceptance of the initial problem and social norms for the target health behavior; increased centrality of community leader and inter-agency communications and cooperation; increased community leader and resident perceptions of empowerment *and* capacity to empower other leaders and agencies for long-term health initiatives through policy change; and institutionalization of prevention programs in the community.

RESEARCH METHODS AND CONDUCT

Role of the Researcher

The role of the researcher may differ according to stage of preparation for research in multi-ethnic communities. Specific stages and roles are discussed below.

Acknowledging Need for Prevention

Through informal discussions with contacts in the proposed community and review of archival records and local print media coverage, the prevention researcher should determine the most culturally familiar and acceptable method of approaching the community for prevention. The methods may include but are not limited to: word of mouth, designated information seeking, and support/resource seeking. In almost all cases, these communication models assume self-recognition or a strong sense of identity by the multi-ethnic community. All three assume that the first approach for prevention is from inside of the community out toward the researcher. The prevention researcher should determine, then, not only the best method of communication approach but also a means for the community to initiate the approach.

Selecting/Planning Intervention

In assisting the community to select and plan the most appropriate prevention program, the researcher takes on the role of information sharer or broker. The researcher can translate the results of epidemiological research on drug use development and key mediators of effective drug abuse prevention programs to the terms, situational contexts, and resources of the community. Some researchers have developed risk profile models by which each community can gauge its relative risk and protective factors for drug use (Hawkins, et al., 1985). Such models are intended to be generalizable for use by any community, yet flexible enough to enable a community to tailor a prevention program to its own risk profile.

Adopting/Implementing Intervention

Ready adoption by community leaders is a key factor in diffusing a prevention program across a community (Rogers, 1987), and high-quality implementation is a critical factor in determining whether that program is likely to be effective in changing youth drug use (Pentz and Trebow, 1997). After assisting communities to select the appropriate program, a researcher takes on the role of information sharer and resource provider or networker to help promote early adoption and high quality implementation. In multi-ethnic communities that have parallel groups of influential leaders and implementors representing each ethnic interest, the researcher may have to repeat information-sharing and resource-provision across each ethnic group and tailor these accordingly. For example, in an inner city area of African-American families, resource provision might consist of providing an appropriate setting for parent training, for example, local churches; in another area of the same community, a smaller ethnic group of Hispanic families might require translation of printed materials.

Disseminating Intervention

Finally, the researcher facilitates dissemination of the community prevention program across different ethnic groups in a community by acting as advisor to each group and to community leaders as a whole regarding the best use of their existing resources for dissemination, including donated media, business support, and volunteers. The mechanisms for dissemination may be the same as those discussed earlier to initiate approach to a community, but the particular mechanism may vary across ethnic groups and density of the groups within the community. For example, dissemination among a tight-knit group of Hispanic families living in the same neighborhood may be accomplished through word of mouth or through a trusted church or family leader. Dissemination among individuals of the same ethnic group living in isolation from one another or in a large widespread area might require use of a communication channel that easily reaches those individuals and is used exclusively and respected by that group, for example, a local language community newsletter.

Formative Evaluation

Formative evaluation is a crucial step in adapting existing theories and community organization models to multi-ethnic communities. At a minimum, formative evaluation should include: the early use of focus groups to generate or validate cultural themes, procedures, and content; measures, intervention, and design development; piloting; and early revision.

Based on the discussion in previous sections, the types, procedures, settings, and themes of focus groups used in formative evaluation in multi-ethnic communities can be expected to differ from other communities. Questions about the meaning of health and prevention, normative communication patterns, empowerment and other predictors of community readiness, and perceptions of research can be used to develop focus group content. However, based on the selective review of studies of drug abuse prevention in multi-ethnic communities, only five of the twenty used focus groups to develop methods or program materials (Butterfoss, et al., 1996; Schorling, et al., 1997) and only eight assessed readiness for prevention (Amodeo, 1995; Butterfoss, et al., 1996; Galbraith, et al., 1996; Groth-Marnat, 1996; Hernandez, 1996; Johnson, et al., 1990; Schorling, et al., 1997). These findings suggest that few community prevention research studies include formative evaluation for identifying potential ethnic group differences, although the need for formative evaluation in planning prevention research in multi-ethnic communities is widely acknowledged.

Summative Evaluation

Conducting an appropriate summative or outcome evaluation of intervention in multi-ethnic communities requires attention to all aspects of research methodology to eliminate the potential for a biased estimate or interpretation of intervention effect. These aspects include measurement, intervention, and analysis. The most typical drug abuse prevention research measure is the self-report survey, usually administered to large numbers of subjects in group settings such as a school, or through the mail. However, if the language, format, or administration of a survey is unfamiliar to a particular ethnic group, or produces different degrees of comprehension among ethnic groups in the same community, any ethnic group differences found in drug use before or after preventive intervention might be biased by the survey. Such concerns have led to inclusion of ethnographic survey methods to aid in developing appropriate self-report surveys, or to replace traditional survey techniques where they are not feasible for a large scale administration, for example, with homeless youth.

In addition to concerns about measurement, the dependent variable and analysis method selected for outcome evaluation may bias estimation and interpretation of community prevention program effectiveness. For example, in a community represented by both white and African-American youth, daily smoking is apt to be very low in the latter group. If the major dependent variable for analysis is daily smoking prevalence, intervention effects on daily smoking among African-American youth are likely to be non-significant, simply because of the very low prevalence rates (low variability) at baseline. A combination of dependent variables that collectively represent the variation in drug use and relevance to each ethnic group in a community is warranted. Then analyses focus on patterns of change across the community as a whole, as well as across each ethnic group, to determine program effectiveness. Similarly, the analysis method or methods used must be relevant to different ethnic groups. For example, survival analysis used to determine how long one stays a non-user is not appropriate for a population with a sporadic use pattern.

ETHNIC/RACIAL COMMUNITY CONSIDERATIONS

The proposed models for community organization and community prevention research are intended to apply to all communities, with individual differences determined by the presence or absence or levels of specific variables representing constructs of readiness, type of community, and impetus for prevention (community or research). As an example, Table 3 shows four case examples of communities that vary in their minority make-up, with realistic goals and directions for community organization and research. Although the community organizational strategies for each are hypothetical, the communities themselves are based on real examples encountered in prevention studies. The rural, Native-American community is based on communities participating in the Tri-Ethnic Center at Colorado State University (Altman, 1986). The rapid in-migration of Vietnamese and other Asian groups along a major interstate that crosses a White community is based on a pilot prevention project in Tustin, California (Pentz, et al., 1986). The primarily Hispanic community within a larger mixed minority metropolitan area is based on a proposed cervical cancer prevention study in East Los Angeles (Pentz, et al., in preparation). The primarily Black city with community units organized as blocs is based on initial efforts by Corporations Against Drug Abuse (CADA) to disseminate portions of the Midwestern Prevention Project programs in wards of Washington, D.C. (CADA, in progress). Note that law enforcement cooperation, grass roots organization, volunteer resources, minimal demands for professional training, and late-stage involvement of researchers predominate in these community examples in order to match organizational strategies to existing resources and minimize further stress on day-to-day community functioning.

CONTRAINDICATIONS TO A GENERAL MODEL OF COMMUNITY ORGANIZATION

It could be argued that the general model described here is a rational decision-making model built on Western (primarily Anglo-Saxon) principles of leadership and community organization; culture-free concepts of behavior change, most notably behavior modification concepts from social learning theory; and initial prevention education strategies that rely on person-level predictors of and solutions to drug abuse. Evidence is growing to support adaptations of this type of general model to diverse populations. The most recent example may be the current organizational efforts of communities participating in the Robert Wood Johnson Fighting Back program. Two years after planning community-wide drug abuse prevention, culturally and ethnically diverse communities that initially attempted to organize from the perspective of community vs. expert-driven initiatives have evolved through organizational, process, and structural models very similar to those presented here (Pentz, 1993). Nevertheless, at least three exceptions should be noted for which any adaptation of a general model may be contraindicated.

The first contraindication is a community with a negative history, if not outright failure, of previous researcher involvement in community organization for prevention. The negative history would go far beyond simple distrust of government services or professional involvement as discussed earlier, to outright refusal of the community to adopt or follow any protocol that is specified a priori. In this case, the community should anticipate a development period that is characterized by multiple regular challenges from competing interest groups as they vie for attention and support.

The second contraindication is a community with such diverse interest groups that consensual, organized leadership for prevention is not possible. In this case, it is conceivable that diverse groups develop their own separate agendas for prevention within the community, and meet only temporarily for the purpose of agreeing to principles of least harm or infringement to each other and to the community. A community may be expected to progress through several slow stages before organization for prevention can be attempted, from a temporary alliance for least harm, to some community healing after harm has been reduced, to tentative consideration of proposals that promote positive growth of separate interest groups while maintaining least harm to others.

The third contraindication is a community with perceptions about drug abuse, prevention, and treatment that are radically different from rational, intra personal, time-limited, and expert-dependent theories and research of Western, white culture. Researchers attempting to work in such communities are advised to conduct a thorough formative evaluation before determining whether any rational, deterministic model can be applied to prevention. Rather than a prevention needs and resources assessment based on available services, a formative evaluation would first consist of evaluating how the population identifies or labels drug abuse and its symptoms, attributes causality, anticipates consequences, and expects a course and duration of "cure" (Landrine and Klonoff, 1992). If the formative evaluation yields findings that do not fit current theoretical and research schemas of drug abuse prevention, the researcher's subsequent role may be observer and documenter of a community process that may or may not develop into an organizational model, and may or may not be generalizable to other minority communities.

Table 3. The General Model Applied to Hypothetical Case Examples of Minority Communities: Organizational and Research Directions

Phase of Community Organization	County, Rural Native American	Small City, White w/ Vietnamese Corridor	Hispanic Community within Metropolitan Area	Primarily Black City
Baseline Community Characteristics	• Low mobility • Low SES* • No business - N • Low density reservation clusters • Community unit = tribe • Adult/youth acculturation conflict - Y • Sense as victim - Y* • Isolated - Y • Empowerment - N* • Affiliation - N	• High mobility • Mixed SES • Small business - Y • Mixed density • Small neighborhoods • Community unit = city • White equation - N • Isolated - Y • Empowerment - N • Affiliation - N	• Low mobility • Low SES • Small business - Y • High density • Large neighborhood • Community unit = city section • Minority integration - N • Isolated - Y • Empowerment - N* • Minority subgroup acculturation conflict - N • Isolated - N • Empowerment - Y • Affiliation - Y	• High mobility • Low SES • Own business - N • High density • Small blocs • Community unit = street block • Minority equation - N • Isolated - Y • Empowerment - N • Affiliation - N
Initiating Event/ Condition	• High rate of youth alcohol abuse	• Youth drunk driving death	• Multiple gang shootings	• Drug-related crimes, youth deaths, poor housing"
Community Leader Identification and Preparation	• N/A - Formal tribal leadership	• Identify formal and informal (parent) leaders through local ads, government/ school nomination, self nomination • Assessment - Y • Introductory training - Y • Decide to organize - Y	• Formal leadership already developed; develop informal parent and peer leaders through neighborhood "hangouts" • Assessment - Y • Introductory training - N • Decide to organize - Y	• Identify informal church, parent leaders through church, resident blocks, teen centers • Assessment - Y • Introductory training - N • Decide to organize - Y

Community Organization Development	• Community development • Assess tribe/government interactions • Initial focus = ↓ alcohol demand • Organization = topdown	• Community organization for alcohol/drug abuse prevention • Community/school cooperation for prevention education • Initial focus = ↑ community awareness of problem • Develop campaign and education tasks • Mass media preparation meetings • Organization = bottom-up parent grass roots initiation with topdown follow-up	• Community organization for juvenile delinquency prevention • Assess law enforcement/ school cooperation • Initial focus = school education • Organization = bottom-up neighborhood grass roots and top down Hispanic organizations	• Community development • Assess volunteer efforts, law enforcement cooperation • Initial focus = clean-up campaign • Organization = bottom-up neighborhood/church grass roots*
Implementation	• Train indigenous parents/ peer leaders in supportive counseling • Peer monitoring • Special events*	• Plan community campaign *with local media in order to commerce, minority leader representatives volunteers independent	• Train teachers/peer leaders • Train parent volunteers to increase parent awareness in neighborhoods	• Mobilize adult/youth volunteers*
Maintenance	• Research assistance for feedback • Long-term focus = development of alternative leisure activities • Acquire resources - N/A • Dissemination - N/A • Gov't involvement - Y	• Research assistance for feedback and maintaining local interest • Long-term focus = regular prevention education in schools • Acquire resources from White and Vietnamese businesses and initial volunteer support • Dissemination - N/A • Gov't involvement - Y	• Research assistance for feedback and maintaining local interest • Long-term focus = regular prevention education in schools/court and counseling assistance for indicted youth • Acquire local business, law enforcement, Hispanic organization resources • Dissemination - Y • Gov't Involvement - N* • Law enforcement - Y*	• Researcher assistance in evaluating effective use of social services • Long-term focus = ↑ education, leisure activities for youth • Acquire job training and job support resources • Dissemination - N/A • Gov't involvement - N • Law enforcement - Y

Table 3. (Cont'd.)

Phase of Community Organization	County, Rural Native American	Small City, White w/ Vietnamese Corridor	Hispanic Community within Metropolitan Area	Primarily Black City
Outcomes	↓ Youth alcohol use ↓ Acceptance of youth alcohol use ↑ Trainer empowerment	↑ Community awareness of alcohol/drug problems ↑ Community leader acceptance of minority groups ↑ Adoption of school prevention program cultural content	↑ Family responsibility for keeping neighborhoods gang free ↑ Mainstreaming of indicted youth into community service ↑ Student peer leader counseling	↑ Residential/safe zone* ↑ Protection/avoidance of gangs, crime ↑ Neighborhood* empowerment
Future Directions for Organization	• Negotiating more control over government resources • Lobby to remove alcohol outlets	• Increasing minority access to local health care and resources	• Integrating law enforcement officers as educators • Changing school policy about drugs/crime free zones • Developing family/sibling alternative models for gang members	• Acquire health care, counseling for youth • Maintaining crime/drug free zones • Developing housing construction resources, volunteers
Future Directions for Research	• Evaluate youth pressure on adults to ↓ alcohol use	• Evaluate community acceptance of minority groups, empowerment of minority groups	• Evaluate effectiveness of community vs. law enforcement control of gang behavior	• Evaluate effects of clean up and safe zones on residential stress, physical illness, employment

Note: Asterisks (*) denote variables that represent common minority community issues and responses. Choice points are indicated by Y (Yes) or N (No) for each variable within each construct represented in Figure 1; variables without Y or N represent continuous variables that are not expected to moderate community organization.

Reprinted with permission from M.A. Pentz, "Alternative models of community prevention research in ethnically and culturally diverse communities," In Langton, P., Epstein, L.G. and Orlandi, M.A. (Eds.), *Challenge of Participatory Research: Preventing Alcohol-related Problems in Ethnic Communities.* CSAP Cultural Competence Series 3, Rockville, MD: Center for Substance Abuse Prevention, 1996.

SUMMARY

The general models described here are, for the most part, rational decision-making models built on culture-adaptable concepts of behavior change, most notably, behavior modification concepts from social learning theory. Evidence is growing to support adaptations of these types of general models to multi-ethnic communities. However, in multi-ethnic communities with perceptions about drug abuse, prevention, and treatment that are radically different from rational theory—another concept from Western, white culture—some of these models may not hold. Researchers attempting to work in such communities are advised to conduct a thorough formative evaluation before determining whether any rational, deterministic, sequential models can be applied to prevention.

REFERENCES

Altman, D. G. (1986). A framework for evaluating community-based heart disease prevention programs. *Social Sciences and Medicine*, 22:479-487.

Amodeo, M., Wilson, S., and Cox, D. (1995). Mounting a community-based alcohol and drug abuse prevention effort in a multicultural urban setting: Challenges and lessons learned. *The Journal of Primary Prevention*, 16(2):165-185.

Bachman, J. G., Johnston, L. D. and O'Malley, P. M. (1991). Explaining the recent decline in cocaine use among young adults: Further evidence that perceived risk and disapproval lead to reduced drug use. *Journal of Health and Social Behavior*, 31(290): 173-184.

Baldwin, J. A., Rolf, J. E., Johnson, J., Bowers, J., Benally, C. and Trotter, R. T. (1996). Developing culturally sensitive HIV/AIDS and substance abuse prevention curricula for Native American youth. *Journal of School Health*, 66(9):322-327.

Bandura, A. (1977). *Social Learning Theory*. Prentice Hall: Englewood Cliffs, New Jersey.

Baranowski, T. (1992). Interpersonal models for health behavior intervention with minority populations: Theoretical, methodologic, and pragmatic issues. In D. M Becker, D. R. Hill, J. S. Jackson, D. M. Levin, F. A. Stillman and S. M. Weiss (Eds.), *Health Behavior Research in Minority Populations: Access, Design, and Implementation* (pp. 112-121). NIH National Heart, Lung, and Blood Institute, NIH Publication No. 92-2965, U.S. Government Printing Office: Washington, D.C.

Boruch, R. F. and Shadish,W. R. (1983). Design issues in community intervention research. In E. Seidman (Ed.), *Handbook of Social Intervention* (pp. 73-98). Sage Publications: Beverly Hills, CA.

Botvin, G. J., Batson, J. W., Witts-Vitale, S., Bess, V., Baker, E. and Dusenburg, L. (1989). A psychosocial approach to smoking prevention for urban Black youth. *Public Health Reports*, 104:5783-5758.

Botvin, G. J. and Botvin, B. M. (1992). Adolescent tobacco, alcohol, and drug abuse: prevention strategies, and empirical findings, and assessment issues. *Journal of Developmental and Behavioral Pediatrics*, 13(4):2990-3301.

70 / SUBSTANCE ABUSE PREVENTION

Brown, L. S., Jr. (1993). Alcohol abuse prevention in African-American communities. *Journal of the National Medical Association*, 85(9):665-673.

Butterfoss, F. D., Goodman, R. M. and Wandersman, A. (1996). Community coalitions for prevention and health promotion: Factors predicting satisfaction, participation and planning. *Health Education Quarterly*, 23(1):65-79.

Caetano, R. and Medina-Mora, M. E. (1988). Acculturation and drinking among people of Mexican descent in Mexico and the U.S. *Journal of Studies on Alcohol*, 49:462-471.

Chavis, D. M. and Wandersman, A. (1990). Sense of community in the urban environment: A catalyst for participation and community development. *American Journal of Community Psychology*, 18(1):55-81.

Cheadle, A., Pearson, D., Wagner, E., Psaty, B.M., Diehr, P. and Koepsell, T. (1995). A community-based approach to preventing alcohol use among adolescents on an American Indian reservation. *Public Health Reports*, 110(4):439-447.

Clark, P. B. and Wilson, J. Q. (1961). Incentive systems: A theory of organizations. *Administrative Science Quarterly*, 6:129-166.

Delgado, M. (1996). Implementing a natural support system AOD project: Administrative considerations and recommendations. *Alcoholism Treatment Quarterly*, 14(2):1-14.

Ellis, G. A., Reed, D. F. and Scheider, H. (1995). Mobilizing a low-income African American community around tobacco control: A force field analysis. *Health Education Quarterly*, 22(4):443-457.

Fisher, E. B., Auslander, W., Sussman, L., Owens, N. and Jackson-Thompson, J. (1992). Community organization and health promotion in minority neighborhoods. In D. M. Becker, D. R. Hill, J. S. Jackson, D. M. Levin, F. A. Stillman and S. M. Weiss (Eds.), *Health Behavior Research in Minority Populations: Access, Design, and Implementation* (pp. 53-72). NIH National Heart, Lung, and Blood Institute, NIH Publication No. 92-2965, U.S. Government Printing Office: Washington, D.C.

Florin, P. and Wandersman, A. (1990). An introduction to citizen participation, voluntary organizations, and community development: Insights for empowerment through research. *American Journal of Community Psychology*, 18(1):41-53.

Freeman, L. (1978) Centrality in social networks: Conceptual clarification. *Social Networks*, 1:215-239.

Galaskiewicz, J. (1979). The structure of community organizational networks. *Social Forces*, 57:1346-1364.

Galbraith, J., Ricardo, I., Stanton, B., Black, M., Feigelman, S. and Kaljee, L. (1996). Challenges and rewards of involving community in research: An overview of the "Focus on Kids" HIV Risk Reduction Program. *Health Education Quarterly*, 23(3): 383-394.

Giachello, A. L. (1992). Reconciling the multiple scientific community needs. In D. M. Becker, D. R. Hill, J. S. Jackson, D. M. Levin, F. A. Stillman and S. M. Weiss (Eds.) *Health Behavior Research in Minority Populations: Access, Design, and Implementation* (pp. 237-241). NIH National Heart, Lung, and Blood Institute, NIH Publication No. 92-2965, U.S. Government Printing Office: Washington, D.C.

Goodman, R. M. and Steckler, A. (1990). A model for the institutionalization of health promotion programs. *Family and Community Health*, 11(4):63-78.

Goodman, R. M., Wandersman, A., Chinman, M., Imm, P. and Morrissey, E. (1996). An ecological assessment of community-based interventions for prevention and health promotion: Approaches to measuring community coalitions. *American Journal of Community Psychology.* 24(1):33-61.

Green, D. W., Kreuter, M, Deeds, S. G. and Partridge, K. B. (1980). *Health education planning: A diagnostic approach.* Mayfield Publishing Co.: Palo Alto, CA.

Greene, L. W., Smith, M. S. and Peters, S. R. (1995). "I have a future," Comprehensive adolescent health promotion: Cultural considerations in program implementation and design. *Journal of Health Care for the Poor and Under-Served,* 6(2):267-281.

Groth-Marnat, G., Leslie, S. and Renneker, M. (1996). Tobacco control in a traditional Fijian village: Indigenous methods of smoking cessation and relapse prevention. *Social Science and Medicine,* 43(4):473-477.

Hancock, L., Sanson-Fisher, R. W., Redman, S., Burton, R. and Burton, L., et al. (1997). Community action for health promotion: A review of methods and outcomes 1990-1995. *American Journal of Preventive Medicine,* 13(4):229-239.

Hansen, W.B. (1992). School-based substance abuse prevention: A review of the state of the art in curriculum, 1980-1990. *Health Education Research,* 7(3):403-430.

Hawkins J. D., Catalano R. F. and Miller J. Y. (1992). Risk and protective factors for alcohol and other drug problems in adolescence and early adulthood: Implications for substance abuse prevention. *Psychological Bulletin,* 11(1):64-105.

Hawkins, J. D., Lishner, D. M. and Catalano, R. F. (1985). Childhood predictors and the prevention of adolescent substance abuse. In C. L. Jones and R. J. Battjes (Eds.), *Etiology of Drug Abuse: Implications for Prevention* (pp. 75-126). National Institute on Drug Abuse Research Monograph, 56.

Hernandez, L. P. and Lucero, E. (1996). DAYS La Familia Community Drug and Alcohol Program: Family-centered model for working with inner-city Hispanic families. *The Journal of Primary Prevention,* 16(3):255-272.

Javier, R. A. (1992). Design and implementation as a function of models: Critical assessment of models. In D. M. Becker, D. R. Hill, J. S. Jackson, D. M. Levin, F. A. Stillman and S. M. Weiss (Eds.), *Health Behavior Research in Minority Populations: Access, Design, and Implementation* (pp. 141-44). NIH National Heart, Lung, and Blood Institute, NIH Publication No. 92-2965, U.S. Government Printing Office: Washington, D.C.

Johnson, C. A., Pentz, M. A., Weber, M. D, Dwyer, J. H., MacKinnon, D. P., Flay, B. R., Baer, N. A. and Hansen, W.B. (1990). The relative effectiveness of comprehensive community programming for drug abuse prevention with risk and low risk adolescents. *Journal of Consulting and Clinical Psychology,* 58(4):4047-4056.

Katz, D. and Kahn, R. L. (1978). *The Social Psychology of Organizations.* John Wiley and Sons: New York.

Kaufman, J. S., Jason, L. A., Sawlski, L. M. and Halpert, J. A. (1994). A comprehensive multi-media program to prevent smoking among black students. *Journal of Drug Education,* 24(2):95-108.

Landrine, H. and Klonoff, E. A. (1992). Culture and health-related schemas: A review and proposal for interdisciplinary integration. *Health Psychology,* 11(4):2667-2676.

Landrine, H., Richardson, J. L., Klonoff, E. A. and Flay, B. (1994). Cultural diversity in the predictors of adolescent cigarette smoking: The relative influence of peers. *Journal of Behavioral Medicine*, 17(3):331-346.

Legge, C. and Sherlock, L. (1990-91). Perception of alcohol use and misuse in three ethnic communities: Implications for prevention programming. *International Journal of the Addictions*, 25(5A-6A):629-653.

Murray, D. M., Jacobs, D. R., Perry, C. L., Pallonen, U., Harty, K. C., Griffin, G., Moen, M. E. and Hanson, G. (1988). A statewide approach to adolescent tobacco-use prevention: The Minnesota-Wisconsin Adolescent Tobacco-Use Research project. *Preventive Medicine*, 17:461-474.

Oetting, E. R. and Beauvais, F. (1991). Critical incidents: Failure in prevention. *International Journal of the Addictions*, 26(7):797-820.

Pentz, M. A. (1986). Community organization and school liaisons: How to get programs started. *Journal of School Health*, 56:382-388.

Pentz, M. A. (1989). A model public/private collaborative program for drug abuse prevention among adolescents: The Midwestern Prevention Project. In *Evaluating School-Based Prevention Strategies: Alcohol, Tobacco and Other Drugs* (pp. 31-35). University of California at San Diego: San Diego, CA.

Pentz, M. A. (1993). Comparative effects of community-based drug abuse prevention. In J. S. Baer, G. A. Marlatt and R. J. McMahon (Eds.), *Addictive Behaviors Across the Lifespan: Prevention, Treatment, and Policy Issues* (pp. 69-87). Sage Publications: Thousand Oaks, CA.

Pentz, M. A. (1994). Target populations and interventions in prevention research: What is high risk? In B. Bukowski and Z. Amzel (Eds.), *NIDA Research Monograph* (pp. 75-94). NIH Publication No. 94-3631, U.S. Government Printing Office: Washington, D.C.

Pentz, M. A. (1995a). Prevention research in multiethnic communities: Developing community support and collaboration, and adapting research methods. In G. J. Botvin, S. Schinke and M. A. Orlandi (Eds.), *Drug Abuse Prevention with Multiethnic Youth*. Sage Publications: Thousand Oaks, CA.

Pentz, M. A. (1995b). A comprehensive strategy to prevent the abuse of alcohol and other drugs: Theory and methods. In R. Coombs and C. Ziedonis (Eds.), *Handbook on Drug Abuse Prevention*. Allyn & Bacon: Boston.

Pentz, M. A. (1996). Alternative models of community prevention research in ethnically and culturally diverse communities. In P. Langton, L. G. Epstein and M. A. Orlandi (Eds.), *Challenge of Participatory Research: Preventing Alcohol-Related Problems in Ethnic Communities* (pp. 69-104). CSAP Cultural Competence Series 3, Center for Substance Abuse Prevention: Rockville, MD.

Pentz, M. A. and Montgomery, S. B. Research-based community coalitions for drug abuse prevention: Guidelines for replication. Unpublished manuscript.

Pentz, M. A., Alexander, P., Cormack, C. and Light, J. (1990). Issues in the development and process of community-based alcohol and drug prevention: The Midwestern Prevention Project. In N. Giesbrecht, P. Consley, R. W. Denniston, et al. (Eds.), *Research, Action, and the Community: Experiences in the Prevention of Alcohol and Other Problems*, OSAP Prevention Monograph 4, USDHHS: Washington, D.C.

Pentz, M. A., Cormack, C., Flay, B. R., Hansen, W. B. and Johnson, C. A. (1986) Balancing program and research integrity in community drug abuse prevention: Project STAR. *Journal of School Health*, 56:389-393.

Pentz, M. A., Dwyer, J. H., MacKinnon, D. P., Flay, B. R., Hansen, W. B., Wang, E. Y. I. and Johnson, C. A. (1989). A multi-community trial for primary prevention of adolescent drug abuse: Effects on drug use prevalence. *Journal of the American Medical Association*, 261(22):3259-3266.

Pentz, M. A., Peters, R. and MacKinnon, D. P. Cervical cancer prevention for high-risk Hispanic populations (in preparation).

Pentz, M. A. and Trebow, E. (1997). Implementation issues in drug prevention research. *Substance Use and Misuse*, 32(12&13):1665-1670.

Pentz, M. A. and Valente, T. (1993). Effects of community organization on a drug abuse prevention campaign. In T. E. Backer, E. Rogers, M. Rogers and R. Denniston (Eds.), *Impact of Organizations on Mass Media Health Behavior Campaigns*. Sage Publications: Thousand Oaks, CA.

Perkins, D. D., Florin, P., Rich, R. C., Wandersman, A. and Chavis, M. (1990). Participation in the social and physical environment of residential blocks: Crime and community context. *American Journal of Community Psychology*, 18(1):83-115.

Prestby, J. and Wandersman, A. (1985). An empirical exploration of a framework of organizational viability: Maintaining block organizations. *Journal of Applied Behavioral Science*, 2(13):287-305.

Rappaport, J. (1995). Empowerment meets narrative: Listening to stories and creating settings. *American Journal of Community Psychology*, 23(5):795-807.

Reitsma-Street, M. and Arnold, R. (1994). Community-based action research in a multi-site prevention project: Challenges and resolutions. *Canadian Journal of Community Mental Health*, 13(2):229-240.

Roberts, R. N. (1993). Early education as community intervention: Assisting an ethnic minority to be ready for school. *American Journal of Community Psychology*, 21(4): 521-535.

Rogers, E. M. (1987). The diffusion of innovations perspective. In N. D. Weinstein (Ed.), *Taking Care: Understanding and Encouraging Self-Protective Behavior* (pp. 79-94). Cambridge University Press: New York.

Romer, D. and Kim, S. (1995). Health interventions for African American and Latino youth: The potential role of mass media. *Health Education Quarterly*, 22(2):172-189.

Rothman, J. (1979). Three models of community organization practice, their mixing and phasing. In F. M. Cox, et al. (Eds.), *Strategies of Community Organization: A Book of Readings*, 3rd ed. (pp. 25-45). F. E. Peacock Publishers: Itasca, IL.

Sarason, S. B. (1974). *The Psychological Sense of Community: Prospects for a Community Psychology*. Jossey-Bass: San Francisco, CA.

Sarason, S. B. (1983). Psychology and public policy: Missed opportunity. In: R. E. Felner, L. A. Jason and J. M. Moritsugu (Eds.). *Preventive Psychology: Theory, Research, and Practice*. Pergamon Press: New York.

Scheier, L. M., Botvin, G. J., Diaz, T. and Ifill-Williams, M. (1997). Ethnic identity as a moderator of psychosocial risk and adolescent alcohol and marijuana use: Concurrent and longitudinal analyses. *Journal of Child and Adolescent Substance Abuse*, Special Issue, 6(1).

Schilling, R. F., Schinke, S. T., Nichols, S. E. and Botvin, G. J. (1989). Developing strategies for AIDS prevention research with Black and Hispanic drug users. *Public Health Reports*, 104(1):2-11.

Schinke, S., Jansen, M., Kennedy, E. and Shi, Q. (1994). Reducing risk-taking behavior among vulnerable youth: An intervention outcome study. *Community Health*, 16(4): 49-56.

Schinke, S. P., Orlandi, M. A. and Cole, K. C. (1992). Boys and girls clubs in public housing developments: Prevention services for youth at risk. *Journal of Community Psychology*, Special Issue:118-128.

Schorling, J. B., Roach, J., Siegel, M., Baturka, N., Hunt, D. E., Guterbock, T. M. and Stewart H. L. (1997). A trial of church-based smoking cessation interventions for rural African Americans. *Preventive Medicine*, 26:92-100.

Shea, S., Basch, C. E., Wechsler, H. and Lantigua, R. (1996). The Washington Heights-Inwood Healthy Heart Program: A 6 year report from a disadvantaged urban setting. *American Journal of Public Health*, 86(2):166-171.

St. Pierre, T. L., Kaltreider, D. L., Mark, N. N. and Aikin, K. J. (1992). Drug prevention in a community setting: A longitudinal study of the relative effectiveness of a three-year primary prevention program in boys and girls clubs across the nation. *American Journal of Community Psychology*, 20(6):673-706.

Sussman, L. K. (1992). Critical assessment of models. In D. M. Becker, D. R. Hill, J. S. Jackson, D. M. Levin, F. A. Stillman and S. M. Weiss (Eds.), *Health Behavior Research in Minority Populations: Access, Design, and Implementation* (pp. 145-148). NIH National Heart, Lung, and Blood Institute, NIH Publication No. 92-2965, U.S. Government Printing Office: Washington, D.C.

Tobler, N. S. (1992). Drug prevention programs can work: Research findings. *Journal of Addictive Diseases*, 11(3):1-28.

Valente, T. W. and Pentz, M. A. (1990). *Communication networks as predictors of perceived program efficacy*. Paper presented at the Sunbelt X International Social Network Conference, February 15-18: San Diego, CA.

Wallerstein, N. and Berstein, E. (1988). Empowerment education: Friere's ideas adapted to health education. *Health Education Quarterly*, 15(4):379-394.

Walton, F. R., Ackiss, V. D. and Smith, S. N. (1991). Education versus schooling—Project Lead: High expectations! *Journal of Negro Education*, 60(3):441-453.

Wandersman, A. (1981). A framework of participation in community organizations. *Journal of Applied Behavioral Sciences*, 17:27-58.

Wandersman, A. and Giamartino, G. A. (1980). Community and individual difference characteristics as influences on initial participation. *American Journal of Community Psychology*, 8(2):217-228.

Weiner, R. L., Pritchard, C., Frauenhoffer, S. M. and Edmonds, M. (1993). Evaluation of a drug free schools and community program. *Evaluation Review*, 17(5):488-503.

Yin, R. K. and Kaftarian, S. J. (1996). What the national cross-site evaluation is learning about CSAP's community partnerships. In: N. R. Chavez and S. J. O'Neill (Eds.), *Secretary's youth substance abuse prevention initiative: Resource papers* (SAMSHA Pre-publication documents, pp. 179-196). U.S. Department of Health and Human Services: Washington, D.C.

Zimmerman, M.A. and Rappaport, J. (1988). Citizen participation, perceived control, and psychological empowerment. *American Journal of Community Psychology*, 16: 725-750.

CHAPTER 3

Engaging Women/Mothers in Multicultural Community Organizing to Prevent Drug Abuse*†

Gauri Bhattacharya

A recent survey on drug abuse among schoolchildren documented that the current use (within the past 30 days) of cigarettes and marijuana increased significantly among eighth graders (Monitoring the Future Survey, 1996).[1] Between 1995 to 1996, the use of cigarettes increased from 19.1 percent to 21 percent; marijuana use increased from 9.1 percent to 11.3 percent; the percentage who reported having been "drunk" in the past month increased from 8.3 percent to 9.6 percent. Another national survey (National Household Survey on Drug Abuse, 1996) found that, during the same time period, more teenagers in the twelve- to seventeen-year-old age group tried heroin for the first time; that children's perception of cocaine as risky was down; and that the use of hallucinogens continued an upward trend. Although the rate of use for all illicit drugs in the twelve to

*An earlier version of this chapter was presented at the 124th Annual Meeting of the American Public Health Association, New York, NY, in 1996.

†This study was supported by a grant from the National Institute on Drug Abuse (DA 009982; Gauri Bhattacharya, Principal Investigator). The views expressed herein do not necessarily reflect the positions of the granting agency or of the institute by which the author is employed.

[1] Throughout, the term drug abuse refers to the abuse of all drugs including alcohol, unless a specific substance is being discussed.

seventeen age group declined from 10.9 percent in 1995 to 9 percent in 1996, this survey reported that in 1996, 4.1 million smoked cigarettes in this age group, and there were about nine million current alcohol drinkers under age twenty-one. Youths age twelve to seventeen who currently smoked cigarettes were about nine times as likely to use illicit drugs and sixteen times as likely to drink heavily as non-smoking youths. In another survey, America's children and their parents identified drugs as the biggest problem they face (National Center on Addiction and Substance Abuse, 1996).

Empirically based longitudinal studies have shown that the onset, severity, and pattern of drug abuse are linked with risk factors present in both the individual and the environment (Blum and Richards, 1979; Hawkins, et al., 1992; Jessor and Jessor, 1977; Jones and Battjes, 1985; Newcomb, 1995). Studies have also indicated that early intervention programs can significantly delay the onset of tobacco, alcohol, and marijuana use by adolescents and can slow down the progression of drug use (Hansen, 1992; Pentz, 1995). Consistent with these findings, the field of drug abuse prevention emphasizes early childhood intervention programs to reduce risk factors and build resistance to drug use even before children enter school. Furthermore, since studies have also found that children's behaviors are positively associated with their families' predominant behaviors, cultural orientations, norms, and values, families are recognized as critical partners with other organizations in these prevention programs (Brook and Brook, 1992; Kandel, 1982; Kumpfer and Avarado, 1995).

In addition to educating children *early* about the negative effects of drug use/abuse and helping them acquire the social competence skills to resist drugs, a pro-active community that reinforces individuals' attitudes and norms, and strengthens skills, and works to eradicate the availability of drugs is critical to the success of any drug prevention program. Unless the demand and supply components are successfully integrated, education about the dangers of drug use alone, in a social environment that facilitates the availability of drugs, will fail (Brown, 1996). Thus, partnerships between families and the community are considered essential for reducing the demand for and the supply of drugs (Wechsler and Weitzman, 1996).

Although parents may unite around their concern for the destructive consequences of drug abuse by their children, the nature and characteristics of drug abuse problem also present unique barriers to the organizing at the community level. The legal consequences of drug use, parents' feelings of guilt over having failed to keep their children off drugs, and parents' denial of their children's addiction present unique impediments to the organizing process.

Policy makers, program planners and funding institutions in both the federal government and private have been promoting grass-roots organizations for family-community partnerships. However, the mechanism for translating individual-level concerns to collective efforts in multicultural communities is not yet well developed. This chapter proposes a new strategy for expanding these individual-level concerns for organizing family-based community programs.

This strategy is based on the author's study (1) of the characteristics of cultures that support parents' desire to care for their children and to extend that individual-level desire to all children in the context of *community organizing*, and (2) of three organizations that have based their interventions on those characteristics, and to use that framework as an effective approach to preventing drug abuse among children and adolescents. Consistent with this approach, the chapter focuses on strengthening the involvement of families, particularly mothers and other concerned women, as *change agents* in community organizing in multicultural communities.

This chapter is divided into five sections. The *first section* reviews the state-of-the-art research on the family's role in preventing drug abuse and in multicultural community organizing. The *second section* discusses the theoretical concepts on which the author's analysis of the organizations are based. Guided by the sociopsychological perspectives embedded in the cultural competence paradigm, this framework is grounded in the relevant literature on community organizing and research on drug abuse.[2] The *third section* presents the methods of analysis. The *fourth section* describes three organizations, initiated in three distinctively diverse cultures, whose strategies are based on cultural strengths that honor the values of caring and commitment. The *fifth section* develops a theory-driven drug prevention strategy in which parental concerns about drug abuse problems can be translated into collective actions via the community organizing process. The conclusion presents policy implications for the societal acceptance and operationalization on those values in the context of preventing drug abuse by children and adolescents. The author emphasizes that although women, especially mothers, have historically been associated with nurturing and the provision of care, such qualities are not their exclusive domains. The society as a whole should accept and operationalize these values in the context of drug abuse prevention among children and adolescents.

ROLES OF THE FAMILY IN DRUG ABUSE PREVENTION AND COMMUNITY ORGANIZING

In this chapter, families are viewed broadly as both biological and affinal (e.g., legal, common-law, informal) entities whose members supposedly care about one another. Within this broad framework, the structure and dynamics of the family are adapting to economic and social changes, and family roles and responsibilities are reconfigured; for example, single fathers are parenting their children and more and more mothers are entering the labor force (Klein and White, 1996).

---

[2] Tobacco is considered a gateway drug and is included in this study.

In whatever family forms children are raised, they are socialized by their parents according to certain traditions, mores, and beliefs, and by schools, their communities, and their environments. Their parents' cultural orientations influence their values, which, in turn, affect the manner in which they view the world (Bhattacharya, 1998). Thus, parents, individually and collectively, in collaboration with other organizations, can be instrumental for reducing both the demand for and the supply of drugs.

Reducing the Demand for Drugs

A "healthy" family is more likely to transmit non-drug-using behavior, both verbally and non-verbally, by (1) integrating pro-social values and beliefs, (2) providing supportive parenting, and (3) fostering psychological nurturance and adjustment (for an extensive literature on Family Strengths, see Kumpfer and Alvarado, 1995). A strong bond between parents and children ensures pro-social values and beliefs that can protect adolescents from and mediate against their children's formation of bonds with deviant peers. The length of the time spent with a child, however, is not the proxy for parent-child bonding. Rather, the communication of consistent, clear messages regarding commitment to school, academic success, and friends who have conventional values influences behavior directly through the social reinforcement of pro-social behavior and the positive consequences and the development of values and attitudes against drug use. Parents' roles in the family supervision, monitoring, and encouragement are important in reducing the demand for drugs and effectively applying drug prevention strategies. In contrast, a chaotic family environment results in adolescents' defying family rules, disrupting the powerbase in terms of family, and threatening the family's cohesiveness. This situation may lead to weakened family bonds and the lack of communication, which, in turn, may alienate parents and children and lead to bonds with deviant peers. Because adolescence is the period of socialization or the transition from childhood to adulthood, when emotional, psychological, and sociocultural skills are learned, it is also a critical time for implementing interventions that protect adolescents from using drugs (for an extensive literature on protective and risk factors, see: Newcomb, 1995).

Reducing the Supply of Drugs

A national survey (CASA, 1996) revealed that more than 70 percent of fifteen to seventeen years olds and their parents know that drugs are used and sold in high schools. According to this survey, children find that buying marijuana is easier than beer and admit that they can buy marijuana within a few hours. The supply of drugs can be reduced by (1) physically controlling the availability of drugs and (2) intervening early in the process of abusing drugs. Studies have found that children start using drugs at home, at friends' home, and in cars (Kumpfer and

Alvarado, 1995). Parents' supervision and monitoring of adolescents' activities at home and in the community can physically control the availability of drugs and thus can directly affect the supply. Drug abuse, however, is only one indicator of a multifaceted risk behavior; others include dropping out of school, associating with deviant peers, and engaging in promiscuous sexual behavior. Parents are often the first persons to notice any behavioral changes in adolescents (e.g., cutting classes, isolating from family, and bonding with deviant peers). They are often also the first ones to find out if those changes are related to drug abuse and then to be able to intervene immediately in the process. Parents' efforts to teach children skills to deal with the social environment (e.g., not to do drugs even when friends say it is the "in" thing to do) will be bolstered by their close supervision and monitoring of children's activities.

Although partnerships between families and the community are crucial for preventing drug abuse, this chapter focuses on involving parents, particularly mothers, more in community organizing. In this regard, participation is not restricted exclusively to biological mothers. Rather, other concerned women in the community such as neighbors of families with children and grandmothers who are worried for their grandchildren's use of drugs are encouraged to get involved in community organizing. Hence, throughout the remainder of this chapter the terms *mothers* and *women* are used interchangeably

Involvement of Women

Instead of confining themselves to their caretaking roles in their families, women may be empowered to build on their practice as caretakers to unite in the community for the cause of preventing abuse of drugs. Involvement of women in community organizing is conceptualized in this chapter from this broad perspective.

The empowerment of mothers and other women is considered as a *tool* in the community organizing process. The *empowerment* concept addresses the individual's capacity to recognize his/hers potential skills and to believe in his/her ability to change bad situations instead of coping with or accepting them (Gutierrez, 1995). Empowerment enables individuals to utilize their existing resources (e.g., caring and commitment) to initiate changes at both the individual and the community levels. The empowerment approach discussed here has been successfully applied in community organizing among the elderly poor persons in Tenderloin Senior Organizing Project in San Francisco (Minkler, 1992).

Organizing mothers to initiate sociobehavioral changes at the community level is a strategy that has not been fully utilized in drug prevention programs. However, the role of mothers in voluntary organizations as advocates for various political, economic, and legislative changes is increasingly being recognized. Three organizations that were started by mothers are described on p. 86.

COMMUNITY ORGANIZING IN MULTICULTURAL COMMUNITIES

A Multicultural Community

From a demographic perspective, a multicultural community is a place where people from different cultural groups live (Orlandi, 1992). However, residence is not the sole or crucial criterion of connectedness and a common interest or concern among community members—the basic requirement for community organizing. Drug problems may further exacerbate the sense of "disconnectedness" by increasing distrust among neighbors (Chavis and Wandersman, 1990). Thus, the description of a multicultural community entails the need to define the specific characteristics of each community (e.g., ethnicity and socioeconomic status) and also to understand the extent of connectedness (or disconnectedness) among the various ethnic groups in the community.

Culture is a system of interrelated values that influence and condition perceptions, judgment, communication, and behavior in a given society (Mazrui, 1986). Cultural beliefs and practices also influence the nature, extent, and context of drug use. Culture, however, is *not* only of past values and practices. Rather, cultural practices change over time in accordance with the interpretative values, beliefs, norms, and practices of a group in new environments. To change drug-use behavior, the need to examine health beliefs and actions at both the micro (individual) and macro (environmental) levels within a changed context are emphasized (Airhihenbuwa, 1995; Bhattacharya, 1998; Orlandi, 1992).

Community Organizing

Community organizing is a process that initiates "a purposive planned change in the community" (Green and Kreuter, 1991). In community organizing, the community is viewed as the medium for change and the goal—in this case, to prevent drug abuse—is considered as both the means (not to use drugs) and the end (drug abuse prevention) of the process. The community organizing process for preventing drug abuse among young adolescents described in this chapter is specially relevant for developing *universal* drug abuse prevention programs for the general population. Although the purpose of universal programs is to reduce the overall prevalence of drug use, such programs can increase the community's awareness of the problem by widely disseminating information on the availability of treatment services among those who are at risk (homeless youths and children in drug-abusing families). To be effective, however, universal programs must be comprehensive and their individual, familial, and environmental components must be well coordinated. Translating individual concerns into collective actions requires changes at different levels. At the individual level, for an adolescent, it requires changes in attitudes toward the use and abuse of drugs, and then the motivation to follow up with behavior; for parents it requires changes to take actions for changing the situation; for environments it requires changes to encourage forces that inhibit drug abusing behaviors and promote alternate pro-social behaviors.

THEORETICAL CONCEPTS

A public health perspective to health promotion is particularly relevant to examine the change process translating individual level concerns to the collective efforts to prevent children from drug abuse. Three principles espoused in this perspective are: (1) to understand the interrelationships between a person, situation, and the environment on behavior development; (2) to examine the impact of social norms, the cultural values, and the environmental circumstances surrounding and supporting the individual on health-related behavior; (3) to integrate changes at the individual level with the community level to monitor, reinforce, and sustain healthy and pro-social behavior. These three principles are also crucial to develop any program to prevent drug abuse among children and adolescents.

Theoretical Approaches to the Change Process

Theories of Community Change

Theories of community changes, like theories of individual changes, emphasize two components of change: attitudinal and structural. Attitudinal variables encompass shared interests or concerns, recognition of individual responsibility for initiating change, and affiliation with and acceptance of group membership. Structural variables include community resources—leadership, guidance, and skills in monitoring and/or modifying activities during the implementation process to complete tasks and achieve goals.

Previous research has emphasized changing community environments in order to initiate and sustain changes in individual's behavior (Cottrell, 1976). Two elements identified critical in community changes are (1) social changes require changes in the social context and (2) changes are more likely to occur if people are involved at the grass-roots level. Research has focused on the identification of needs and the competence of the community to address those issues. An approach that focuses on enabling the community as both the means to achieve goals and as a goal in itself is particularly relevant for community organizing to prevent drug abuse (O'Reilly and Piot, 1996; Tawail, et al., 1995). This approach postulates that to initiate community-level changes, program planners must identify both the strengths and risks/barriers to adoption of changes in the community and then develop strategies to foster the participation of individuals and groups to address those specific needs.

Three techniques are generally used in community organizing. (1) The *social action approach* depends on professionals as change agents to advocate the redistribution social resources to disadvantaged, oppressed persons (Rothman, 1995). (2) The *social planning approach* relies on expert planners to deliver the goods and services the community needs. (3) In contrast, the *locality development approach* relies on grass-roots development and actions for addressing problems in the community. Proper guidance and leadership to unite members of the community, develop strategies, and maintain the momentum of the process are essential in all three approaches. To develop programs to address the extent, dimension, and nature of the drug abuse problem, which varies from community to community and often within a community, the locality development approach is considered the most appropriate.

Integrating a Social-Psychological Perspective into a Culturally Competence Approach

The need to build a social norm for resilient behavior that is conducive to protecting children from drug abuse justifies the relevance of adapting the social-psychological perspective to the prevention of drug abuse among adolescents. Individual's behavior is viewed as socially conditioned, culturally embedded, and economically impacted acts. Health-related behavior is embedded in this overall behavior construct, and changing that behavior requires attention to social norms, the cultural values, and the economic and environmental circumstances surrounding and supporting that individual (Allen and Allen, 1990). The concept of building a social norm for behavior conducive to health is crucial in the social-psychological perspectives and justifies community approaches to health promotion. Following this perspective, empowerment is viewed as the mechanism and community organizing as the process to draw out and connect families on the basis of their shared concern and to promote and disseminate the desirable norms continuously to all segments of the community. To develop strategies to unite families in a multicultural community, community organizers must view competence in relation to values, purposes, and knowledge, which translate into effective performance. A culturally competent approach is multidimensional; it entails recognition, understanding, and appreciation of the similarities and the unique differences among different cultural groups in the community. To maximize the success of their efforts in multicultural communities, community organizers must develop culturally competent skills at the grass-roots, community advocacy, and professional community levels. They must also understand the efficacy of beliefs and practices related to the use of drugs that are prevalent in different cultures, some of which may be beneficial, some neutral, and some harmful in the context of drug use among adolescents. For example, Asians generally drink alcohol with their friends in recreational settings but consider getting drunk a personal deficit that indicates the loss of personal control (Bhattacharya, 1998).

Cultural competence is not a static notion, however. As cultural beliefs and practices change with changes in the environment, cultural competence should reflect the changed cultural perspectives of the people over time for which the programs are developed.

Cultural Themes

Parents' desire to protect their children from drug abuse may unite them across various cultural groups. To translate the individual-level concern to the community level, however, community organizers must understand the factors that are associated with community organizing in multicultural communities and the cultural factors that are relevant to the use and abuse of drugs. The factors related to community organizing include knowledge of symbolic-linguistic communication patterns; the underlying attitudes, values, and belief systems of different ethnic groups in the community; and knowledge of the interactional processes of different systems (family, peer, and community) in an ethnic group. The cultural factors related to the use and abuse of drugs include the similarities and differences in the etiologies of drug use in various ethnic and cultural groups and implications of the uniqueness of an etiology in a particular culture (e.g., drug addiction as a moral problem or religious sanctions against drinking alcohol). Practically, fulfillment of the above requirements necessitates involvement of multi-ethnic persons in a community organizing team. Particularly, at the grass-roots level, members of a multi-ethnic team may identify themselves culturally with the various cultural groups in the community. Furthermore, team members' familiarity with the customs, traditions, and kinship rules of the various groups may gain them access to social networks in the community, often predicting drug use/abuse pattern of the group. In addition to these factors, community organizers must become acquainted with the geographic area, the leaders, and the residents of the multicultural community (for a detailed discussion, see Pentz, 1995; Recio Adrados, 1993).

METHODS OF ANALYSIS

Eligibility

Organizations were eligible for inclusion in the analysis if they included the following elements: (1) parents' concern for the well-being of their children was translated from an individual-level to community organizing, (2) mothers and other women were united as change agents, (3) community organizing occurred in diverse cultures, (4) various strategies were interrelated but not constrained to one dimension (political, legal, economic, or cultural), and (5) the goals were measurable.

Procedure

In a review of the literature on women in community organizing, three organizations were found that satisfied the eligibility criteria and were included in the study. A content contingency analysis (Carney, 1972; Holsti, 1968; Krippendorf, 1980) was used to define each domain; to expand, identify, and clarify the items in each domain; and to ascertain differences among the organizations. Factors related to three broad domains—issues on which women united, characteristics of the community organizing process, and factors related to the outcomes—were examined.

Data Analysis

A thematic analysis of each domain identified items that were specifically associated with explaining a particular domain. Two independent coders identified themes for each narrative, and discrepancies were resolved in consultation with the author. Using content contingency analysis, it was determined if the item was consistent or inconsistent among the organizations. The resulting list of consistent or inconsistent items was documented. The responses for the items were coded as either dichotomous or categorical. For such items as, Was the issue related to a collective concern? That is, did all members of a family benefit? was dichotomized as yes or no. For such items as, Did the community organizing process involve a multilevel coalition? the responses were coded no, somewhat, to a certain extent, to a great extent, and extensively. Table 1 presents a comparison of the items in each domain across the three organizations and the characteristics that may define drug abuse prevention programs.

THREE ORGANIZATIONS IN THREE CULTURALLY DIVERSE COMMUNITIES

Given the diversity of social, cultural, economic, and political environments and their influences on the structure and dynamics of the communities, a single model would not sufficiently address the needs and elements that are unique to each community. Furthermore, different community organizers use different styles of functioning to ensure that their coalitions work. However, community organizers can use experiences with models tested in the field to guide their multifaceted plans for initiating changes and can adapt these models for use with specific communities or groups. Three organizations described here—Madres de Plaza de Mayo in Argentina, the Grameen Bank in Bangladesh, and Mothers Against Drunk Driving in the United States—were organized by mothers of

Table 1. Three Organizations Initiated by Women in Three Cultures

Elements	Madres	Grameen Bank	MADD	Drug Prevention
ISSUE				
Social approval	Humanitarian	Economic	Humanitarian	Social crisis
Focused goal	Missing children	Loan for work	Stop drunk driving	Stop drug use
Noncontroversial aspect	Family issue	Family issue	Social issue	National issue
Collective concern	All benefit	All benefit	All benefit	All benefit
PROCESS				
Task Performance				
Nature	Nonpolitical	Nonpolitical	Nonpolitical	Nonpolitical
Leadership	Mothers and women	A man	Mothers	Mothers and women
Membership	Mothers and women	Women	All	All
Level of public respect	International	International	International	Community/national
Multicoalition	A certain extent	Extensively	Extensively	Extensively
OUTCOME				
Goal Achievement				
Response to changing needs	Not effective	Shifted	Shifted	Need to shift
Ability to expand activity	Not effective	Effective	Effective	Need to broaden

© 1997 Gauri Bhattacharya, DSW, NDRI.

different socioeconomic classes, but the binding force was their genuine concern for the safety of their children. Their efforts illustrate the diversity of the community organizing processes, strategies that were used, and the outcomes that were achieved.

Madres de Plaza de Mayo

The Madres de Plaza de Mayo began in Argentina after the civilian government was overthrown by a military coup in 1976. Before the coup, paramilitary forces wanted to suppress the emergence of leftist idealism. In this process, suspected "rebels," including many university teachers, lawyers, and students, began to disappear. After the coup, terror tactics were used to create fear among the people and to suppress political activities that challenged the military government. From March 1976 through October 1979, according to estimates by the Amnesty International, 15,000 people disappeared. Later estimates were 30,000 who disappeared during the military regime—from 1976 to 1983 (Bonder, 1983). The government denied any responsibility for these disappearances and even denied that they occurred. The mothers were given no information about what happen to their children. At the same time, the military promoted the family values, the supremacy of God, loyalty to the government, obeying orders, and maintaining tranquillity (Buckles, 1988).

The Madres de Plaza de Mayo was the most prominent movement that developed as a result of the 1976-1983 repressive military dictatorship. The unique characteristic of this movement was the emergence of the idea of mothers as *change agents*. These women neither challenged nor condoned their gender-specific, stereo-typical roles as mothers; were not political activists; and used peaceful means to defy the military junta.

The movement began in mid-1977, when a group of mothers gathered in the Plaza de Mayo in Buenos Aires and silently protested the disappearance of their loved ones, thus openly defying the military rule of the country. This protest received a great deal of national and international publicity during the World Cup Soccer Tournament in Argentina. The Madres' members consisted primarily of middle-aged mothers, many of whom had not previously been involved in political activities. Their activities were supported by people from all walks of life. Although the Madres was not the only group that was responsible for the return of democracy in Argentina in 1983, Madres represented the most visible example of female political activism in their defiance of the military regime. The Madres was successful with the help of the civilian government to persecute the military, to investigate the status of their disappeared children, and a repeal of the general amnesty for the armed forces (Feminia,1987).

By 1987, however, the Madres lost its support from the public. After the return of the civilian government, the restructuring of the economy was considered to be the highest priority in Argentina and the group's activities were no longer considered "relevant to contemporary needs" and was declared as anti-democratic by the new government. The downfall of The Madres' was the result of the fact that they were essentially a one-issue organization. When democracy was restored, that issue wasn't so important and the group did not expand its activities. Furthermore, the organization suffered from ideological conflicts, was divided into two separate groups, and consequently lost power.

The Grameen Bank

The Grameen (Village) Bank, an alternative approach to noncorporate finance in Bangladesh, was started in 1976 to help landless, poor women who could not provide normal bank collateral to obtain credit to start small businesses. In 1994, it had more than two million borrowers—94 percent of whom were women who belonged to the poorest 50 percent of the population. Each month the bank extends new loans totaling $30 million to $40 million; 97 percent of the loans are repaid—a repayment rate that is comparable to that of the Chase Manhattan Bank (Bornstein, 1996). Since each borrower is self-employed and represents one family, almost ten million persons have benefited from these loans.

The success of the Grameen Bank is attributed to three factors. First, the common link among women is the goal of generating regular incomes and improving the financial situation of their entire families. The bank provides small loans—around $100 each—to mothers to start small businesses (e.g., owning a milking cow and selling milk, or making and selling costume jewelry at a profit) that they can manage on their own and combine with their housework. The *family-friendly* nature of this approach, which has brought immediate benefits to the recipient families (including more nourishing food and winter clothes for children) has been supported by both male and female members of the families. Second, "group decision"—the approval and repayment of loans as a group responsibility—is an important component of the bank's approach. There are five members in each lending group. The bank gives a loan to an individual woman who must be a member of a group. The availability of future loans depends on the repayment of previously borrowed funds by each member of the group. Solidarity, trust, and belief within each group after an evaluation of the capacity of each potential borrower to pay the loans are the key elements of this approach. The third and the most crucial factor in the bank's success is that, in sharp contrast to charitable and not-for-profit ideologies of helping women, the Grameen Bank functions as a "socially conscious capitalist enterprise" (Bornstein, 1996, p. 342). It charges interest four points above the prevailing commercial banking rate and never exempts anyone from repaying a loan, even after a natural calamity such as flood or cyclone, but will restructure payment schedules if necessary. The management of the entire banking operation is characterized by the efficient guidance that integrated social development into a commercially oriented, cost-effective framework; the close supervision of field operations; and the dedicated service of bank officials.

This model for providing small loans to village women for self-employment has gained recognition all over the world. It has been adapted in both developing countries (e.g., Ghana) and developed countries (e.g., the United States) with different levels of success (Bornstein, 1996).

Mothers Against Drunk Driving (MADD)

MADD was founded in California in 1980 after Candy Lightner's thirteen-year-old daughter was killed by a drunk, hit-and-run driver who had three previous drunk driving arrests and two convictions and plea bargained the charge down to vehicular manslaughter. Although the driver was sentenced to two years in prison, the judge allowed him to serve time in a work camp and later a halfway house (MADD brochure). MADD is a nonprofit grass-roots organization with more than 600 chapters and community action teams nationwide. Its members include both men and women who are injured victims, bereaved family members, and others. The mission of MADD is to stop drunk driving and to support the victims of this violent crime. Candy Lightner left MADD in 1985. After her departure, MADD pursued the efforts she and others had initiated. Two-thirds of the members of the National Board of Directors of MADD are representatives of local chapters and state organizations. All members are volunteers. Elections for board offices are held annually.

The continued mission of MADD can be best described as propagating a cause that is emotionally, legally, economically, and politically relevant to people. MADD is not a crusade against alcohol consumption. Rather, its *multi-component strategy* focuses on finding effective solutions to drunk driving and underage drinking. It engages in public awareness activities (e.g., publicity in the mass media, newsletter, and speakers), providing support to victims and their families (e.g., a victim hotline, support groups, and candlelight vigils), and legislative advocacy to strengthen existing laws (e.g., the enforcement of sobriety check points) and to pass new laws that include sanctions (e.g., the administrative revocation of driver's licenses).

Each of the three organizations illustrates the significant roles that mothers have played in developing and implementing organizational activities in the community. The success of these organizations is attributed not only to the community organizing capacity of the women but also to the issues that unite them in their accomplishment of tasks. The elements that are crucial for mothers' successful organization of community programs are described next.

ESSENTIAL ELEMENTS FOR COMMUNITY ORGANIZING IN DIVERSE CULTURES

Social, cultural, economic, and political environments influence community structures and dynamics, which, in turn, determine the mechanisms that are adapted in community organizing. Despite the diversities of these environments, several elements were identified as essential for the success of the three organizations (see Table 1).

Appealing Power of the Issue

Two characteristics of an issue are crucial for organizing mothers: (1) it must have high social approval and (2) should have a focused goal. Madres, Grameen Bank, and MADD all promulgated issues that the society as a whole acknowledged to be important. The goals of each organization were specific, simple, and noncontroversial. For Madres, the goal was to find missing children; for the Grameen Bank, it is to give loans for self-employment; and for MADD, it is to stop drunk driving.

Collective Concern and Engagement

Raising the consciousness of individuals and emphasizing the benefits of collective action for achieving goals are essential for mobilizing mothers. Family-oriented issues give mothers a sense of emotional attachment—the feeling of bonding for a cause. Mothers who have been exposed to the consequences of the problem (e.g., violence including drug dealing-related shooting) can visualize the benefits to be gained from changes. The Madres, Grameen Bank, and MADD each shared issues that affected their families directly.

The members' desire to unite for a humanitarian cause and the non-controversial nature of the activities are extremely important factors for engaging others in collective action. The women in Madres gained respect from the public because of their credibility as nonpolitical human beings who simply wanted to find their missing children; the Grameen Bank members were supported because they wanted to raise income via self-employment and sought bank loans on regular terms and conditions; and MADD was supported because its members raised the public's awareness about drunk driving and did not take part in controversial political drug-related issues (e.g., the legalization of drugs).

Implementing the Process

Mothers' efforts to develop projects and achieve goals should be supplemented by guidance and leadership from experts. Often guidance from professionals of various disciplines—administration, finance, and the law—and of both genders is sought. For example, Muhammad Yunus, a male, Harvard-educated economist, is the mastermind behind the development of the Grameen Bank. Mothers learn by experience during the process and come to realize that success does not happen overnight—social change is a long-term process.

Task Performance and Goal Accomplishment

Mothers' organizations must regularly monitor the progress toward meeting the goal(s), and, if necessary, should shift priorities during this process. Often, they may need to adapt strategies to incorporate changing needs especially in changed economic and political situations. Programs based solely on feminist issues or gender stereotypes, unless integrated into political, economic, and social contemporary needs, may not succeed.

APPLYING THE FRAMEWORK TO DRUG ABUSE PREVENTION IN MULTICULTURAL COMMUNITIES

The social-psychological perspective in a culturally competent context is an effective framework for community organizing to prevent drug abuse among adolescents. Drug abuse and its destructive effects are of concern to mothers, irrespective of their ethnicity and socioeconomic status. These individual-level concerns may be extended to the community level to unite women in community organizing.

The Individual Level

Raising Women's Awareness

The empowerment of mothers begins with the realization that they, with support from others, can change the situation and that action should be taken immediately. Instead of being overwhelmed and paralyzed by their constant fear of the consequences of drug use on their children, mothers are encouraged to have the *ability* to change a negative situation. The notion of *responsibility* is adapted to enhance their role as *change agents,* not as victims or perpetrator of the problem. Community-based meetings, distribution of the fact sheets on the extent of the problem and available prevention services, and discussions in the media of examples successful community organizations may facilitate this process. The mothers are also taught that some cultural norms are tolerant of drug-use behavior and may be harmful; for example, smoking tobacco is not only accepted but is expected in some cultures (Oetting, 1992).

Overcoming Denial of the Problem

Mothers may deny that their children and/or other family members use or abuse drugs. To overcome their denial, it must be emphasized that the causes of drug abuse among adolescents are multiple and interactive. Mothers whose children are abusing drugs should not be labeled failures; they can share their frustrations and provide their experiences in observing the early signs of drug abuse and can be taught about the different aspects of drug abuse, including the legal consequences. In their roles as enablers and facilitators, community workers, including social workers and public health professionals, need to provide information on how to identify relevant deviant behaviors and to use tools, such as group dynamics principle.

Linking Perceived and Collective Self-Efficacy

The overwhelming nature of the task of preventing drug abuse among adolescents may lead mothers to feel hopeless. However, this hopelessness can be alleviated by emphasizing the importance of collective empowerment to achieve the desired goal. Social learning theory (Bandura, 1977) addresses the differences and similarities between the concepts of perceived and collective self-efficacy. Social action strategies to initiate behavioral changes among adolescents may lead to social changes and thus may prevent drug abuse among adolescents.

The Community Level

Gaining Trust

To build a sense of affiliation in the community, it is necessary for mothers to learn to trust each other, as well as *outside experts and community workers.* Mothers whose children are abusing drugs or are themselves abusing drugs may be the most reluctant to develop trusting relationships with others. Other barriers to building trust are differences in cultures, language, and socioeconomic status and fear of the legal consequences of disclosing information about the use and selling of drugs. Connectedness with outside experts is the prerequisite for trusting them and being willing to disclose information to them. Freire's (1973) conscious- raising strategy for initiating dialogue among members of the community may be adapted to suit the context, complexities, and subtleties of the nature of the drug use problem issues. Community workers must assume a leadership role at this stage to build participatory involvement and mutual support. They can use a combination of methods, including social organizing to foster group solidarity, educational approach to provide information on drug treatment and prevention, and professional expertise to inform about the legal process.

Understanding the Comprehensive Nature of the Problem

Adolescence is the period of socialization or transition from childhood to adulthood, when emotional, psychological, and sociocultural skills are learned; therefore, the influences of the family to whom the child is bonded, as well as the peer network to whom the adolescent is attached, need to be considered (Brook and Brook, 1992; Jessor and Jessor, 1977; Kandel, 1978; Kumpfer and Alvarado, 1995). Consequently, the empowerment of mothers and other women needs to focus not only on empowerment at the individual level, but community partnerships to confront the drug abuse problem.

Implementing the Process

Given the multi-ethnic composition of the communities and the prevalent drug culture, which includes the manner in which drugs are bought and sold, implementation will vary.

Identifying and Ranking Needs

Because drug abuse is such a serious and overwhelming problem, it is necessary to establish priorities among the needs to accomplish the overall goals. Early accomplishments are essential to reassure the mothers that large problems can be solved in the future. Two important aspects of this process must be recognized: (1) it is time consuming to initiate changes in any social behaviors and health outcome patterns, particularly drug abuse by adolescents, and (2) it is important to set short-term goals such as the need to provide alternative activities and to make the organization's presence felt. The strategies that can be adapted include: arranging extracurricular activities after school in community centers or schools and to increase the organization's visibility and physical presence on the streets where drugs are sold. The long-term goals can be identified as eliminating the media's and manufacturer's promotion of drugs; two possible strategies that can be adapted are working to remove cigarette vending machines from shopping malls and to prohibit billboards from displaying liquor advertisements.

To achieve the goals, a systematic plan must be prepared, with inputs from both mothers in the community and professionals. This plan must be followed as a guide to the strategies to be used and should be modified as needs change.

Collaborating With Other Organizations

To confront drug abuse and "take back the community," mothers must collaborate with other organizations and establish links between individual and community problems (e.g., drug dealing on street corners). Parents may be intimidated by highly educated professionals, or may have higher expectations of them, or may be dependent on them for actions, whereas, community workers may be highly skeptical of the abilities of uneducated parents. Knowledge of and appreciation for the culture and traditions may help professionals to explain the problem of drug abuse and the need for locality development to the mothers (Rivera and Erlich, 1995). Also actively involving mothers and other concerned women in the process of change is another aspect of empowerment (Gutierrez, 1995). Professionals need to provide training materials on the prevention of abuse, information on relevant research, and other resources that may help mothers' organizations accomplish their goals.

Sustaining the Process and Avoiding Burnout

This phase has two aspects: (1) maintaining the mothers' ongoing enthusiasm for commitment to preventing adolescents from abusing drugs in the face of disappointments and frustrations and (2) redefining priorities for achieving this goal in the context of changing economic, cultural, and political situations. For example, with new immigrant families in the community, mothers may decide to focus also on how acculturative stress (e.g., adaptation to a new culture and language constraints) affects self-esteem and leads to drug use among children. Both process and outcome evaluations need to be carried out at regular intervals. Experience gained from the process needs to be disseminated to the public to publicize the organization's efforts and to develop the models further.

Evaluation of Success

More and more health and human services, as well as funding organizations, are conducting quantitative assessments of the achievement of goals to obtain information on service needs, activities, and outcomes for dissemination of data for adaptation, modification, and improving the delivery of services and the allocation of resources. Although evaluation criteria may vary, depending on the problem and service needs, three issues need to be highlighted here:

1. It is often difficult to evaluate community projects because of residents' general distrust of outside professionals and researchers. In addition, the illegal aspects of drug abuse exacerbate mothers' suspicion of data collection methods. Therefore, it may be unrealistic to try to conduct such assessments using strict scientific research procedures (Minkler, 1992).

2. The lack of capacity building is considered the most common and serious drawback of community organizing. Capacity building encompasses community

residents' sense of individual and collective responsibility for the community operationalized via participatory involvement and mutual support (Pilisuk, et al., 1996).

3. Building community self-reliance is considered one of the most effective criteria for evaluation. Three areas that deserve particular attention are these:

(i) The concept of self-reliancy goes beyond just "solving" the original problem. For example, drug abuse prevention can be extended to developing health check-ups for all residents and sex education to those who want it. Drug prevention training programs can also be broadened as has been done in two of the three community organizations discussed earlier (MADD teaches school-children not to use drugs, as well as not to drive while drunk, and the Grameen Bank teaches vocational skills, as well as giving loans).

(ii) Researchers, sometimes, receive grants from organizations or the government to initiate community organizing for drug prevention programs and hire others with project funds. Grants are funded for a specified period, and their renewal depends on may factors, including progress in achieving goals. Some-times, a group of professionals, though not paid, become extensively involved in implementing a project. Multi-agency collaboration among schools, law enforce-ment agencies, and social service agencies are particularly essential in drug abuse prevention programs. However, the timing of professionals' withdrawal from a program needs to be carefully monitored to maintain continuity and financial solvency. Therefore, a tapering-off of the withdrawal may be helpful for assessing the competence of the mothers' groups for identifying areas that may need support for a longer time.

CONCLUSIONS

The increasing multi-ethnic population in the United States highlights the need to examine issues from a multicultural perspective. Drug abuse among children and adolescents is such an issue that encompasses all ethnic groups, irrespective of their social class and economic status. The cultural competence perspective applied to the community organizing process seems to be an effec-tive approach for preventing drug abuse among adolescents. Parent-community partnerships can reduce the demand for, as well as the supply of, drugs. Strategies that focus on individuals, such as Just Say No and school-based educational programs on the consequences of drug use have had limited success. The indi-vidual approach emphasizes demand-reduction factors (at the individual level), but underestimates the importance of the supply (environmental/social structural) determinants of drug use (Wechsler and Weitzman, 1996).

The approach to empowering women to establish community-based drug abuse prevention programs for adolescents proposed here integrates two key components of the social marketing strategy that are considered crucial for the success of such programs. These two components are: (1) reduction of the supply-availability of drugs in the immediate environment (at home) and in the community (drug selling in the neighborhood) and (2) reduction of the demand for using drugs among adolescents.

Mothers' desire to nurture their children may be extended to the context of community organizing for use as an effective approach to drug abuse prevention among children and adolescents. Although mothers are associated with the provision of care for their children, it is a societal value and must be endorsed by all members of the society. Consistent with this value system, instilling pro-social behaviors including not using drugs is a societal responsibility and must be shared by all members of the community.

REFERENCES

Airhihenbuwa, C. O. (1995). *Health and Culture.* Sage Publications: Thousand Oaks, CA.

Allen, J. and Allen, R. F. (1990). A sense of community, a shared vision, and a positive culture: Core enabling factors in successful culture-based change. In R. D. Patton and W. B. Cissel (Eds.), *Community Organization: Traditional Principles and Applications* (pp. 5-18). Latchpins Press: TN.

Bandura, A. (1977). *A Social Learning Theory.* Prentice Hall: Englewood, NJ.

Bhattacharya, G. (1996). *Communication Strategies to Address the Needs of Asian and Pacific Islander Audiences.* Prevention Brochure. Contributor, Center for Substance Abuse Prevention Communication Team (CSAP Contract No. 277-92-4006).

Bhattacharya, G. (1998). Drug use among Asian-Indian adolescents: Identifying protective/risk Factors. *Adolescence,* 33(129):169-184.

Blum, R. and Richards, L. (1979). Youthful drug use. In R.I. Dupont, A. Goldstein and J. O'Donnell (Eds.), *Handbook on Drug Abuse* (pp. 257-67). US Government Printing Office: Washington, D.C.

Bonder, G. (1983). Women in Power Spheres. *International Social Science Journal,* UNESCO, 35(4):569-583.

Bornstein, D. (1996). *The Price of A Dream.* Simon & Schuster: New York.

Brook, D. W. and Brook, J. S. (1992). Family processes associated with alcohol and drug use and abuse. In E. Kaufman and P. Kaufman (Eds.), *Family Therapy of Drug and Alcohol Abuse* (pp. 15-33). Allyn & Bacon: Boston, MA.

Brown, E. R. (1996). Coalitions for public health (President's column). *The Nation's Health,* American Public Health Association.

Buckles, M. (1988). *Strange Bedfellows: Women and Gender Stereotypes in Argentine Politics,* Master of Arts Thesis (Unpublished) at the University of California, Los Angeles.

Carney, T. F. (1972). *Content Analysis: A Technique for Systematic Inference from Communications.* University of Manitoba Press: Winnipeg, Canada.

Chaloupka, M., Ed. (1996). *MADD In Action.* In *MADD Mission Statement,* 15(1). MADD National Office: TX.

Chavis, D. M. and Wandersman, A. (1990). Sense of community in the urban environment: A catalyst for participation and community development. *American Journal of Community Psychology,* 18:55-81.

Cottrell, L. S. (1976). The competent community. In B. H. Kaplan, R. N. Wilson and A. H. Leighton (Eds.), *Further Exploration in Social Psychiatry* (pp. 195-209). Basic Books: New York.

Femenia, N. A. (1987). Argentina's Mothers of Plaza de Mayo: The mourning process from junta to democracy. *Feminist Studies*, 13(1):9-19.

Freire, P. (1973). *Education for Critical Consciousness*. Seabury Press: New York.

Green, L. W. and Kreuter, M. W. (1991). *Health Promotion Planning: An Educational and Environmental Approach* (pp. 13-25). Mayfield Publishers: CA.

Gutierrez, L. M. (1995). Working with women of color: An empowerment perspective. In J. Rothman, J. L. Erlich, and J. E. Tropman (Eds.), *Strategies of Community Intervention* (pp. 204-10). Peacock Publishers: Itasca, IL.

Hansen, W. B. (1992). School-based substance abuse prevention: A review of the state of the art in curriculum, 1980-1990. *Health Education Research*, 7:403-430.

Hawkins J. D., Catalano. R. F. and Miller, J. L. (1992). Risk and Protective factors for alcohol and other drug problems in adolescence and early adulthood: Implications for substance abuse prevention. *Psychological Bulletin*, 112(1):64-105.

Holsti, O. (1968). Content analysis. In G. Lindzey and E. Aronson (Eds.), *The Handbook of Social Psychology*, Vol. 2. Addison Wesley: Reading, MA.

Jessor, R. and Jessor, G. L. (1977). *Problem Behavior and Psychosocial Development: A Longitudinal Study of Youth.* Academic Press: New York.

Johnston, L. D., O'Malley, P. M. and Bachman, J. G. (1996). *National Survey Results on Drug Use from the Monitoring the Future Study, 1975-1994.* National Institute on Drug Abuse: Rockville, MD.

Jones, C. L. and Battjes, R. J., Eds. (1985). *Etiology of Drug Abuse: Implications for Prevention.* NIDA Research Monograph No. 56, Washington Printing Press: Washington, D.C.

Kandel, D. B. (1978). Convergences in prospective longitudinal surveys of drug use in normal populations. In D. B. Kandel (Ed.), *Longitudinal Research on Drug Use: Empirical Findings and Methodological Issues* (pp. 3-38). Hemisphere: Washington, D.C.

Kandel, D. B. (1982). Epidemiological and psychosocial perspectives on adolescent drug use. *Journal of American Academy on Clinical Psychiatry*, 21:328-347.

Klein, M. D. and White, J. M. (1996). *Family Theories.* Sage Publishers: Thousand Oaks, CA.

Krippendorf, K. (1980). *Content Analysis: An Introduction to its Methodology.* Sage Publications: Beverly Hills, CA.

Kumpfer, K. L. and Alvarado, R. (1995). Strengthening families to prevent drug use in multiethnic youth. In G. J. Botvin, S. Schinke and M. A. Orlandi (Eds.), *Drug Abuse Prevention with Multiethnic Youth* (pp. 255-283). Sage Publications: Thousand Oaks, CA.

Mazuri, A. A. (1986). *The Africans: A Triple Heritage.* Little-Brown: Boston, MA.

Minkler, M. (1992). Community organizing among the elderly poor in the United States: A case study. *International Journal of Health Services,* 22(2):303-316.

National Household Survey on Drug Abuse (1996). Source: SAMHSA, Office of Applied Studies: Rockville, MD.

The National Survey of American Attitudes on Substance Abuse and Addiction II: Teens and Their Parents (1996). Press Release, National Center on Addiction and Substance Abuse at Columbia University, September 9: New York.

Newcomb, M. D. (1995). Drug use etiology among ethnic minority adolescents: Risk and protective factors. In G. J. Botvin, S. Schinke and M. A. Orlandi (Eds.), *Drug Abuse Prevention with Multiethnic Youth* (pp. 105-126). Sage Publications: Thousand Oaks, CA.

Oetting, E. R. (1992). Planning programs for prevention of deviant behavior: A psychosocial model. In J. E. Trimble, C. S. Bolek and S. J. Niemcryk (Eds.), *Ethnic and Multicultural Drug Abuse: Perspectives on Current Research* (pp. 313-344). The Hawarth Press, Inc: New York.

O'Reilly, K. R. and Piot, P. (1996). International perspectives on individual and community approaches to the prevention of sexually transmitted disease and Human Immunodeficiency Virus infection. *Journal of Infectious Diseases*, 174(Suppl. 2):214-221.

Orlandi, M. A. (1992). The challenge of evaluating community-based prevention programs: A cross cultural perspective. In M. A. Orlandi (Ed.), *Cultural Competence for Evaluators*. DHHS Publication No. (ADM) 92-1884, Office of Substance Abuse Prevention.

Pentz, M. A. (1995). Prevention research in multiethnic communities: Developing community support and collaboration, and adapting reserach methods. In G. J. Botvin, S. Schinke and M. A. Orlandi (Eds.), *Drug Abuse Prevention with Multiethnic Youth* (pp. 193-210). Sage Publications: Thousand Oaks, CA.

Pilisuk, M., McAllister, J. and Rothman, J. (1996). Coming together for action: The challenge of contemporary grassroots community organizing. *Journal of Social Issues*, 52(1):15-37.

Recio Adrados, J. L. (1993). Acculturation: The broader view. Theoretical framework of the acculturation scales. In M. R. De La Rosa and J. L. Recio Adrados (Eds.), *Drug Abuse among Minority Youth: Advances in Research and Methodology* (pp. 57-78). NIDA Research Monograph 130, National Institute on Drug Abuse: Rockville, MD.

Rivera, F. G. and Erlich, J. L. (1995) Organizing with people of color. In J. Rothman, J. L. Erlich and J. E. Tropman (Eds.), *Strategies of Community Intervention* (pp. 198-212). Peacock Publishers: Itasca, IL.

Rothman, J. (1995). Approaches to community intervention. In J. Rothman, J. L. Erlich and J. E. Tropman (Eds.), *Strategies of Community Intervention* (pp. 25-45). Peacock Publishers: Itasca, IL.

Tawail O., Verster, A. and O'Reilly, K. R. (1995). Enabling approaches for HIV/AIDS prevention: Can we modify the environment and minimize the risk? *AIDS*, 9: 1299-1306.

Wechsler, H. and Weitzman, E. R. (1996). Community solutions to community problems—preventing adolescent alcohol use (Editorial). *American Journal of Public Health*, 86(7):923-925.

CHAPTER 4

School-Based Substance Abuse Prevention: What Works, For Whom, and How?

Phyllis Ellickson

During the late 1980s and early 1990s, The Drug-Free Schools Act of 1986 fueled the spread of school-based drug prevention across the country. Passed in response to mounting public concern about the high rates of drug use among the nation's youth, the act sharply increased the federal contribution to state and local drug prevention and required schools to show that they have developed a comprehensive drug education plan before they can receive federal education funds. It also reflected the belief that drug use is a problem threatening adolescents from a wide array of communities and sociodemographic backgrounds. Hence it is best addressed by programs targeted at all children, not just those at highest risk of becoming drug users.

However, recent information about the performance of some of the more widely used programs suggests the need for greater guidance about which type of approach is likely to work. A five-year study conducted for the Department of Education concluded that most school-based programs conducted under this act are ineffective and that schools rarely implement the program models that show promise (Research Triangle Institute, 1997). Several evaluation studies have questioned the effectiveness of DARE, a police-led program adopted in communities across the United States (Ennett, Tobler, Ringwalt and Flewelling, 1994; Tobler, 1995). Other popular programs (QUEST: Skills for Living, Project CHARLIE, Here's Looking at You, 2000, Project Adventure, B.A.B.E.S., OMBUDSMAN, Children are People) lack the evaluation data needed to judge their effectiveness (Hansen and O'Malley, 1996).

At the same time, questions have arisen about the appropriateness of a "one size fits all" approach for children from widely different racial/ethnic backgrounds. Some authors have questioned the cultural appropriateness of programs that were originally developed in white, middle class communities (Austin, 1988; Sussman, et al., 1995); others have suggested that different ethnic groups may be more receptive to programs that were developed by members of the same group and use same-race characters (Lopes, et al., 1995; Milburn, et al., 1990; Parker, et al., 1996).

To better gauge the appropriateness of different drug prevention models, we need to understand who uses drugs and why, as well as how the programs actually work in different settings. In this chapter, I seek to address these concerns by examining the following questions:

1. What drugs are most prevalent and who uses them?
2. What are the most important factors contributing to adolescent drug use and which of them can be addressed through prevention programming?
3. Which approaches are most effective and for whom?

In the course of answering these questions, I also assess the degree to which drug use, risk factors, and program effectiveness vary across different racial/ethnic groups.

To preview the highlights of my discussion: No single drug prevention program is likely to be equally effective in addressing the multiple influences on drug use. Instead, programs need to be sensitive to developmental changes in a child's vulnerability, targeting family and school bonds during elementary school or earlier, more proximal influences such as peer pressure and normative beliefs during the shift to adolescence. Developing different prevention programs for different racial/ethnic groups appears to be premature. None of the results of program evaluations to date strongly suggest that such programs are merited. However, future evaluations may identify risk factors or influences for specific groups that could be more effectively countered in special programs. In my discussion, I note those areas in which our understanding of risk factors for certain groups is particularly impoverished.

WHAT DRUGS ARE MOST PREVALENT AND WHO USES THEM?

Among adolescents, alcohol, cigarettes, and marijuana are the main drugs of choice. As Figure 1 shows, alcohol is by far the most widely used drug among both younger and older adolescents. Over 50 percent of eighth graders have tried alcohol; by grade twelve, that number has grown to 81 percent. Cigarettes and marijuana rank second and third for high school seniors, with lifetime use amounting to nearly two-thirds for cigarettes and slightly over two-fifths for

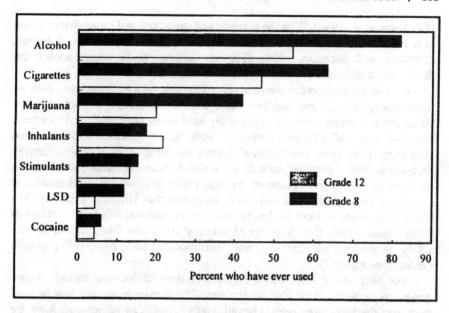

Figure 1. Adolescent drug use in the United States, Grades 8 and 12.
Source: *Monitoring the Future,* 1996.

marijuana (Johnston, O'Malley, and Bachman, 1996). For eighth graders, however, inhalants outrank marijuana in popularity: nearly 22 percent have tried inhalants compared to 20 percent for marijuana. Although not typically classified as drugs, inhalants are often used to get high, especially by younger adolescents. As adolescents grow older, their use of these chemicals tends to drop off: among twelfth graders, lifetime use of inhalants was only 18 percent, substantially lower than the figures for cigarettes and marijuana, but higher than the rates for specific illicit drugs other than marijuana.

Among all the illicit drugs other than marijuana, only stimulants and LSD have been tried by more than 10 percent of high school seniors. Use of other hard drugs (cocaine, crack, tranquilizers, steroids, heroin, and PCP) is substantially lower (Johnston, O'Malley, and Bachman, 1996).

Gender and Racial/Ethnic Differences in Drug Use

Both males and females exhibit high rates of alcohol and cigarette use, and equal proportions of both groups have tried these substances by grade twelve (Johnston, O'Malley, and Bachman, 1996). Alcohol misuse is also quite common among both males and females, but males are more likely to be persistent misusers

(Ellickson, et al., 1996). With the exception of stimulants and tranquilizers, males also tend to have higher prevalence rates for specific illicit drugs (Johnston, O'Malley, and Bachman, 1996). However, among middle school adolescents these gender differences are usually no more than 2 percent.

Data do not support the common perception that African-American youth are more susceptible to drug use and abuse than other groups. In fact, African-American and Asian adolescents generally have lower prevalence and incidence rates for drugs of all kinds compared with Native Americans, Whites, and Hispanics. Data from the National Survey on Drug Abuse, which includes dropouts as well as enrolled students, show that African-American youth between the ages of twelve and seventeen are less likely than Whites or Hispanics to have used most of the licit and illicit drugs and that Hispanic youth are less likely than whites to have used most drugs except cocaine (National Institute of Drug Abuse, 1990). Data from the Monitoring the Future Study, which focuses solely on students enrolled in school, corroborates those findings for twelfth graders (see Figure 2).

The data source from which Figure 2 is derived does not include Asian-American or Native-American adolescents. The former group has low rates of drug use; the latter high rates. Overall, Native-American adolescents have the highest rates of licit and illicit drug use, followed by Whites and Hispanics.

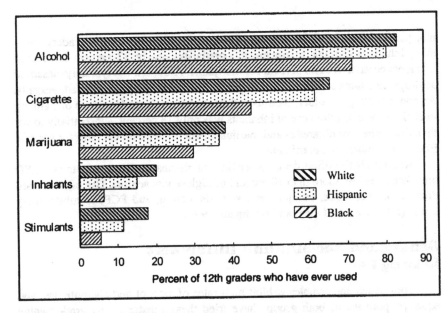

Figure 2. Adolescent drug use by racial/ethnic group, grade 12.
Source: *Monitoring the Future*, 1993 and 1994.

African-American and Asian-American adolescents have the lowest use rates (Bachman, et al., 1991; Wallace, Bachman, O'Malley, and Johnston, 1995).

African-American and Asian youth in grades seven through twelve are also less likely to misuse alcohol than Whites, Hispanics, and Native Americans (Ellickson, et al., 1996; NIDA, 1995; Welte and Barnes, 1987). However, despite lower levels of consumption and high risk drinking, African-American high school seniors and dropouts are as susceptible, and sometimes more so, to some of the more serious consequences of drinking (having an accident, getting into a fight, getting arrested) (Ellickson, et al., 1996). They also experience more alcohol-related problems per ounce consumed than other groups (Welte and Barnes, 1987). Similarly, among Asian-American adolescents in school, males who do drink tend to drink heavily (Welte and Barnes, 1987).

These racial/ethnic differences tend to disappear if we focus on different types of drug misuse and abuse among youth who are already using drugs. For example, a recent examination of drug use among high school seniors and dropouts from California and Oregon found no significant racial/ethnic differences among past year users in several measures of high consumption, high risk use, or drug-related problems—including polydrug use, daily drinking, daily marijuana use, trouble with police, fighting, and getting arrested because of drinking, and six out of seven marijuana consequences (Bell and Ellickson, under review).

As with gender differences, racial/ethnic differences in use rates tend to be substantially smaller in middle school than they are by the end of high school, reflecting in part lower levels of use among younger adolescents. National data indicate that the largest differences between racial/ethnic groups for younger adolescents are for marijuana and inhalant use. At grade eight, both African-Americans and Whites have substantially lower rates of past year marijuana use than Hispanic youth (6% and 8% versus 14%); African-American youth also exhibit substantially lower rates of inhalant use than the other two groups (5% versus 11%) (Hansen and O'Malley, 1996).

Summary and Implications for Drug Prevention

National data indicate that prevention programs for children and adolescents should give the most attention to alcohol, cigarettes, marijuana, and inhalants, the most widely used substances among adolescents. But targeting the substances that young people use first and most widely does not mean that prevention efforts should ignore other substances. For years, the prevention community failed to recognize the threat of inhalants to young people and inhalant use became increasingly popular among adolescents. Children who are likely to be exposed to cocaine, crack, and other "hard" drugs need to know about their dangerous effects.

Moreover, as children mature, their likely exposure to these substances increases. Use of hallucinogens more than doubles between grade eight and grade twelve, rising from 5 percent to over 12 percent. Cocaine use goes up by a third over these years and use of tranquilizers rises by over 50 percent (Johnston, O'Malley, and Bachman, 1996). Regional data suggest that specific hard drugs such as PCP are more common in some cities and neighborhoods than others (Reuter, et al., 1988). Thus, the drugs targeted by specific programs should vary by age, and sometimes by location. Local drug use data can help communities tailor prevention goals to their particular circumstances.

Data on racial/ethnic variations in drug use indicate that there are substantial differences across different groups by age eighteen, with African-American and Asian youth generally exhibiting lower rates for most drugs than Whites, Hispanics, and Native Americans. However, these differences are small during middle school and do not support developing different programs for different groups. Moreover, aggregated data across twelve to seventeen year olds yield few statistically significant differences for Black and Hispanic youth relative to Whites (Flewelling, et al., 1994). In addition, all four groups follow the same initial sequence of drug use initiation—alcohol, then cigarettes, then marijuana (Ellickson, Hays, and Bell, 1992; Welte and Barnes, 1985), information that further supports targeting these substances for all young people.

Nevertheless, the racial/ethnic differences that exist by grade twelve suggest the need for sensitivity to different vulnerabilities in programs targeted at both middle school and high school students. Whites, Hispanics, and Native Americans need to recognize their broad susceptibility to multiple forms of drug use and abuse, while African Americans and Asians need to be aware that generally lower levels of use, particularly lower alcohol consumption and high risk drinking, do not necessarily protect them from some of the more serious consequences of use.

WHAT FACTORS CONTRIBUTE TO ADOLESCENT DRUG USE AND HOW CAN PREVENTION PROGRAMS ADDRESS THEM?

To develop effective drug prevention, we also need to know how drug use starts and continues—what experiences and characteristics put children and adolescents at risk and which ones help protect them from becoming involved with drugs. Research on factors that predict drug use initiation and continuation helps us identify which ones to target.

The major predictors of drug use initiation fall into five categories: (1) pro-drug social influences (parents, peers, and others who use drugs or approve of doing so); (2) pro-drug beliefs and attitudes (intentions to use, positive versus negative outcome expectancies, beliefs that drug use is normative, low resistance self-efficacy); (3) inadequate familial bonds and supervision; (4) weak bonds with school and poor school performance; and (5) prior deviant behavior and susceptibility to deviance.

These influences on drug use also correspond to the factors highlighted in various theories of how drug use begins. *Social learning theory* recognizes that young people are especially vulnerable to social models and pressures from family, peer groups, and the media, stressing the role of significant others as models for, and reinforcers of, deviant or conventional behavior (Bandura, 1977a). The *theory of reasoned action* suggests that intentions determine behavior and that intentions are in turn affected by the individual's attitudes and beliefs about that behavior, its normative status in society, and its likely consequences (Ajzen and Fishbein, 1980). The *self-efficacy theory* of behavior change stresses the belief that one can successfully alter a specific behavior as key to actual behavior change (Bandura, 1977b); while the *Health Belief Model* singles out beliefs about the seriousness of negative consequences and one's susceptibility to them (as well as barriers to action and the benefits of discontinuing, or not beginning, unhealthy habits) as key components of healthy behavior (Becker, 1974).

Social bonding theory stresses attachments to family and school as factors that protect young people from deviant behavior—and inadequate bonds with these institutions as risk factors (Hawkins and Weis, 1985); *social control theory* also focuses on attachment and commitment to conventional social institutions such as families, school, and religion as inhibiting influences (Hirschi, 1969). *Problem behavior theory* focuses on aspects of all of these—the environmental system (influences from parents, peers, other important people in the child's environment) and the personality system (values, expectations, beliefs about self, and attitudes)—while adding an emphasis on the child's own prior behavior as a strong influence on later behavior (Jessor and Jessor, 1977).

Drug use is fostered by multiple influences and no single theory encompasses the phenomenon. Risk factors tend to have a cumulative effect: the more risk factors children have, the more likely they are to use drugs (Newcomb, Maddahian, and Bentler, 1986).

- Weak bonds with family, school, and religious institutions "set the stage" for drug use (Oetting and Beauvais, 1987), but their impact on initiation of both gateway and "hard" drug use is typically smaller than that of the more proximal factors—pro-drug environmental influences and beliefs (Conrad, Flay, and Hill, 1992; Ellickson, Collins and Bell, in press; Ellickson and Hays, 1992; Hansen, 1997; Robinson, et al., 1987).

- Peers, parents, siblings, and other admired role models who use drugs or approve of doing so all contribute to a pro-drug climate in which models for use are plentiful, drugs are readily available, and social norms foster use (Brook, et al., 1988; Chassin, 1984; Conrad, Flay, and Hill, 1992; Kandel,

Kessler, and Margulies, 1978; Oetting and Beauvais, 1987; Petraitus, Flay, and Miller, 1995).

- Adolescents are particularly susceptible to drug use initiation during periods of transition, such as those from elementary to middle school and from middle school to high school (Sloboda and David, 1997). Marked by environmental changes that offer more opportunities for high-risk behavior, these periods also bring developmental changes that challenge adolescents' identity and heighten their vulnerability to pro-drug influences.

- Peer influences become more important after children make the transition into middle or junior high school (Berndt, 1979; Kandel, 1985; Krosnick and Judd, 1982; Silverberg and Gondoli, 1996). Parental drug use and approval tend to be comparatively more influential at earlier ages, but they also contribute to heavy use and progression through the drug sequence during the adolescent years (Ellickson and Hays, 1991a; Kandel and Andrews, 1987; Krosnick and Judd, 1982; Simons, Conger, and Whitbeck, 1988; Wadsworth, et al., under review).

- Beliefs that drugs have positive consequences and pose little harm predict future drug involvement, while high resistance self-efficacy inhibits use (Ellickson and Hays, 1992; Leigh, 1989; Leigh and Stacy, 1991; Stacy, Widaman, and Marlatt, 1990). Beliefs that drug use is acceptable and that most of one's peers use drugs also promote greater use, as do reported intentions to use (Collins, et al., 1987; Ellickson and Hays, 1991b; Hansen, 1997). Beliefs about drugs tend to become more stable as children mature, are exposed to others who use, or use drugs themselves (Chassin, 1984).

- Strong family and school bonds protect children against a variety of problem behaviors, including drug use (Brook, et al., 1990; Dembo, et al., 1981; Hundleby and Mercer, 1987; Resnick, et al., 1997; Selnow, 1987;). Impaired relationships with these institutions have a modest impact on early drug use; they also presage more serious use as the child grows older (Baumrind and Moselle, 1985; Kandel, et al., 1978; Kandel and Andrews, 1987; Newcomb and Bentler 1988; Shedler and Block, 1990; Brunswick and Messeri, 1985; Hundleby and Mercer, 1987; Smith and Fogg, 1978; Robins, 1980; Skinner, et al., 1985).

- Early deviant behavior (acting out in school, stealing, truancy, early drug use) and poor school grades are strong warning signals for later deviance of all kinds, as are predispositions toward unconventionality and rebellion (Barnes and Welte, 1986; Elliott and Morse, 1989; Gottfredson, 1988; Kandel, 1978; Newcomb and Felix-Ortiz, 1992). Early drug use is the single most important predictor of future use and abuse (Bachman, O'Malley, and Johnston, 1984; Fleming, Kellam, and Brown, 1982; Robins and Pryzbeck, 1985; Yamaguchi and Kandel, 1984).

Racial/Ethnic Differences in Risk
and Protective Factors

Research on racial/ethnic differences in risk and protective factors and their links with drug use has been hampered by small samples and insufficient validation or cross-validation of suggestive findings. Studies that compare drug use risk factors across ethnic groups are scarce, and the few that do exist yield conflicting results. Some find little or no difference in important risk factors across different groups, concluding that the results provide little basis for differential prevention strategies (Coreil, et al., 1991; Flannery, et al., 1994; Harford, 1986; Humphrey, Stephens, and Allen, 1983); others highlight both common *and* unique antecedents or correlates (Bettes, et al., 1990, Brook, et al., 1992; Catalano, et al., 1992; Ellickson and Morton, in press; Headen, et al., 1991; Humm-Delgado and Delgado, 1983; Sussman, et al., 1987). Variables that have been singled out as especially important risk or protective factors for different groups are as follows: religion (African Americans), risk-taking (African Americans), education (Asians), and family relationships (Hispanics) (Gfoerer and De La Rosa, 1993; Harford, 1986; Headen, et al., 1991; Landrine, et al., 1994; Sussmán, et al., 1987; Wallace and Bachman, 1991). At least three studies have found fewer significant risk factors and thus less explanatory power for drug use prevalence (including heavy use) among African-Americans and Asian adolescents compared with Whites and Hispanics (Ellickson and Morton, in press; Maddahian, Newcomb, and Bentler, 1988; Sussman, et al., 1987).

One study that did have access to large national samples is Wallace and Bachman's (1991) effort to explain racial/ethnic differences in adolescent drug use by controlling for the impact of background and lifestyle characteristics. They found that background characteristics such as parental education, family structure, region, and urbanicity do *not* account for most racial/ethnic differences in use. The one exception is Native Americans, whose high use rates drop down to those for Whites after controlling for background characteristics. The authors suggest that above average levels of drug use among Native Americans may be linked with their relatively disadvantaged socioeconomic status.

Support for the limited impact of background factors in explaining group differences comes from a recent study of teenage alcohol misuse (Ellickson, et al., 1996). African Americans and Asians still had significantly lower rates of high-risk drinking, high consumption, and alcohol-related problems than Whites and Hispanics after controls for parental income, education, and family structure.

The limited utility of background characteristics in explaining racial/ethnic differences in adolescent drug use may be attributable to different effects for different groups. Ellickson and Morton (in press) found that limited parental education was a risk factor for future "hard" drug use by Whites, but African American and Hispanic adolescents with better-educated parents were actually more likely to become hard drug users than those whose parents lacked a high school degree. Similarly, coming from a disrupted family increased the probability of hard drug use for Whites, decreased it for Asians, and had no effect for Hispanics and African Americans. Thus, using such characteristics as a predictor of drug use not only yields inaccurate predictions, but also perpetuates myths and contributes to stigmatization.

Role of Education, Religiosity, and Family Attachment in Explaining Group Differences

Lifestyle factors play an important role in accounting for racial/ethnic differences in drug use. Wallace and Bachman (1991) found that such differences were sharply reduced or eliminated after they added lifestyle variables to the equations. The key predictors included measures of school bonding and performance (grades, educational aspirations, and truancy), religious commitment, and time spent in peer-oriented activities. The authors suggest that strong educational values and performance help explain lower drug use rates for Asians, while religious commitment is particularly important for African Americans. However, they failed to provide empirical evidence for these hypotheses in the form of differential exposure or sensitivity to these factors in the sample.

Asian-American children tend to do particularly well in school and to go on to college or other post-secondary institutions (Sue and Okazaki, 1990). Strong school bonds and performance might protect comparatively more Asian youth from engaging in deviant behaviors like drug use; conversely, Asian youth who do poorly in school or have low educational aspirations may be more estranged from cultural and societal norms about appropriate behavior and thus more likely to act out in deviant ways. Support for this hypothesis comes from an analysis of predictors of illicit drug use other than marijuana in which being Asian interacted with repeating more grades of school to produce higher rates of use (Ellickson, Collins, and Bell, in press).

African-American adolescents tend to be more committed to religion than White youth (Bachman, Johnston, and O'Malley, 1987) and more likely to belong to fundamentalist denominations that promote abstinence (Herd, 1985). Stark and colleagues (1982) have argued that higher levels of religiosity protect African American youth from drug use and that the relationship between religiosity and drug use resistance may be stronger for African-Americans because the church plays such a prominent role in group social and political life. However, this argument has not been supported in recent analyses. Data from the Monitoring the Future study indicate that the comparatively greater religiosity of African-American youth is not a strong deterrent to drug use; among high school seniors, the expected protective effect of high religiosity is experienced largely by Whites (Amey, Albrecht, and Miller, 1996). However, such an effect may be difficult to detect if there is little variability among African-American youth in religiosity.

Stronger family relationships are frequently cited as an explanation for lower rates of drug use among Hispanics, who report greater ties with family, having more cohesive families, and greater mutual supportiveness among family members (Betancourt and Lopez, 1993; Freeberg and Stein, 1996; Markides, et al., 1986; Mindel, 1980). When these bonds break down, drug use may escalate. Evidence for differential links between family relationship variables and drug use among Hispanics comes from several studies. An analysis of African-American and Puerto Rican seventh to tenth graders found that attachment variables more often served as protective factors for Puerto Ricans than models of nondrug use (Brook, et al., 1992). Similarly, disruptive family events such as parental job loss, remarriage, or hospitalization differentially increased the likelihood of any hard drug use for Mexican-American youth compared to Whites, African Americans and Asians (Ellickson, Collins, and Bell, in press). Acculturation into U.S. society, which may reflect the diminution of family ties, is associated with higher rates of illicit drug use among Hispanics, particularly those with lower educational attainment (Amaro, et al., 1990). Family factors may also be more important for African-American children, especially at younger ages. Among urban fifth graders, attachment to parents and parental influence on friends the child sees are correlated with fewer drugs initiated for Blacks, but not for Whites or Asians (Catalano, et al., 1992).

Research on differential exposure or susceptibility to proximal risk factors (role models for use or nonuse, drug availability, drug-related beliefs) yields variable results. Most studies suggest that pro-drug social influences have fairly consistent effects across different groups, although they may explain more of the variance for some groups than others (Brook, et al., 1992; Flannery, et al., 1994; Gillmore, et al., 1990; Landrine, et al., 1994; Riley, et al., 1991; Vega, et al., 1993).

In sum, explanations for lower rates of drug use among Asian and Hispanic youth compared to Whites find more support than those for lower rates of use among African Americans. Educational ties play a protective role for Asians; family relationships are important for Hispanics, and perhaps for African Americans. Nevertheless, current and past analyses typically explain more of the variance in drug use among Whites and Hispanics than they do among African-Americans and Asians (Sussman, et al., 1996).

Moreover, most studies fail to account for social/environmental risk factors associated with neighborhood environments, which may be particularly important in explaining high levels of use in particular geographic locations. One study that did so found that reported higher levels of crack-cocaine use among African Americans and Hispanics aged twelve years and older became insignificant once respondents were grouped into neighborhood clusters (Lillie-Blanton, Anthony, and Schuster, 1993). More research is needed to fully account for racial/ethnic differences in drug use.

Implications for Prevention

These findings suggest that no single prevention program is likely to address the multiple influences on drug use equally well. Instead, programs need to be sensitive to developmental differences in the child's likely vulnerabilities—addressing the more proximal influences as they shift into adolescence, targeting family and school bonds at earlier ages. In high-risk neighborhoods, efforts aimed at community risk factors are likely to be particularly important as well.

Because pro-drug social influences and beliefs are strong precipitating factors during the transitional stage of adolescence, drug prevention programs for adolescents need to help them identify and resist these sources of pressure, combat beliefs that promote drug use, and develop reasons not to use. Programs aimed at risk factors that heighten vulnerability to pro-drug influences (weak bonds with family and school, impaired family relationships, poor school performance and attitudes, early antisocial behavior) should logically precede those focused on the more proximal causes of use. Addressing these factors during the elementary school years or earlier could yield multiple benefits because they are linked with several other health risks and problem behavior (dropping out, violence, suicide, delinquency).

Empirical findings to date suggest that developing different prevention programs for different racial/ethnic groups is premature. We still have limited insight into the reasons for racial/ethnic differences in drug use; moreover, a broad array of risk factors from different domains is relevant for most groups. Nevertheless, prevention experts should be mindful of the generally heightened risk for Whites and Native Americans for drug use of all kinds and the specific vulnerabilities of Asians who do poorly in school, Hispanics who suffer from disruptive family events and impaired family relationships, and all adolescents who live in high-risk neighborhoods.

I have reviewed what drug-use risk factors imply for prevention programs. Let me now turn specifically to the effects of school-based programs, focusing on the nature of programs appropriate for various developmental stages.

PREVENTION STRATEGIES FOR SCHOOL-BASED PROGRAMS

School-based programs have been the dominant prevention mode for adolescents and children. Most of them focus on helping the child cope with the societal and personal forces that promote drug use, but a few have tried to change the school, the family, or both. The former typically focus on helping children develop motivations not to use and identify and resist pro-drug social influences (social influence programs). The latter are more likely to be implemented in elementary school or kindergarten.

Programs for Elementary School and Kindergarten Children

Social influence programs are generally not appropriate for children in most elementary school grades or kindergarten. Most of these programs have been tested with sixth or seventh graders, when children have made the transition out of elementary school and are becoming particularly vulnerable to peer influences. Hence they capitalize on the child's readiness to understand what social influence means and to profit from lessons on how to identify and resist it. One program, which was tested on both fifth and sixth graders, yielded positive results for the older group, but was ineffective with fifth graders (Dielman, et al., 1989). These results suggest that children at grade five or below are not developmentally ready to acquire effective resistance skills; they are even less equipped to understand the subtle distinctions between internal and external pressure.

However, both elementary school and kindergarten offer appropriate venues for dealing with the family and school factors that make children more or less vulnerable to pro-drug social influences. Because these factors affect a wide variety of problem behaviors (Hawkins, Catalano, and Miller, 1992; Resnick, et al., 1997), school-based programs that improve children's school performance and their attachment to family and school may have multiple payoffs.

Evidence of multiple payoffs from a program that targets both school and family factors comes from the Perry Preschool project, a daily active learning program provided to fifty-eight African-American three and four year olds more than thirty years ago. Several adults trained in early education delivered the program (no more than 5 to 6 children per adult), which also included weekly home visits with parents and child. Those visits involved implementing curriculum activities at home and helping the mother provide the child with educational and emotional support. Results at age twenty-seven indicated that program participants had significantly fewer arrests, including arrests for drug use or drug dealing, a higher level of schooling completed, and higher monthly earnings (Schweinhart, Barnes, and Weikart, 1993).

Head Start, which was loosely based on the Perry Preschool model, involved less interactive learning, lower teacher/child ratios, and no home visits. It was also implemented on a nationwide scale, reaching more than 600,000 three to five year olds between 1964 and 1993. This program has yielded greater access to preventive health services for children of all races, reduced the likelihood of repeating a grade in elementary school for White children, and improved cognitive achievement for both White and African-American children. The test score effects last well into adolescence for White children, but are quickly lost among African Americans (Currie and Thomas, 1995), results that suggest the latter group may need continued special learning activities after they enter elementary school.

A systems approach aimed at changing the entire elementary school environment for children in high-risk schools involved developing a teacher/parent governance group, using mental health staff to provide services to children, staff, and parents, and establishing overall academic goals and strategies for the entire school, with education programs tailored to the individual needs of at-risk students. Program outcomes for this approach have focused solely on school-related behaviors and show improved attendance, better reading and math skills, and greater parent participation in the test schools, whose students were largely African-American (Comer, 1985, 1988). However, this intensive program is difficult to implement in new settings and early evaluations have included only a few schools and lacked rigorous evaluation features such as random assignment.

Another multiple component program for elementary school children aims at preventing juvenile delinquency and drug abuse and includes parent and teacher training, home-school liaison services, and conflict-resolution for high risk children. One analysis of short-term effects in this Seattle-based program revealed significant effects on early antisocial behavior for White boys and less self-destructiveness among White girls. However, no effects were found for African-American children (Hawkins, Von Cleve, and Catalano, 1991).

The Center for Substance Abuse Prevention and the National Institute on Drug Abuse have funded several studies designed to develop and evaluate drug prevention programs for kindergarten and elementary school children, but they have not yet yielded results.

Programs for Adolescents

Prevention models designed for middle school or older adolescents have typically been based on one of three approaches—the information model, the affective model, and the social influence model. However, only the last has demonstrated substantial effectiveness in curbing drug use.

The information model tended to focus on providing children with information about the harmful consequences of drugs and to assume that such knowledge would be enough to promote anti-drug attitudes. Popular in the early 1960s and 1970s, many such programs exaggerated the perils of drugs and lost credibility. They also had limited impact: although many increased knowledge about drugs, few altered attitudes about them, and even fewer affected drug use behavior (Goodstadt, 1978; Swisher, 1974; Tobler, 1986).

The affective model switched the focus to the personality and values of the adolescent, assuming that adolescents turn to drugs because of low self-esteem, inadequate values, or poor communication and decision-making skills. Programs based on this model included efforts to help young people clarify their values, improve communication, decision-making, or assertive skills, and develop higher self-esteem (Carney, 1971, 1972; Kim, 1981). This approach, which focused on characteristics or skills only weakly related to drug use (and frequently failed to mention drugs at all), also had little impact on drug use (Schaps, et al., 1986; Tobler, 1986).

The social influence model, which stresses motivating young people against drug use *and* helping them identify and resist pro-drug influences, has shown the most consistent prevention results (Hansen, 1992; Tobler, 1986; Tobler and Stratton, 1997). Such programs seek to help adolescents identify both internal and external pressures to use, to counter pro-drug arguments and normative beliefs that "everyone uses," and to learn skills for avoiding drug use when faced with pressure situations (Ellickson, 1995). They also explicitly recognize that teaching children how to resist drugs is not enough—programs also need to motivate them to resist.

Motivational strategies used in different social influence programs include exposing young people to role models for nonuse, helping them understand that most people do not use drugs or approve of doing so, building confidence in their ability to resist pro-drug pressures, and increasing their awareness of, and sense of susceptibility to, the consequences of drug use and the benefits of nonuse. Because adolescents often believe that "far-off" harms like liver or lung disease will not happen to them, these programs emphasize how drug use can affect people in their daily lives and social relationships. As a group, the social influence programs tend to be highly interactive, encouraging student participation through small group exercises, socratic methods, and role-playing and deliberately avoiding didactic, lecture-style teaching.

Early Social Influence Programs

Originally developed to combat adolescent smoking, the earliest versions of the social influence model focused on tobacco (Arkin, et al., 1981; Best, et al., 1988; Evans, et al., 1978; McAlister, et al., 1980). Overall, these programs yielded reductions in smoking for 5 to 8 percent of the targeted population, reductions that typically lasted for one to two years after initial program delivery (Cleary, et al., 1988). Because most were tested in largely White middle class communities, they were less successful in targeting high-risk and minority youth (Glynn, 1989). However, a few showed smoking reductions for minority youth as well (Botvin, et al., 1989a, 1989b).

Social Influence Model Extended to Other Substances

During the 1980s and 1990s, several research organizations and prevention practitioners sought to extend the social influence approach to substances besides tobacco. Among the most notable efforts are those based at the University of Michigan and targeted at alcohol misuse (Dielman, et al., 1989; Shope, et al., 1992); the Project Northland program, also focused on alcohol and developed at the University of Minnesota (Perry, et al., 1996); several programs targeted at alcohol, cigarettes, and marijuana and developed at USC (Hansen, Malotte, and Fielding, 1988; Hansen, et al., 1988; Pentz, et al., 1989); and Project ALERT, a multiple substance program developed at RAND (Ellickson and Bell, 1990;

Ellickson, Bell, and McGuigan, 1993). An important variant of the social influence model, Life Skills Training, has been developed at Cornell Medical School: this version adds general skills in communication, problem solving, assertiveness, coping, and dating to the basic social influence curriculum (Botvin, et al., 1995). DARE, a police-led program originally developed by the Los Angeles Police Department, includes elements of the informational approach, the affective approach, and the social influence model.

With the exception of DARE, all of the above programs have yielded reductions in adolescent use of substances besides cigarettes (Botvin, et al., 1995; Ellickson and Bell, 1990; Ellickson, Bell and McGuigan, 1993; Ennett, et al., 1994; Johnson, et al., 1990; Pentz, et al., 1989; Perry, et al., 1996; Shope, et al., 1992, 1994). DARE's poor results are probably attributable to the hybrid nature of the curriculum and the didactic style in which it is implemented (Tobler, 1986; Tobler and Stratton, 1997).

Recent meta-analyses confirm the superiority of the social influence model over the informational and affective approaches (Hansen and O'Malley, 1996; Tobler and Stratton, 1997). Overall, results from multiple studies indicate that this approach can effectively reduce both cigarette and marijuana use, that it works in communities with diverse racial/ethnic populations and socioeconomic backgrounds, and that it can curb both experimental and more regular use (Ellickson, 1995).

Nevertheless, the social influence approach is not a panacea. It tends to be more effective at preventing cigarette and marijuana use than drinking behavior (Ellickson and Bell, 1990; Hansen, Malotte and Fielding, 1988; Johnson, et al., 1990), although it has prevented alcohol misuse among previously unsupervised drinkers (Shope, et al., 1992). In addition, the prevention impact is modest, yielding reductions that average around 30 percent, and the effects fade after the lessons are discontinued (Institute of Medicine, 1994). Booster programs in high school help extend prevention gains (Botvin, et al., 1995) and, adding community and parent components to the school-based curriculum, appears to enhance program effects on alcohol (Perry, et al., 1996).

Effect of Parent and Community Components

Because they target additional risk factors such as parental attitudes about drugs, community norms, and media messages, the addition of peer and community components to school-based programs should enhance the effectiveness of the social influence model. To date, however, there is little hard data to support this expectation. Efforts to involve parents in drug prevention activities typically suffer from inability to attract parents whose involvement with their children is limited (Rohrbach, Hansen, and Pentz, 1992). Assessing the added effect of parent participation activities has been hampered by these biases in who participates.

The best evidence for the effectiveness of parent and community programs comes from Project Northland, a program tested in largely rural and small communities. Although the evaluation did not test the *added* impact of adding parent and community components to a school-based curriculum, it did yield prevention gains for baseline drinkers and baseline users of cigarettes and marijuana that lasted up to three years (Perry, et al., 1996). Project STAR has demonstrated the feasibility of adding media components, as well as community organization effort and parent intervention to a school-based effort (Pentz, et al., 1989). The Center for Substance Abuse Prevention, which funded 251 community coalitions or partnerships aimed at drug prevention across the United States, reports that over 60 percent include schools as members (Kaftarian and Hansen, 1994). However, programmatic activities varied widely across different communities and the national evaluation shows little impact of these partnerships on adolescent substance use.

Program Effectiveness Across Different Racial/Ethnic Groups

Although the social influence model was originally developed for children in White, middle class communities, recent evidence suggests that it is effective with children from widely different racial, ethnic, and socioeconomic backgrounds. One example, Project ALERT, was tested in thirty California and Oregon schools: eighteen drew from neighborhoods with household incomes below the median for their state and nine had minority populations of 50 percent or more. Results showed that the program was effective in both high and low minority schools: indeed, where there were differences between the two groups of schools, the results tended to favor the high minority schools (Ellickson and Bell, 1990). Graham and colleagues (1990) found consistent effects for Project SMART among African-American, Hispanic, Asian, and White subgroups. A test of Life Skills Training in inner-city (New York) schools that have predominantly minority students indicated lower rates of drinking, smoking, and using marijuana among intervention students compared to controls after three months (Botvin, et al., 1997).

Why are these programs effective with adolescents from different backgrounds? One explanation may lie in their highly interactive approach. Because social influence programs encourage student participation, they also provide the opportunity for students to bring their life experiences and knowledge into the classroom. Using question and answer exercises, teachers can ascertain what children believe about drugs, correct myths and misperceptions, and add in information that students have not yet acquired. Group discussions give students a chance to talk about what kind of pressures they face in their own neighborhoods. Role-playing exercises allow students to come up with solutions to pressure situations that reflect their own experiences and background. Hence the lessons change in subtle ways from classroom to classroom, reflecting the different backgrounds and capabilities of each student group. The interactive nature of these programs allows teachers to address the issues and concerns of both heterogeneous and homogeneous populations without undermining the basic guidelines of the overall prevention model.

WAYS TO IMPROVE SCHOOL-BASED DRUG PREVENTION

Research to date indicates that school-based prevention programs can and do work. Nevertheless, we can strengthen their effectiveness by using what we have learned about their strengths and weaknesses as guidelines for curriculum modification. We also need to do better at disseminating results about proven programs and supporting their implementation on a national basis.

The most effective school-based approach for adolescents is the social influence model. Because its impact fades after the lessons stop, this approach should be reinforced by high school boosters through the tenth grade or later. To date, however, few programs offer such extenders. Exceptions include Life Skills Training, Project STAR, Project Northland, and Project ALERT; the latter has launched a test of an integrated middle school and high school program in forty-eight South Dakota school districts.

The social influence approach has also been somewhat less effective at reducing alcohol use than reducing use of cigarettes and marijuana. Drinking is both widespread and socially acceptable in American society, and programs that are constantly counteracted by societal messages face tougher odds than those that are reinforced by parents, communities, and media efforts. Adding parent and community components to school-based prevention has yielded better results for alcohol use (Perry, et al., 1996), but the limited results of community partnership programs suggests that much needs to be learned about how to develop and implement effective community-based programs.

Social influence programs target proximal risk factors that are most strongly linked with drug use initiation and continuation. They do not address the more distal factors that increase the child's likely vulnerability to pro-drug social influences and beliefs. Hence programs that seek to improve the child's school performance and attachment to school, as well as those that foster greater family attachment and supervision, can provide a solid base for later drug prevention efforts aimed at adolescents. Programs that seek to change schools and families in ways that provide climates in which children flourish are especially appropriate for elementary school and younger children. Because they address risk factors that have been implicated in unhealthy or unproductive behavior more generally, they may also have broad payoffs across several societal problems.

Even a comprehensive school-based approach with a solid middle-school prevention curriculum, high school boosters, parent and community components, and early prevention efforts aimed at schools and families is unlikely to be successful if the people responsible for putting it in place lack the motivation, skills, and resources to implement it effectively. Insufficient teacher training and staff time is a major factor in the failure of most school-based programs conducted under the Drug-Free Schools Act; many teachers also report that the programs are not given priority within the school and that they themselves are not comfortable with interactive teaching methods (Research Triangle Institute, 1997). Moreover, despite the availability of federal funding, resources for comprehensive programs are still limited. Hence, key components of effective prevention also include appropriate teacher training, top level support for prevention, selection of motivated teachers, and adequate resources.

FOCUS FOR FUTURE RESEARCH AND EVALUATION EFFORTS

Clearly we must continue empirical evaluations of the effectiveness of our drug prevention efforts and use the insights we derive to improve what we do. In this chapter, I have discussed a comprehensive strategy that uses schools as the basic venue for drug prevention. These recommendations are grounded in both theory and empirical research, but the overall strategy has not been empirically tested. Until it is, our knowledge about what makes for effective drug prevention and how to improve existing efforts will remain limited. In an era of increasingly constrained budgets for prevention activities, we need more than ever to know what we are about.

Well designed evaluations of school-based programs could also enhance our ability to design and implement programs that give greater attention to the needs of different racial/ethnic groups. Although empirical results to date do not support the design of separate programs, they do support making programs more sensitive to clearly documented differences in risk factors across these groups. Future research is needed to pinpoint risk and protective factors that are unique to (or particularly important for) specific racial/ethnic groups and to establish whether culturally sensitive programs are more effective for them.

REFERENCES

Amaro, H., Whitaker, R., Coffman, G. and Heeren, T. (1990). IX. Acculturation and marijuana and cocaine use: Findings from HHANES 1982-1984. *American Journal of Public Health*, 80(Supplement):54-60.

Amey, C. H., Albrecht, S. L. and Miller, M. K. (1996). Racial differences in adolescent drug use: The impact of religion. *Substance Use and Misuse*, 31(10):1311-1132.

Ajzen, I. and Fishbein, M. (1980). *Understanding Attitudes and Predicting Social Behavior*. Prentice-Hall: Englewood Cliffs, NJ.

Arkin, R. M., Roemhild, H. F., Johnson, C. A., Luepker, R. V. and Murray, D. M. (1981). The Minnesota smoking-prevention program: A seventh-grade health curriculum supplement. *The Journal of School Health*, 51(9):611-616.

Austin, G. (1988, Fall). *Prevention Goals, Methods, and Outcomes (Prevention Research Update 1)*. Southwest Regional Laboratory: Los Alamitos, CA.

Bachman, J. G., Johnston, L. D. and O'Malley, P. M. (1987). *Monitoring the Future: Questionnaire Responses From the Nation's High School Seniors*. Institute for Social Research: Ann Arbor, MI.

Bachman, J. G., O'Malley, P. and Johnston, L. (1984). Drug use among adults: The impacts of role status and social environment. *Journal of Personality and Social Psychology*, 47(3):629-645.

Bachman, J. G., Wallace, J., O'Malley, P., Johnston, L., Kurth, C. and Neighbors, H. (1991). Racial/ethnic differences in smoking, drinking, and illicit drug use among American high school seniors, 1976-1989. *American Journal of Public Health*, 81:372-377.

Bandura, A. (1977a). Self-efficacy: Toward a unifying theory of behavioral change. *Psychology Review*, 84:191-215.

Bandura, A. (1977b). *Social Learning Theory*. Prentice Hall: Englewood Cliffs, NJ.

Barnes, G. M. and Welte, J. W. (1986). Patterns and predictors of alcohol use among 7-12th grade students in New York State. *Journal of Studies on Alcohol*, 47:53-62.

Baumrind, D. (1983, October). *Why Adolescents Take Chances—And Why They Don't*. Paper presented at the National Institute for Child Health and Human Development, Bethesda, MD.

Baumrind, D. and Moselle, K. A. (1985). A developmental perspective on adolescent drug abuse. *Advances in Alcohol and Substance Abuse*, 4(3-4):41-67.

Becker, M. H., Ed. (1974). The health belief model and personal health behavior. *Health Education Monographs*, 1:324-473.

Bell, R. M. and Ellickson, P. L. (under review). *Patterns of Substance-use and Consequences-of-use Measures for White, Hispanic, Asian, and Black Adolescents*.

Berndt, T. (1979). Developmental changes in conformity to peers and parents. *Developmental Psychology*, 15:608-616.

Best, J., Thomson, S., Santi, S., Smith, E. and Brown, K. (1988). Preventing cigarette smoking among school children. *Annual Review of Public Health*, 9:161-201.

Betancourt, H. and Lopez, S. R. (1993). The study of culture, ethnicity, and race in American psychology. *American Psychologist*, 48:629-637.

Bettes, B. A., Dusenbury, L., Kerner, J., James-Ortiz, S. and Botvin, G. J. (1990). Ethnicity and psychosocial factors in alcohol and tobacco use in adolescence. *Child Development*, 61:557-565.

Botvin, G. J., Baker, E., Dusenbury, L., Botvin, E. M. and Diaz, T. (1995). Long-term follow-up results of a randomized drug abuse prevention trial in a white middle-class population. *Journal of the American Medical Association*, 273(14):1106-1112.

Botvin, G. J., Baston, J. W., Witts-Vitale, S., Bess, V., Baker, E. and Dusenbury, L. (1989a). A psychosocial approach to smoking prevention for urban Black youth. *Public Health Reports*, 104:573-582.

Botvin, G. J., Dusenbury, L., Baker, E., James-Ortiz, S. and Kerner, J. (1989b). A skills training approach to smoking prevention among Hispanic youth. *Journal of Behavioral Medicine*, 12:279-296.

Botvin, G. J., Epstein, J. A., Baker, E., Diaz, T. and Williams, M. I. (1997). School-based drug abuse prevention with inner-city minority youth. *Journal of Child and Adolescent Substance Abuse*, 6:5-20.

Brook, J. S., Brook, D. W., Gordon, A. S., Whiteman, M. and Cohen, P. (1990). The psychological etiology of adolescent drug use: A family interactional approach. *Genetic, Social, and General Psychology Monographs*, 116(Whole No. 2).

Brook, J. S., Whiteman, M., Balka, E. B. and Hamburg, B. A. (1992). African-American and Puerto Rican drug use: Personality, familial, and other environmental risk factors. *Genetic, Social, and General Psychology Monographs*, 118(4):417-438.

Brook, J. S., Whiteman, M., Gordon, A.S. and Brook, D. W. (1988). The roles of older brothers in younger brothers' drug use viewed in the context of parent and peer influences. *Journal of Genetic Psychology*, 151:59-75.

Brunswick, A. and Messeri, P. (1985). *Causal Factors in Onset of Adolescent's Cigarette Smoking*. Haworth Press: New York.

Carney, R. E. (1971). *An Evaluation of the Effect of a Values-Oriented Drug Abuse Education Program Using the Risk Taking Attitude Questionnaire*. Coronado Unified School District: Coronado, CA.

Carney, R. E. (1972). *An Evaluation of the Tempe, Arizona 1970-71 Drug Abuse Prevention Education Program Using the RTAQ and B-VI: Final Report*. Tempe School District: Tempe, AZ.

Catalano, R. F., Morrison, D. M., Wells, E. A., Gillmore, M. R., Iritani, B. and Hawkins, J. D. (1992). Ethnic differences in family factors related to early drug initiation. *Journal of Studies on Alcohol*, 53(3):208-217.

Chassin, L. (1984). Adolescent substance use and abuse. In P. Karoly and J. J. Steffen (Eds.) *Advances in Child Behavioral Analysis and Therapy*, Vol. 3. (pp. 99-153). Lexington Books: Lexington, MA.

Cleary, P. D., Hitchcock, J. L., Semmer, N., Flinchbaug, L. J. and Pinney, J. M. (1988). Adolescent smoking: Research and health policy. *Milbank Quarterly*, 66(1): 137-171.

Collins, L. M., Sussman, S., Rauch, J. M., Dent, C. W., Johnson, C. A., Hansen, W. B., et al. (1987). Psychosocial predictors of young adolescent cigarette smoking: A sixteen-month, three-wave longitudinal study. *Journal of Applied Social Psychology*, 17(6):554-573.

Comer, J. P. (1985). The Yale-New Haven Primary Prevention Project: A follow-up study. *Journal of the American Academy of Child Psychiatry*, 24:154-160.

Comer, J. P. (1988). Educating poor minority children. *Scientific American*, 259:42-48.

Conrad, K. M., Flay, B. R. and Hill, D. (1992). Why children start smoking cigarettes: Predictors of onset. *British Journal of Addiction*, 87(12):1711-1724.

Coreil, J., Ray, L. and Markides, K. S. (1991). Predictors of smoking among Mexican-Americans: Findings from the Hispanic HANES. *Preventive Medicine*, 20:508-517.

Currie, J. and Thomas, D. (1995). Does Head Start make a difference? *The American Economic Review*, 85(3):361-364.

Dembo, R., Farrow, D., Jarlais, D. C. D., Burgos, W. and Schmeidler, J. (1981). Examining a causal model of early drug involvement among inner-city junior high school youths. *Human Relations*, 34:169-193.

Dielman, T. E., Shope, J. T., Leech, S. L. and Butchart, A. T. (1989). Differential effectiveness of an elementary school-based alcohol misuse prevention program. *Journal of School Health*, 59:255-282.

Ellickson, P. L. (1995). Schools. In R. Coombs and D. Ziedonis (Eds.), *Handbook of Drug Abuse Prevention*. Prentice Hall: Englewood Cliffs, NJ.

Ellickson, P. L. and Bell, R. M. (1993). Preventing adolescent drug use: The effectiveness of Project ALERT: A response. *American Journal of Public Health*, 84(3):500-501.

Ellickson, P. L., Bell, R. M. and McGuigan, K. A. (1993). Preventing adolescent drug use: Long term results of a junior high program. *American Journal of Public Health*, 83(6):856-861.

Ellickson, P. L., Collins, R. L. and Bell, R. M. (in press). Adolescent use of illicit drugs other than marijuana: How important is social bonding and for whom? *Substance Use and Misuse*.

Ellickson, P. L. and Hays, R. D. (1991a). Antecedents of drinking among young adolescents with different alcohol use histories. *Journal of Studies on Alcohol*, 52(5): 398-408.

Ellickson, P. L. and Hays, R. D. (1991b). Beliefs about resistance self-efficacy and drug prevalence: Do they really affect drug use? *International Journal of the Addictions*, 25(11a):1353-1378.

Ellickson, P. L. and Hays, R. D. (1992). On becoming involved with drugs: Modeling adolescent drug use over time. *Health Psychology*, 11(6):377-385.

Ellickson, P. L., Hays, R. D. and Bell, R. M. (1992). Stepping through the drug use sequence: Longitudinal and scalogram analysis of initiation and regular use. *Journal of Abnormal Psychology*, 101(3):441-451.

Ellickson, P. L., McGuigan, K. A., Adams, V., Bell, R. M. and Hays, R. D. (1996). Teenagers and alcohol misuse: By any definition, it's a big problem. *Addiction*, 91(10): 1489-1503.

Ellickson, P. L. and Morton, S. (in press). Identifying adolescents at risk for hard drug use: Racial/Ethnic variations. *Journal of Adolescent Health*.

Elliott, D. S. and Morse, B. J. (1989). Delinquency and drug use as risk factors in teenage sexual activity. *Youth and Society*, 21(1):32-60.

Ennett, S. T., Tobler, N. S., Ringwalt, C. L. and Flewelling, R. L. (1994). How effective is drug abuse resistance education? A meta-analysis of project DARE outcome evaluations. *American Journal of Public Health*, 84(9):1394-1401.

Evans, R. I., Rozelle, R. M., Mittelmark, M., Hansen, W. B., Bane, A. and Havis, J. (1978). Deterring the onset of smoking in children: Knowledge of immediate psychological effects and coping with peer pressure, media pressure, and parent modeling. *Journal of Applied Social Psychology*, 8:126-135.

Flannery, D. J., Vazsonyi, A. T., Torquati, J. and Fridrich, A. (1994). Ethnic and gender differences in risk for early adolescent substance use. *Journal of Youth and Adolescence*, 23(2):195-213.

Fleming, J. P., Kellam, S. G. and Brown, C. H. (1982). Early predictors of age at first use of alcohol, marijuana, and cigarettes. *Drug and Alcohol Dependence*, 9:285-303.

Flewelling, R. L., Ennett, S. T., Rachal, J. V. and Theisen, A. C. (1994). *National Household Survey on Drug Abuse: Race/Ethnicity, Socioeconomic Status, and Drug Abuse: 1991.* Research Triangle Institute, Center for Social Research and Policy Analysis. US Department of Health and Human Services.

Freeberg, A. L. and Stein, C. H. (1996). Felt obligation towards parents in Mexican-American and Anglo-American young adults. *Journal of Social and Personal Relationships*, 13(3):457-471.

Gersick, K. E., Grady, K., Sexton, E. and Lyons, M. (1981). Personality and sociodemographic factors in adolescent drug use. In D. J. Lettieri and J. P. Ludford (Eds.), *Drug Abuse and the American adolescent, Research Monograph 38.* National Institute on Drug Abuse: Rockville, MD.

Gfoerer, J. and De La Rosa, M. (1993). Protective and risk factors associated with drug use among Hispanic youth. *Journal of Addictive Disease*, 12(2):87-107.

Gillmore, M. R., Catalano, R. F., Morrison, D. M., Wells, E. A., Iritani, B. and Hawkins, J. D. (1990). Racial differences in acceptability and drugs and early initiation of substance use. *American Journal of Drug Alcohol Abuse*, 16(3 and 4):185-206.

Glynn, T. J. (1989). Essential elements of school-based smoking prevention programs. *Journal of School Health*, 59(5):181-188.

Goodstadt, M. S. (1978). Alcohol and drug education: Models and outcomes. *Health Education Monographs*, 6:263-279.

Gottfredson, D. C. (1988). *Issues in Adolescent Drug Use.* Unpublished final report to the U.S. Department of Justice, Johns Hopkins University, Center for Research on Elementary and Middle Schools: Baltimore, MD.

Graham, J. W., Johnson, C. A., Hansen, W. B., Flay, B. R. and Gee, M. (1990). Drug use prevention programs, gender, and ethnicity: Evaluation of three seventh-grade Project SMART cohorts. *Preventive Medicine*, 19:305-313.

Hansen, W. B. (1992). School-based substance abuse prevention: A review of the state of the art in curriculum, 1980-1990. *Health Education Research*, 7:403-430.

Hansen, W. B. (1997). Prevention programs: Factors that individually focused programs must address. In *Resource Paper for the Secretary's Youth Substance Abuse Initiative.* SAMHSA/CSAP Teleconference, October 22. Pre-Publication Document.

Hansen, W. B., Johnson, C. A., Flay, B. R., Graham, J. W. and Sobel, J. (1988). Affective and social influences approaches to the prevention of multiple substance abuse among seventh grade students: Results from Project SMART. *Preventive Medicine*, 17(2):135-152.

Hansen, W. B., Malotte, C. K. and Fielding, J. E. (1988). Evaluation of a tobacco and alcohol abuse prevention curriculum for adolescents. *Health Education Quarterly*, 15:93-114.

Hansen, W. B. and O'Malley P. M. (1996). Drug use. In R. J. DiClemente, W. B. Hansen and L. E. Ponton (Eds.), *Handbook of Adolescent Health Risk Behavior.* Plenum Press: New York.

Harford, T. C. (1986). Drinking patterns among Black and nonblack adolescents. Results of a national survey. *Annals of the New York Academy of Sciences*, 472:130-141.

Hawkins, J. D., Catalano, R. E. and Miller, J. Y. (1992). Risk and protective factors for alcohol and other drug problems in adolescence and early adulthood: Implications for substance abuse prevention. *Psychological Bulletin*, 112(1):64-105.

Hawkins, J. D., Von Cleve, E. and Catalano, R. F. (1991). Reducing early childhood aggression: Results of a primary prevention program. *Journal of the American Academy of Child and Adolescent Psychiatry*, 30:208-217.

Hawkins, J. D. and Weis, J. G. (1985). The social development model: An integrated approach to delinquency prevention. *Journal of Primary Prevention*, 6:73-97.

Headen, S. W., Bauman, K. E., Deane, G. D. and Koch, G. G. (1991). Are the correlates of cigarette smoking initiation different for black and white adolescents? *American Journal of Public Health*, 81(7):854-857.

Herd, D. (1985). Ambiguity in Black drinking norms. In L. Bennett and G. Ames (Eds.), *The American Experience with Alcohol: Contrasting Cultural Perspectives* (pp. 143-69). Plenum Press: New York.

Hirschi, J. (1969). *Causes of Delinquency*. University of California Press: Berkeley, CA.

Huba, G. J. and Bentler, P. M. (1984). Casual models of personality, peer culture characteristics, drug use and crucial behavior over a five-year span. In D. Goodwin, K. Van Dusen and S. Mednick (Eds.), *Longitudinal Research in Alcoholism*. Kluwer-Nijhof: Boston, MA.

Humm-Delgado, D. and Delgado, M. (1983). Hispanic adolescents and substance abuse: Issues for the 1980s. *Child and Youth Services*, 6:71-87.

Humphrey, J. A., Stephens, V. S. and Allen, D. F. (1983). Race, sex, marijuana use and alcohol intoxication in college students. *Journal of Studies on Alcohol*, 44(4):733.

Hundleby, J. D. and Mercer, G. W. (1987). Family and friends as social environments and their relationship to young adolescents' use of alcohol, tobacco, and marijuana. *Journal of Clinical Psychology*, 44:125-135.

Institute of Medicine (1994). *Growing Up Tobacco Free: Preventing Nicotine Addiction in Children and Youths*. Committee on Preventing Nicotine Addiction in Children and Youths. Division of Biobehavioral Sciences and Mental Disorders. National Academy Press: Washington, D.C.

Jessor, R., Donovan, J. E. and Windmer, K. (1980). *Psychosocial Factors in Adolescent Alcohol and Drug Use: The 1980 National Sample Study and the 1974-78 Panel Study*. Unpublished final report, University of Colorado, Institute of Behavioral Science: Boulder, CO.

Jessor, R. and Jessor, S. L. (1977). *Problem Behavior and Psychosocial Development: A Longitudinal Study of Youth*. Academic Press: New York.

Johnson, C. A., Pentze, M. A., Weber, M. D., Dwyer, J. H., Baer, N., MacKinnon, D. P. and Hansen, W. B. (1990). Relative effectiveness of comprehensive community programming for drug abuse prevention with high-risk and low-risk adolescents. *Journal of Consulting and Clinical Psychology*, 58(4):1-10.

Johnston, L. D., O'Malley, P. M. and Bachman, J. G. (1996). National survey results on drug use from the monitoring the future study, 1975-1995, Vol. 1, Secondary School Students. In *National Institute on Drug Abuse, USDHHS, NIH Pub. No. 96-4139*. U.S. Government Printing Office: Washington, D.C.

Kaftarian, S. J. and Hansen, W. B. (1994). Improving methodologies for the evaluation of community-based substance abuse prevention programs. In Community Partnership

Program Center for Substance Abuse Prevention. [Monograph series CSAP special issue]. *Journal of Community Psychology*, 3-5.

Kandel, D. (1985). On processes of peer influences in adolescent drug use: A developmental perspective. In J. S. Brook, D. J. Lettieri and D. W. Brock (Eds.), *Alcohol and Substance Abuse in Adolescence*. Haworth Press: New York.

Kandel, D. B. (1982). Epidemiological and psychosocial perspectives on adolescent drug use. *Journal of American Academic Clinical Psychiatry*, 21:328-347.

Kandel, D. B., Ed. (1978). *Longitudinal Research on Drug Use: Empirical Findings and Methodological Issues*. Hemisphere-Wiley: Washington, D.C.

Kandel, D. B. and Andrews, K. (1987). Processes of adolescent socialization by parents and peers. *International Journal of the Addictions*, 22:319-342.

Kandel, D. B., Kessler, R. and Margulies, R. (1978). Antecedents of adolescent initiation into stages of drug use: A developmental analysis. *Journal of Youth and Adolescence*, 7:13-40.

Kim, S. (1981). An evaluation of ombudsman primary prevention program on student drug abuse. *Journal of Drug Education*, 11:27-36.

Krosnick, J. and Judd, C. (1982). Transitions in social influence at adolescence: Who induces cigarette smoking? *Developmental Psychology*, 18:359-368.

Landrine, H., Richardson, J. L., Klonoff, E. A. and Flay, B. (1994). Cultural diversity in the predictors of adolescent cigarette smoking: The relative influence of peers. *Journal of Behavioral Medicine*, 17(3):331-346.

Leigh, B. C. (1989). Attitudes and expectancies as predictors of drinking habits: A comparison of three scales. *Journal of Studies on Alcohol*, 50:432-444.

Leigh, B. C. and Stacy, A. W. (1991). On the scope of alcohol expectancy research: Remaining issues of measurement and meaning. *Psychological Bulletin*, 110:147-154.

Lillie-Blanton, M., Anthony, J. C. and Schuster, C. R. (1993). Probing the meaning of racial/ethnic group comparisons in crack cocaine smoking. *Journal of the American Medical Association*, 269(8):993-997.

Lopes, C. E., Sussman, S., Galaif, E. R. and Crippens, D. L. (1995). The impact of a videotape on smoking cessation among African-American women. *American Journal of Health Promotion*, 9:257-260.

Maddahian, E., Newcomb, M. D. and Bentler, P. M. (1988). Adolescent drug use and intention to use drugs: Concurrent and longitudinal analyses of four ethnic groups. *Addictive Behaviors*, 13:191-195.

Markides, K. S., et al. (1986). Sources of helping and inter-generational solidarity: A three generation study of Mexican Americans. *Journal of Gerontology*, 41:506-511.

McAlister, A. L., Perry, C., Killen, J., Slinkard, L. A. and Maccoby, N. (1980). Pilot study of smoking, alcohol, and drug abuse prevention. *American Journal of Public Health*, 70(7):719-721.

Milburn, N. G., Gary, L. E., Booth, J. A. and Brown, D. R. (1990). Conducting epidemiologic research in a minority community: Methodological considerations. *Journal of Community Psychology*, 19:3-11.

Mindel, C. H. (1980). Extended familism among urban Mexican Americans, Anglos, and Blacks. *Hispanic Journal of Behavioral Sciences*, 2:21-34.

National Institute of Drug Abuse, (1990). *U.S. Department of Health and Human Services Publication No. (ADM) 90-1682.* U.S. Government Printing Office: Washington, D.C.

National Institute of Drug Abuse, (1995). *Drug Use Among Racial/ethnic Minorities.* U.S. Department of Health and Human Services, Public Health Service, National Institutes of Health, NIH Publication, No. 95-3888.

Newcomb, M. D. and Bentler, P. M. (1988). *Consequences of Adolescent Drug Use: Impact on Psychosocial Development and Young Adult Role Responsibility.* Sage Publications: Beverly Hills, CA.

Newcomb, M. D., Maddahian, E. and Bentler, P. M. (1986). Risk factors for drug use among adolescents; Concurrent and longitudinal analyses. *American Journal of Public Health,* 76:525-531.

Newcomb, M. D. and Felix-Ortiz, M. (1992). Multiple protective and risk factors for drug use and abuse: Cross-sectional and prospective findings. *Journal of Personality and Social Psychology,* 63(2):289-296.

Oetting, E. and Beauvais, F. (1987). Peer cluster theory, socialization characteristics, and adolescent drug use: A path analysis. *Journal of Counseling Psychology,* 34: 205-213.

Parker, V. C., Sussman, S., Crippens, D. L., Elder, P. and Scholl, D. (1996). *The Relation of Ethnic Identification with Cigarette Smoking Among Urban Minority Youth.* Unpublished manuscript, University of Southern California, Institute for Prevention Research, Department of Preventive Medicine: Los Angeles, CA.

Pentz, M. A., Dwyer, J., MacKinnon, D., Flay, B., Hansen, W., Yang, E. and Johnson, C. (1989). A multi-community trial for primary prevention of adolescent drug abuse: Effects on drug use prevalence. *Journal of American Medical Association,* 261: 3259-3266.

Perry, C. L., Williams, C. L., Veblen-Mortenson, S., Toomey, T. L., Komro, K. A., Anstine, P. S., McGovern, P. G., Finnegan, J. R., Forster, J. L., Wagenaar, A. C. and Wolfson, M. (1996). Project Northland: Outcomes of a Communitywide Alcohol Use Prevention Program during Early Adolescence. *American Journal of Public Health,* 86(7): 956-965.

Petraitus, J., Flay, B. R. and Miller, T. Q. (1995). Reviewing theories of adolescent substance use: Organizing pieces of the puzzle. *Psychological Bulletin,* 117(1): 67-86.

Research Triangle Institute (1997). *School-based Drug Prevention Programs: A Longitudinal Study in Selected School Districts.* Executive Summary, Research Triangle Institute.

Resnick, M. E., Bearman, P. S., Blum, R. W., Bauman, K. E., Harris, K. M., Jones, J., Tabor, J., Beuhring, T., Sieving, R. E., Shew, M., Ireland, M., Bearinger, L. H. and Urdry, R. (1997). Protecting adolescents from harm: Findings from the National Longitudinal Study on adolescent health. *Journal of the American Medical Association,* 278(10):823-832.

Reuter, P., Haaga, J., Murphy, P. and Praskac, A. (July 1988). *Drug Use and Drug Programs in the Washington Metropolitan Area.* The RAND Corporation, R-3655-GWRC: Santa Monica, CA.

Riley, W. T., Barenie, J. T., Mabe, P. A. and Myers, D. R. (1991). The roles of race and ethnic status on the psychosocial correlates of smokeless tobacco use in adolescent males. *Journal of Adolescent Health*, 12:15-21.

Robins, L. N. (1980). The natural history of drug abuse. *Acta Psychiatrica Scandinavia*, 62(Suppl. 284):7-20.

Robins, L. N. and Przybeck, T. (1985). Age of onset of drug use as a factor in drug and other disorders. In C. Jones and R. Battjes (Eds.), *Etiology of Drug Abuse: Implications for Prevention*. NIDA: Rockville, MD.

Robinson, T. N., Killen, J. D., Taylor, C. B., Telch, M. J., Bryson, S. W., Saylor, K. E., Maron, D. J., Maccoby, N. and Farquhar, J. W. (1987). Perspectives on adolescent substance use: A defined population study. *Journal of the American Medical Association*, 258(15):2072-2076.

Rohrbach, L. A., Hansen, W. B. and Pentz, M. A. (1992). Strategies for involving parents in drug abuse prevention: Results from the Midwestern Prevention Program. *American Public Health Association Abstracts*, 120:263.

Schaps, E., Moskowitz, J., Malvin, J. and Schaeffer, G. (1986). Evaluation of seven school-based prevention projects: A final report on the Napa Project. *International Journal of the Addictions*, 21:1081-1012.

Schweinhart, L. J., Barnes, H. V. and Weikart, D. P. (1993). Significant benefits: The High/Scope Perry Preschool study through age 27. In *Monographs of the High/Scope Educational Research Foundation, Number Ten*. The High/Scope Press: Ypsilanti, MI.

Selnow, G. W. (1987). Parent-child relationships and single and two parent families: Implications for substance usage. *Journal of Drug Education*, 17: 315-326.

Shedler, J. and Block, J. (1990). Adolescent drug use and psychological health: A longitudinal inquiry. *American Psychologist*, 45(5):612-630.

Shope, J. T., Dielman, T. E., Butchart, A. T., Campanelli, P. C. and Kloska, D. (1992). An elementary school-based alcohol misuse prevention program: A follow-up evaluation. *Journal of Studies on Alcohol*, 53(2):106-121.

Shope, J. T., Kloska, D. D., Dielman, T. E. and Maharg, R. (1994). Longitudinal evaluation of an enhanced Alcohol Misuse Prevention Study (AMPS) curriculum for grades 6 through 8. *Journal of School Health*, 64:160-166.

Silverberg, S. and Gondoli, D. (1996). Autonomy in adolescence: A contextualized perspective. In G. Adams, R. Montemayor and T. Gullotta (Eds.), *Psychosocial Development During Adolescence: Progress in Developmental Contextualism* (pp. 12-61). Sage Publications: Thousand Oaks, CA.

Simons, R. L., Conger, R. D. and Whitbeck, L. B. (1988). A multistage social learning model of the influences of family and peers upon adolescent substance abuse. *Journal of Drug Issues*, 18(3):293-315.

Skinner, W., Massey, J., Krohn, M. and Lauer, R. M. (1985). Social influences and constraints on the initiation and cessation of adolescent tobacco use. *Journal of Behavioral Medicine*, 8:353-375.

Sloboda, Z. and David, S. L. (1997). *Preventing Drug Use among Children and Adolescents: A Research-based Guide*. NIDA: Rockville, MD.

Smith, G. M. and Fogg, C. P. (1978). Psychological predictors of early use, late use, and non-use of marijuana among teenage students. In D. Kandel (Ed.), *Longitudinal Research on Drug Use: Empirical Findings and Methodological Issues.* Hemisphere-Wiley: Washington, D.C.

Stacy, A. W., Widaman, K. F. and Marlatt, G. A. (1990). Expectancy models of alcohol use. *Journal of Personality and Social Psychology,* 58:918-928.

Stark, R., Kent, L. and Doyle, D. P. (1982). Religion and delinquency: The ecology of a "lost" relationship. *Journal of Research in Crime and Delinquency,* 19:4-24.

Sue, S. and Okazaki, S. (1990). Asian-American educational achievements: A phenomenon in search of an explanation. *American Psychologist,* 45:913-920.

Sussman, S., Dent, C. W., Flay, B. R., Hansen, W. B. and Johnson, C. A. (1987). Psychosocial predictors of cigarette smoking onset by white, black, Hispanic, and Asian adolescents in Southern California. *Mortality and Morbidity Weekly Report,* 36(4S):11S.

Sussman, S., Parker, V. C., Lopes, C., Crippens, D. L., Elder, P. and Scholl, D. (1995). Empirical development of brief smoking prevention videotapes which target African-American adolescents. *International Journal of the Addictions,* 30: 1141-1164.

Sussman, S., Stacy, A. W., Dent, C. W., Simon, T. R. and Johnson, C. A. (1996). Marijuana use: Current issues and new research directions. *Journal of Drug Issues,* 26:695-733.

Swisher, J. D. (1974). The effectiveness of drug education: Conclusions based on experimental evaluation. In M. Goodstadt (Ed.), *Research on Methods and Programs of Drug Education.* Addiction Research Foundation: Toronto, Canada.

Tobler, N. S. (1986). Meta-analysis of 143 adolescent drug prevention programs: Quantitative outcome results of program participants compared to a control or comparison group. *Journal of Drug Issues,* 16:537-567.

Tobler, N. S. (1995). *Meta-Analysis of Adolescent Drug Prevention Programs.* Doctoral Dissertation, State University of New York at Albany, June, 1994. Dissertation Abstracts International 55(11a):UMI-Order Number 9509310.

Tobler, N. S. and Stratton, H. H. (1997). Effectiveness of school-based drug prevention programs: A meta-analysis of the research. *The Journal of Primary Prevention,* 18(1):71-128.

Vega, W. A., Zimmerman, R. S., Warheit, G. J., Apospori, E. and Gil, A. G. (1993). Risk factors for early adolescent drug use in four ethnic and racial groups. *American Journal of Public Health,* 83:185-189.

Wadsworth, K. N., Schulenberg, J., Deilman, T., Shope, J. and Zucker, R. A. (under review). *Developmental Models of Parent and Peer Influences on Adolescent Alcohol Misuse.*

Wallace, J. M. and Bachman, J. G. (1991). Explaining racial/ethnic differences in adolescent drug use: The impact of background and lifestyle. *Social Problems,* 38(3): 333-357.

Wallace, J. M., Bachman, J. G., O'Malley, P. M. and Johnston, L. D. (1995). Racial/ethnic differences in adolescent drug use: Exploring possible explanations. In G. Botvin, S. Schinke and M. Orlandi (Eds.), *Drug Abuse Prevention with Multi-Ethnic Youth.* Sage Publications: Thousand Oaks, CA.

Welte, J. W. and Barnes, G. M. (1985). Alcohol: The gateway to other drug use among secondary school students. *Journal of Youth and Adolescence*, 14:487-498.

Welte, J. W. and Barnes, G. M. (1987). Youthful smoking: Patterns and relationships to alcohol and other drug use. *Journal of Adolescence*, 10:327-340.

Yamaguchi, K. and Kandel, D. (1984). Patterns of drug use from adolescence to young adulthood: II. Sequences of progression. *American Journal of Public Health*, 74: 668-672.

CHAPTER 5

Ethnic Identity as a Protective Factor in the Health Behaviors of African-American Male Adolescents*

Chris Ringwalt, Phillip Graham,
Kathy Sanders-Phillips, Dorothy Browne,
and Mallie J. Paschall

The high prevalence of violence and other risk behaviors among African-American male adolescents has generated considerable interest in preventive approaches that target this population. Although programs like Rites of Passage and manhood training, often coupled with adult mentoring, have proliferated nationwide (Gabriel, et al., 1996; Ringwalt, et al., 1996; Warfield-Coppock, 1992), their efficacy in preventing high risk behaviors in African-American males has not been sufficiently explored. Such programs seek to develop in young males an understanding of and appreciation for their ethnic history, culture, and accomplishments, and to recreate for them the traditional manhood initiation rites of their African forebears. These programs are predicated on the assumption that the risk behaviors these youth manifest are in part a function of a multi-generational legacy of prejudice, discrimination, and denigration by a dominant White culture that at best has left these youth detached from, and at worse ashamed of, their ethnicity. Instilling in these youth a strong sense of ethnic pride and providing them with information pertaining to the achievements of their

*This chapter was supported by Grant No. R49/CCR411632-03 from the Centers for Disease Control and Prevention (CDC). Its contents are solely the responsibility of the authors and do not necessarily represent the official views of the CDC.

ethnic group, it is argued, will decrease the likelihood that they will behave in ways that are destructive to themselves and others.

In seeking a conceptual literature supportive of this approach to prevention, practitioners have turned to the burgeoning literature on ethnic identity. Over the last four decades, and often working in isolation from one another, the major contributors to this literature have described ethnic identity not as a static construct but as an ongoing process. This process involves a sequential series of fairly well-defined stages as individuals progress from an uninformed, naive sense of their ethnic identity, through a period of active and sometimes tumultuous searching and questioning, and finally to a mature understanding and appreciation that encompasses both themselves as members of their ethnic group and their relationships to members of the dominant culture. Implicit in this conceptual schema is the assumption that the successful completion of this quest is essential to an individual's full self-actualization.

While the theory of ethnic identity development has considerable intuitive appeal, as do the programmatic approaches that are based on it, the theory and its application to the prevention of risk behaviors has only recently begun to be subjected to empirical investigation and validation. We have at present only a rudimentary understanding of the relationship between ethnic identity and risk behaviors in minority adolescents, and what position ethnic identity may occupy in the constellation of risk and protective factors thought to determine risk behavior in this population. In this chapter we will summarize our current understanding of the stages of ethnic identity development, assess the potential of ethnic identity as a protective factor that might inhibit or constrain the expression of risk behaviors, and then set forth a research and practice agenda. To set the stage for these discussions, we begin by describing the commonality of risk behaviors in adolescents and specifying the differential mechanisms by which risk and protective factors affect risk behaviors.

RISK BEHAVIORS AMONG AFRICAN-AMERICAN ADOLESCENTS

Approximately one youth in four are at risk of engaging in multiple problem behaviors such as substance use, violence, unprotected sexual activity, and other behaviors that enhance the likelihood of negative social and health consequences both for themselves and for the individuals with whom they come into contact. These problem behaviors are generally more prevalent among minorities, and particularly among African Americans (Dryfoos, 1990). Most salient in this regard are rates of violence within the African-American community. Homicide is the leading cause of death for African-American males aged fifteen through twenty-four (Eron, Gentry, and Schlegel, 1994; Rosenberg and Finley, 1991), and African-American males between the ages of fifteen and nineteen are homicide victims at a rate approximately six times that of their white male counterparts.

Elliott (1994) reported approximately 50 percent higher rates of serious violent offenses among African American relative to White adolescents.

Rates of sexual activity are also rising rapidly among African-American adolescents. In a 1992 survey of students in grades nine through twelve, 72 percent of African Americans reported having had intercourse relative to 52 percent and 53 percent of White and Hispanic students, respectively (CDC, 1992). Sexual activity represents a particularly salient problem among young adolescents; Coker, et al. (1994) found that 49 percent of Black males and 12 percent of Black females in their sample, relative to 18 percent of White males and 5 percent of White females, reported having had sexual intercourse before the age of thirteen. In contrast to violence and sexual activity, Black adolescents initiated substance use later, and manifest lower prevalence rates, than their White and Hispanic counterparts (Bachman, et al., 1991; Flewelling, et al., 1993; OAS, 1993). However, this difference begins to attenuate in early adulthood, disappears altogether in middle adulthood, and is followed by a crossover that accounts for the observed greater prevalence of heavy drinking among older Black adults (Flewelling, et al., 1993; Herd, 1989; Kandel, 1992). Trend analyses are beginning to indicate recent increases in the prevalence of heavy alcohol use among African-American adolescents, while the opposite is true for whites (Flewelling, et al., 1993). Indeed, substance use among African-American males may be highly polarized, clustering around either end of a continuum from abstinence to abuse (Herd, 1993; Kandel, 1992; Wallace and Bachman, 1991).

It is becoming increasingly apparent that key risk behaviors, including substance use, violence, and risky sexual behaviors, are associated among adolescents in general and African-American male adolescents in particular (Bachman, et al., 1991; Dembo, et al., 1992; Elliott, et al., 1989; Hays and Ellickson, 1996; Jessor and Jessor, 1977; Osgood, et al., 1988; Parker and McDowell, 1986; Welte and Barnes, 1987). A number of theoretical frameworks support the notion that adolescent risk behaviors tend to cluster together in what Jessor and his colleagues have called a "syndrome" (Donovan and Jessor, 1985; Jessor and Jessor, 1977; Donovan, Jessor, and Costa, 1988), although this perspective is not universally held (e.g., Kaplan and Peck, 1992; White and Burke, 1987). Those who do believe that risk behaviors are associated in adolescents tend also to believe that such behaviors share a common etiology, although Osgood (1995) reminds us that the notion of shared causes only partially explains problem behavior. For Jessor, the central predisposing factor is a tendency to unconventionality, or a lack of successful integration into such key social institutions as the family, school, and neighborhood. Some theorists have posited different explanations; for example, risk taking and impulsiveness (Arnett, 1992; Caspi, et al., 1994, Irwin and Millstein, 1986), sensation seeking (White, Labovie, and Bates, 1985; Zuckerman, 1979, 1983), and a combination of low self-control, weak bonds to other people and to conventional goals, and available opportunities to engage in risky behaviors (Gottfredson and Hirschi, 1990).

THE RISK AND PROTECTIVE FACTOR MODEL

The social development model developed by Hawkins and Weis (1985) constitutes a more general or ecological (Bronfenbrenner, 1979) approach to an understanding of the common etiology of risk behaviors in adolescents (Hawkins, Catalano, and Miller, 1992). This model, which is in part an integration of control theory (Hirschi, 1969) and social learning theory (Bandura, 1977), suggests that a wide variety of risk factors may in aggregate be responsible problem behaviors among adolescents. Risk factors, which are precursors to problem behaviors and increase the likelihood of their onset, severity, and duration, are typically categorized in one of the following domains. These domains are often labeled as intra-individual (both biological and psychological), inter-individual (relationships with families and peers), the school, neighborhood and wider community, and broader societal and cultural conditions. Inventories of risk factors are now commonplace in the literature (e.g., Hawkins, Catalano, and Miller, 1992; Newcomb, 1995). Key to the paradigm is the understanding that factors in these various domains are interdependent and multiplicative (or at least additive) (Newcomb, 1995), and that behaviors are the result of reciprocal relationships between factors within individuals and their social contexts (Cassel, 1976; Noack, 1988; Sclar, 1980).

As related to the issue of violence, the ecological perspective provides a mechanism for examining the interaction of the individual with other levels of the environment. The largest environment—that is, the macrosystem—contains some of the most important factors that affect individual behaviors, but these are also among the most difficult to measure. For example, stereotypes of ethnic groups often emanate from the macrosystem and are given structure and reality as they permeate the levels of the ecological system more proximal to the African-American adolescent. A failure to understand and assess these stereotypes and their ill-effects (e.g., chronic stress) will lead to an incomplete understanding of the causes of risk behaviors among minority adolescents (Gouges, 1986; Moritsugu and Sue, 1983).

Also key to an understanding of the risk and protective factor model, but less well understood and intuitively obvious (Richters and Weintraub, 1990; Smith, et al., 1995), is the notion of protective factors. Protective factors refer to characteristics that improve individuals' resistance to risk factors by at least partially negating or inhibiting the effects of exposure to these risk factors on health and social outcomes (e.g., Resnick, et al., 1997; Rutter, 1985). In essence, they provide a potential answer to the question of why some adolescents are able to surmount the difficult personal and environmental characteristics to which they are exposed, while others follow the negative life trajectories that might be expected of them (Engle, Castle, and Menon, 1996). As Hawkins and his colleagues (1992) have suggested, protective factors thus help decrease individuals' vulnerability to risk factors or increase their resiliency in the presence of these factors.

The exact mechanism by which protective factors affect the relationship between risk factors and behaviors has yet to be fully resolved; some posit both a mediating or moderating model (e.g., Hawkins, Catalano, and Miller, 1992), while others appear to limit the model to a moderating one. In mediating relationships the mediating variable explains, at least in part, the relationship between an independent and dependent variable. On the other hand, a moderating variable affects a given outcome in interaction with an independent variable; as a moderating variable, a protective factor can be said to "potentiate" or enhance (or suppress) the effects of an independent variable by strengthening (or attenuating) its relationship with a dependent variable (Brooke, et al., 1990; Newcomb and Felix-Ortiz, 1992).[1] As Rutter (1987) points out, protective factors are not simply the polar opposite of risk factors. Instead, they should be understood as mechanisms that have an effect on behaviors *in the presence of risk*, such that the protective factor is responsible for differentiating those individuals who subsequently remain healthy from those who manifest deviant or otherwise destructive outcomes (Garmezy, Masten, and Tellegen, 1984; Rutter, 1985; Smith, et al., 1995).

In other words, the preponderance of the theoretical literature appears to favor a moderating model alone, as opposed to a paradigm that suggests that protective factors may operate through both mediating and moderating mechanisms. Empirical evidence of this conclusion has recently been provided by Fitzpatrick's (1997) analyses of data from three nationally representative samples of youth in different age groups. He reports that the protective factors tested proved, as expected, to have only a trivial direct or mediating effect on aggressive behavior but instead operate in interaction with the risk factors tested. Stacy, et al. (1992) found that in conditions of high self-acceptance there was no relationship between respondents' reports of drug use and those of their peers, while that relationship was strong in conditions of low self-acceptance. Similar findings for protective factors have been reported by Newcomb and Felix-Ortiz (1992). Other tests of the protective factor model are beginning to suggest that the effects of such factors may be cumulative, as is the case for risk factors (Scheier, et al., 1997; Smith, et al., 1995).

In summarizing the literature on protective factors, Hawkins (1995) identified several major categories of such factors specifically relevant to adolescents. These include, first, a resilient temperament, characterized by a positive attitude and good coping and social problem-solving skills (Rutter, 1987) in response to adverse or stressful life events, and a positive social orientation, characterized by good social interaction skills. A second category of protective factors includes connectedness to at least one key adult, such as a family member or teacher, who

---

[1] As an example of a moderating variable, consider the buffering effects of red wine on the relationship between cholesterol and heart disease.

provides a nurturing and valuing relationship (see also, Garmezy, 1985; Werner and Smith, 1992); indeed, resilient youth may actively seek out surrogate parents if their own are unavailable (Werner, 1984). The role of connectedness to parents as a key protective factor has recently been validated by analyses of data from the National Longitudinal Study on Adolescent Health (Resnick, et al., 1997) as (to a lesser extent) has connectedness to school. It should be noted, however, that close involvement with adults has not been empirically validated as a protective factor in at least one study (Smith, et al., 1995). A third set of protective factors includes a clear understanding of standards and norms governing behavior in both the family and at school (see also, Snyder and Patterson, 1987; Steinberg, 1996), and a belief in one's self-efficacy to succeed in a variety of environments (see also Rutter, 1987). In addition, religiosity and spirituality are also often identified as protective factors (Jessor and Jessor, 1977; Resnick, et al., 1997; Werner and Smith, 1992), and others will certainly be added as the literature on this subject emerges.

The inventory of risk factors known to have an adverse effect on such behaviors as juvenile delinquency, substance use, and violence, is now substantial, and has received abundant empirical support in the research literature (e.g., Hawkins, Catalano, and Miller, 1992). However, the catalog of protective factors is much more tenuous and incomplete, in part because this field has received considerably less conceptual and empirical attention. Indeed, as has been noted, the definition of what constitutes a protective factor and how such factors may operate to ameliorate or negate risk remains somewhat nebulous. Nevertheless, the pragmatic applications of protective factors are legion, especially if they can be demonstrated through programmatic interventions to buffer the effects of key risk factors, which for many high risk youth are both numerous and largely unmalleable. Ethnic identity, in African American as well as other populations of color, appears to hold considerable promise as one such factor. In subsequent sections we will articulate and examine the key properties of ethnic identity, provide some preliminary evidence as to its efficacy as a protective factor, and lay out an agenda for research and practice. This agenda will serve both to determine the mechanisms by which ethnic identity operates to buffer the effects of risk and how it may be developed through programmatic interventions.

ETHNIC IDENTITY AS A PROTECTIVE FACTOR

The term "ethnic" derives from the Greek word meaning "nation" (Trimble, 1995), and issues concerning ethnicity have been described as critical to interpersonal relationships (Barth, 1969). Ethnic identity can most easily be defined as an individual's attitude toward or affiliation with, and perception of sharing a common heritage and culture with, his or her own ethnic group (Helms, 1990; Hutnik, 1991). However, no consensus as to the definition of this elusive concept has yet emerged. Phinney's (1990) review article suggests a number of key elements to this definition. Ethnic identity forms an important component of one's overall self-concept, involves one's understanding, positive acceptance, and adoption of the values and behaviors of that group, and represents a developmental rather than a static process (see also, Trimble, 1995). Ethnic identity is seen as critical to the social and psychological functioning of minority populations who live in societies in which their group and culture are politically and socially marginalized and disparaged (Phinney, 1990; Weinreich, 1983). Oetting (1993) writes of the importance of inculcating a strong sense of ethnic identity in children as a means to help them understand and negotiate their cultural environment and thus develop a sense of self-mastery, competence, and self-esteem. Concern about ethnic identity among African Americans can be traced to the ethnic revitalization movement of the 1960s, writings concerning "Nigrescence" (which Parham and Helms (1985a) define as the process by which a person "becomes Black"), and the numerous literary works of African Americans about their efforts to develop an understanding of and appreciation for their ethnicity (e.g., DuBois, 1983).

Current models of ethnic identity owe much to the developmental framework of Erikson's (1968) theory of ego identity and development, and, indeed, much of our present understanding of ethnic identity development has its roots in the counseling and pyschotherapy literature (Helms, 1990). According to Erikson, identity is achieved through a process of exploration that typically occurs during adolescence. Exploration, as epitomized in Malcolm X's celebrated autobiography (1965), constitutes a key unifying theme across several models of ethnic identity development (e.g., Cross, 1991; Marcia, 1966, 1980; Phinney, 1989, 1992). A second unifying but not universally accepted (Helms, 1990) theme is that such development proceeds through a number of fairly clearly defined stages and is multi- (as opposed to uni-) dimensional (Felix-Ortiz and Newcomb, 1995; Phinney, 1990). While there are a variety of such models that were conceptualized by theorists working largely in isolation from one another, the characteristics of these models are remarkably similar. For the sake of simplicity, the stages of ethnic identity development may be classified as *pre-encounter, encounter,* and *post-encounter.*

In the *pre-encounter* stage, African Americans view the world as they have been taught or otherwise acculturated by society, often from a Euro-American frame of reference that devalues Blackness and values Whiteness while denying racism (Akbar, 1979). This state has been described by Thomas (1971, 1987) as "Negromachy;" that is, seeking recognition and approval from Whites and failing to develop an understanding of oneself and one's own racial identity. Alternately, African-American youth may adopt with little personal reflection the perspective of their parents or peers. This perspective may vary widely from a Black to a White cultural orientation, which Marcia (1966) terms a "foreclosed" (in the sense of prematurely closed) status. Or they may have no particular ethnic paradigm and be dissociated from, or apathetic about, their racial identity (Cross, 1991), a condition described as "diffuse" (Marcia, 1966). Regardless, feelings of self-worth may be low, since the individual depends upon external sources for self-definition (Thomas, 1971).

In the *encounter* stage, African-American adolescents abandon the perspective on their ethnic identity that they have received from others, often as a consequence of a precipitating or "shattering" (Gay, 1985) personal or social event, such as personal contact with a charismatic Black leader. The consequence of this encounter is that the individual is stripped of his or her ethnic identity (Helms, 1984) and begins an often frenetic quest for a new one that may be "obsessive" in nature (Cross, 1991). This stage is characterized by alternating confusion, clarity, depression, and euphoria (Helms, 1990), and often leads to an "immersion" (Thomas, 1971) in Black culture and an idealization of and militant identification with Blackness and Black ethnic and cultural identity (Jackson, 1975). It is also typically accompanied by high risk taking (Cross, 1991) and deeply negative or hostile feelings about other ethnic groups (and especially the dominant ethnic group). Indeed, Helms (1990) describes this phase as characterized by a "generalized anger," not only at Whites but at other Blacks who do not appear to be similarly radicalized. In addition, feelings of anger may also be turned inwards, as individuals berate themselves for their prior lack of awareness to these issues. This Black-oriented perspective at first is governed by what the individual imagines other African Americans typically believe, but it then gradually comes to be characterized by a period of thoughtful questioning or exploration, during which time the individual is said to be in "emersion" (Cross, 1991) or "moratorium" (Marcia, 1966). In this phase the individual may be assisted by a supportive group of friends within the Black community or through conversations with elders, in which the process of exploration can continue in an environment that is more calm and tolerant of open inquiry and assessment.

In the third and final, or *post-encounter*, stage African-American youth or young adults come to terms with their ethnic identity, taking from their culture those elements with which they feel personally comfortable and developing a new sense of self that combines optimally their personal characteristics with those of their race (Cross, 1991; Helms, 1990). In this stage they find or "achieve" (Marcia, 1966) a measure of healthy, balanced understanding of their Blackness accompanied by a growing appreciation for and security with what is healthy and constructive in other ethnic groups, as well as for individuals from those groups. It is at this stage that individuals "transcend" racism and racial stereotypes, no longer judge others on the basis of their race, and are free to become themselves (Cross, 1991; Thomas, 1971). They also become able to operate fully in both their minority and the majority cultures, becoming in effect "bicultural." That is, they develop the ability to function within the normative and behavioral framework of the dominant ethnic group as well as within one's own, without giving up their own identity (Oetting, 1993; Rotheram-Borus, 1990). At this stage they may become actively involved in their ethnic group's struggle for social justice, or may detach themselves from issues relating to race and go their own way (Phinney, 1990).

As mentioned above, the three major stages of the development of ethnic identity in minority populations may be seen as multidimensional. As has been pointed out by Phinney (1990) and Oetting (1993), two key dimensions of this model are one's attitudes toward one's own group and one's attitudes toward the dominant ethnic group. These dimensions are conceptually orthogonal (i.e., independent), in that a given individual may be high, low, or neutral, on each. The *source* of these attitudes may be considered yet a third dimension, itself orthogonal to the other two: that is, these attitudes may be internally derived or may be adopted (typically with only minimal consideration) from those of one's parents, peers, or the greater society.

Figure 1 depicts the manner in which the three stages of ethnic development may be located within these three dimensions. Notice that in the first, or pre-encounter, stage individuals' senses of ethnic identity may be located almost anywhere on the two attitude-related dimensions that constitute the plane of the Figure. That is, they may feel positively (or negatively) toward their own ethnicity and the dominant White race; or they may be completely indifferent to issues of their ethnic identity. Key to an understanding of this phase, however, is that their

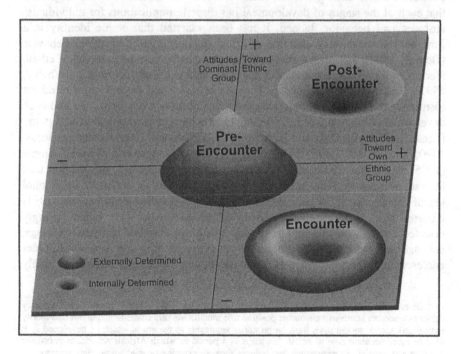

Figure 1. Stages of ethnic identity development.

beliefs tend to be superficial insofar as they have adopted the perspectives of those by whom they have been socialized and with whom they have come into the most contact (typically their parents). In the encounter stage, their attitudes move rapidly to the bottom right quadrant of the Figure, adulatory to their own ethnic group and hostile to the dominant group. As indicated, while they begin this stage by adopting, again with only minimal consideration, the often militant stance of a charismatic figure.[2] However, theorists of ethnic identity development suggest that they then proceed along a path that becomes internal, as they develop their own personal understanding of their ethnic identity. In the final post-encounter stage depicted in the Figure's top right quadrant, they have moved to a position of appreciation of both ethnic groups and relative tranquility and security within their own.

EMPIRICAL INVESTIGATIONS OF THE RELATIONSHIP BETWEEN ETHNIC IDENTITY AND RISK BEHAVIORS

Key to an understanding of the role that ethnic identity may play as a protective factor among African-American male adolescents is the recognition that each of the stages of development has discrete implications for individuals' attitudes and behavior. Indeed, it has been asserted that ethnic identity is a fundamental personality characteristic that organizes and determines behavior (Oetting, 1993), and several researchers have remarked on the potential of ethnic identity to serve as a potential inhibitor of the effects of risk factors (e.g., Whaley, 1992). However, the relationships between behavior and the trajectory of ethnic identity development, and particularly the links between risk behaviors and each developmental stage, are only beginning to be subjected to empirical investigation (Cross, 1991; Felix-Ortiz and Newcomb, 1995; Phinney, 1990; Rotheram-Borus, 1990; Scheier, et al., 1997). In his study of Native-American adolescents, Trimble (1995) found that ethnic identity was not directly associated with alcohol use; instead, he suggested that ethnic identity might mediate the influence on alcohol use of risk factors in the peer and family domains. Oetting and Beauvais (1991) reported that young Native-American adolescents who were either strongly oriented toward their own culture or were bicultural were less likely to use drugs, but that there was no relationship between ethnic identity and drug use in older adolescents. A positive sense of ethnic identity has been reported to be inversely

---

[2] Given the rapidly emerging African-American middle class, many contemporary African-American youth will encounter positive role models who are charismatic but not necessarily radicalized. Cross' model may, thus, be primarily applicable to the era in which he developed it. It may be more accurate now to recast this stage as a period in which African Americans encounter some person, writing, or experience that induces them to examine or re-examine their assumptions concerning their ethnicity and leads to a transformation.

associated with respondents' attitudes toward alcohol use (Gary and Berry, 1985), and a strong racial identity has also been found to be negatively associated with crimes that Blacks commit against other Blacks (Whaley, 1992). However, other studies have reported a positive association between drug use and both cultural identity (Markides, Krause, and Mendes de Leon, 1988) and biculturalism (Amaro, et al., 1990), although Felix-Ortiz and Newcomb (1995) suggests that these findings may be suspect due to the unidimensional nature of the ethnic identity measures used.

Only three studies to date have investigated within minority adolescents the relationship between ethnic identity and other risk and protective factors, as well as a variety of risk behaviors including violence and drug use. In their study of high school students, Gabriel and Larson (1997) used Phinney's (1990) Ethnic Identity scale, a multi-dimensional instrument that included subscales tapping both attitudes toward one's own group and toward other groups (which includes, but is not limited to, the dominant ethnic group). They found that ethnic identity was associated with prosocial norms, self-concept, self-efficacy, confidence, cooperation, and nurturance. However, ethnic identity was generally not associated with behaviors relating either to violence or drug use. In another study, Arbona, et al. (1997) reported that ethnic pride (as measured by three items from Phinney's scale) was related to prosocial norms concerning violence.

The most comprehensive study to date of the role played by ethnic identity as a moderator of the effects of a series of risk factors on substance use was recently reported by Scheier, et al. (1997). In their study, in which they conceptualized ethnic identity as a component of social support, they analyzed self-reported data from a prospective investigation of substance use by inner-city adolescents. However, they used a unidimensional model of ethnic identity, including only the subscale of Phinney's (1990) instrument that tapped respondents' attitudes toward their *own* ethnic group. Scheier and his colleagues found general support for their hypothesis that while high levels of ethnic identity decreased the relationship between risk behaviors and drug use, low levels of ethnic identity did not have that effect, hence supporting the moderating model of ethnic identity. They also found from their longitudinal data analyses that ethnic identity made a unique contribution to alcohol use independent of early use and a variety of risk behaviors.

Several investigators have also examined the relationship between experiences of racial discrimination and risk behaviors in minority populations. Since experiences of racial discrimination may reasonably be expected to affect the development of ethnic identity it is important to examine relationships between experiences of racial discrimination and risk behaviors in minority groups. In a study of alcohol use among Black women, Taylor, Henderson, and Jackson (1991) found that internalized racism accounted for a significant proportion of the variance in alcohol assumption. Internalized racism was defined as the degree to which individuals internalized negative racial stereotypes. Higher levels of internalized racism were associated with higher alcohol use and greater levels of depression.[3] These findings are consistent with Singleton et al. (1986), who reported that smoking among Black women is also related to experiences of racism and racial oppression.

IMPLICATIONS FOR RESEARCH

Perhaps the first task for researchers, and for the entire community interested in the topic of ethnic identity development, is to reach a degree of consensus concerning the definition of ethnic identity, and agreement on the major stages by and through which it develops. We need to reach a shared understanding of the underlying dimensions of ethnic identity, and where each of the various stages is positioned on this multi-dimensional map. Once this key task has been accomplished, researchers can turn their attention to developing and refining measures that can specify in which stage, or along which dimensions, individuals may be located. While considerable progress has already been made in this area by Phinney (1989, 1992) and others, much work remains to be done. For example, we do not yet know how adequately a scale like Phinney's Multigroup Ethnic Identity Measure performs across various racial groups, although it was designed to be applicable to all. That is, we do not know whether any one scale can suffice, or whether discrete scales need to be developed for each racial group.

As we gain greater confidence in our instrumentation, we can begin to address a series of research questions concerning the nature of ethnic identity development and whether this construct develops along differential developmental trajectories for key subgroups. One of the first tasks inherent in validating the model displayed in Figure 1 is to determine if the two attitudinal dimensions are truly orthogonal. It would also be helpful to verify the placement of the three stages specified, and to learn where individuals tend to cluster in each; for instance, what proportion of African-American youth feel negatively toward their own identity and positive about Whites? What proportion feel neutral in that they have no particular opinions one way or the other? We should also develop an understanding of how ethnic identity developmental trajectories may differ across the nation's major minorities, if males differ from females in this regard, and if the ethnic identity model applies to the experiences of other suppressed minorities (e.g., gays and people with special needs). Also useful, especially for the design of age-appropriate ethnic identity development programs, would be an understanding of whether and how different stages are linked to specific age groups; for example, at what age adolescents tend to enter the critical encounter stage.

---

[3] Researchers should be careful to discriminate between internalized racism that is acknowledged relative to that which remains unacknowledged. The former is presumably more health promoting than the latter.

The above discussion relates to developing and promoting an understanding of ethnic identity for its own sake. That is, we as a society may believe that there is intrinsic value in developing within ethnic minorities, and especially those that have a history of discrimination, prejudice, and displacement by the dominant white culture, the life skills they will require to be fully functioning adults. Such efforts will doubtless garner more widespread support if ethnic identity development in minority adolescents is shown to be inversely related to such risk behaviors as violence, substance abuse, and unprotected sexuality. To that end we should investigate the multiple relationships between the various dimensions that constitute ethnic identity and key risk behaviors in adolescents in both a cross-sectional and longitudinal context, adding questions tapping these dimensions to such large scale, ongoing data collection efforts as the Adolescent Health study (Resnick, et al., 1997) cited above. In so doing we can determine which dimensions of ethnic identity development are most closely associated with risk behaviors, and whether that relationship is causal or merely correlational.

It may be particularly important to examine the degree to which relationships between ethnic identity and risk behaviors vary as a function of one's ethnicity. That is, the importance of ethnic identity to individual functioning and the relationship between ethnic identity and risk behaviors may differ considerably across ethnic groups in the United States depending on their history and culture, degree of racial oppression, and desire to assimilate into the dominant culture Ogbu (1983). As a result of these factors, the degree to which ethnic identity may be salient to one's social and psychological functioning may differ and, consequently, its relationship to risk behaviors may vary. This possibility may explain some of the variability in findings regarding relationships between ethnic identity and risk behaviors when different ethnic groups are examined (e.g., Amaro, et al., 1990; Markides, et al., 1988). Given these findings, it is entirely possible that ethnic identity may be a better predictor of risk behaviors for some ethnic groups than for others.

Research is also needed to investigate the relationships between ethnic identity and the key risk and protective factors thought to be associated with youth problem behaviors, as well as the pathways by which ethnic identity, as nested within these factors, affects these behaviors. Do the dimensions and stages that constitute ethnic identity have a protective effect, buffering the relationship between a variety of risk factors and behaviors? As a protective factor, are the effects of ethnic identity "potentiated" (Brooke, et al., 1990; Newcomb and Felix-Ortiz, 1992), i.e., do they interact with, other protective factors such as a resilient personality? With which protective factors specified earlier is ethnic identity most closely related? For example, there are well-documented relationships between self-efficacy and health behaviors (Weinstein, 1993) and between ethnic identity and self-efficacy (Phinney, 1990). Perhaps one of the primary means by which ethnic identity may affect risk behaviors in some ethnic groups is through its influence on self-efficacy. Yet another question to be addressed is whether the putative buffering effects of ethnic identity are more germane to certain conceptually related risk factors (e.g., discrimination resulting in perceived lack of educational or economic opportunity) and risky behaviors (e.g., violence) than others. Further, how do the potential buffering effects of ethnic identity differ across ethnic minorities, especially in those populations of color in which cultural practices that appear to promote risk behaviors may be normative, for example alcohol use among Native Americans (Oetting, 1993)?

Finally, there is a need to clarify whether ethnic identity may be a better predictor of prosocial norms, attitudes, or behaviors and less predictive of risk behaviors or negative attitudes. Existing data suggest that ethnic identity may be related to prosocial norms and behaviors which, in turn, may promote healthier behaviors of reduce risk behaviors. This conclusion is consistent with the role of ethnic identity as a protective factor that moderates the impact of risk factors. However, as Kazdin (1993) points out, the effect of prosocial competence on the prevention of risk behaviors is not clear. In fact, prosocial competence may not be the inverse of risk behaviors (Kazdin, 1993). Therefore, a more accurate prediction of risk behaviors in adolescent groups may depend on the identification of other factors that may be more directly related to risk factors. Though limited, current findings suggest that experiences of racial discrimination and/or internalized negative stereotypes may be more directly related to risk behaviors, although the mechanisms by which these variables may affect risk behaviors have not been identified. Future research should be directed toward identifying those aspects of ethnic identity and its development that promote the development of prosocial attitudes and behaviors among adolescents.

IMPLICATIONS FOR PRACTICE

As mentioned earlier, researchers and practitioners are currently mining the ethnic identity literature to buttress claims of the potential effectiveness of Rites of Passage and manhood training programs targeting minority, and particularly African-American adolescents (e.g., Ringwalt, et al., 1996). If an empirical link between the development of ethnic identity and adolescent risk behaviors can be convincingly demonstrated, the credence of such programs would be greatly increased. Further, a deeper understanding of the discrete and interactive effects on risk behaviors of youths' positions along the three dimensions of ethnic identity specified in Figure 1 would have direct implications for the design of such programs. Most Rites of Passage programs, as well as Afrocentric curricula in the schools, currently concentrate on developing an appreciation of Black history and culture, and so would presumably affect most the dimension relating to attitudes toward the youths' *own* culture. If it were to be shown that youth risk behaviors were linked to positive attitudes toward the *dominant* culture, such curricula might place a greater emphasis on enhancing minority youths' appreciation of other ethnic groups through teaching cross-ethnic appreciation and understanding.

On the other hand, it may be demonstrated that the third dimension specified in Figure 1, the source of attitudes toward one's own and the dominant ethnic group, is also an important consideration for risk behaviors. If so, this would imply a somewhat different perspective for ethnic identity development programs. If youth in the third, post-encounter stage (i.e., with positive attitudes toward both ethnic groups) were least likely to manifest risk behaviors, it might be helpful to include curricula emphasizing the bicultural adaptation skills that are associated with this stage. Alternately, if the rage that appears to be associated with the second, encounter stage is particularly salient as a correlate of risk behaviors, it may be useful to assist adolescents in developing an understanding of the roots and manifestations of their anger (at both Whites and their fellow African Americans, and perhaps toward themselves as well), as well as teaching skills to manage their anger successfully.

A key component of successful ethnic identity programs may be providing an environment in which youth can move expeditiously through the three developmental stages. That is, such programs could offer youth opportunities to discuss among themselves what they know and are taught about their own and the dominant culture, and assist in the acquisition of skills to sort through and clarify their attitudes toward and beliefs about each in a considered and thoughtful manner. Oetting (1993), for example, speaks of the need to provide youth opportunities for cultural enrichment, reflection, and growth in a safe atmosphere in the family, school, and community.

In conclusion, universal or selective (IOM, 1994) and carefully tailored interventions could then be targeted to minority youth in each stage (or critical dimension), to assist them in moving through a process of ethnic identity development that has substantial implications for their perceptions of and behavior within their social environment.

REFERENCES

Akbar, N. (1979). African roots of Black personality. In W.D. Smith, K. Burlew, M. Mosley and W. Whitney (Eds.), *Reflections on Black Psychology*. University of American Press: Washington, D.C.

Amaro, H., Whitaker, R., Coffman, G. and Heeren, T. (1990). Acculturation and marijuana and cocaine use: Finding from HHANES 1982-1984. *American Journal of Public Health*, 80:54-60.

Arbona, C., Jackson, R. H. and Blakeley, C. (1997). *Ethnic pride as a predictor of violent and non-violent conflict resolution attitudes among Black and Hispanic adolescents.* Paper presented at the Third National Conference on Family and Community Violence Prevention, October 12-14: New Orleans, LA.

Arnett, J. (1992). Reckless behavior in adolescence: A developmental perspective. *Developmental Review*, 12:339-373.

Bachman, J. G., Wallace, J. M., O'Malley, P. M., Johnston, L. D., Kurth, C. L. and Neighbors, H. W. (1991). Racial/ethnic differences in smoking, drinking, and illicit drug use among American high schools seniors, 1976-1989. *American Journal of Public Health*, 81:372-377.

Bandura, A. (1977). Self-efficacy: Toward a unifying theory of behavioral change. *Psychological Review*, 84:191-215.

Barth, F. (1969). *Ethnic Groups and Boundaries.* Little, Brown: Boston, MA.

Bronfenbrennder, U. (1979). *The Ecology of Human Development.* Harvard University Press: Cambridge, MA.

Brook, J. S., Brook, D. W., Gordon, A. S., Whiteman, M. and Cohen, P. (1990). The psychosocial etiology of adolescent drug use: A family interactional approach. *Genetic, Social, and General Psychology Monographs, 116* (whole No. 2).

Caspi, A., Moffitt, T. E., Silva, P. A., Stouthamer-Loeber, M., Krueger, R. F. and Schmutte, P. S. (1994). Are some people crime-prone? Replications of the personality-crime relationship across countries, genders, races, and methods. *Criminology*, 32: 163-195.

Cassel, J. (1976). The contribution of the social environment to host resistance. *American Journal of Epidemiology*, 104:107-123.

Centers for Disease Control (1992). *HIV/AIDS Surveillance Report.* U.S. Department of Health and Human Services, Public Health Service, October: Atlanta, GA.

Coker, A. L., Richter, D. L., Valois, R. F., McKeown, R. E., Garrison, C. Z. and Vincent, M. L. (1994). Correlates and consequences of early initiation of sexual intercourse. *Journal of School Health*, 64:372-377.

Cross, W. E. (1971). The Negro-to-Black conversion experience: Towards a psychology of black liberation. *Black World*, 20:13-27.

Cross, W. E. (1978). The Cross and Thomas models of psychological nigrescence. *Journal of Black Psychology*, 5:13-19.

Cross, W. E. (1991). *Shades of Black: Diversity in African-American Identity.* Temple University Press: Philadelphia, PA.

Dembo, R., Williams, L., Wothke, W., Schmeidler, J., Getreu, A., Berry, E. and Wish, E. D. (1992). The generality of deviance replication of a structural model among high-risk youths. *Journal of Research in Crime and Delinquency*, 29:200-216.

Donovan, J. E. and Jessor, R. (1985). Structure of problem behavior in adolescence and young adulthood. *Journal of Consulting and Clinical Psychology*, 53:890-904.

Donovan, J. E., Jessor, R. and Costa, F. M. (1988). Syndrome of problem behavior in adolescence: A replication. *Journal of Consulting and Clinical Psychology*, 56: 762-765.

Dryfoos, J. (1990). *Adolescents at Risk: Prevalence and Prevention.* Oxford University Press: New York.

DuBois, W. E. B. (1983). *Autobiography of W.E.B. DuBois.* International Publishing: New York.

Elliott, D. (1994). Serious violent offenders: Onset, developmental course, and termination—The American Society of Criminology 1993 Presidential Address. *Criminology*, 32:1-21.

Elliott, D., Huizinga, D. and Menard, S. (1989). *Multiple Problem Youth: Delinquency, Substance Abuse, and Mental Health Problems.* Springer-Verlag: New York.

Engle, P. L., Castle, S. and Menon, P. (1996). Child development: Vulnerability and resilience. *Social Science Medicine,* 43:621-35.

Erikson, E. (1968). *Identity: Youth and Crisis.* Norton: New York.

Eron, L. D., Gentry, J. H. and Schlegel, P., Eds. (1994). *Reason to Hope: A Psychological Perspective on Violence and Youth.* American Psychological Association: Washington, D.C.

Felix-Ortiz, M. and Newcomb, M. D. (1995). Cultural identity and drug use among Latino and Latina adolescents. In G. J. Botvin, S. Schinke and M. A. Orlandi (Eds.), *Drug Abuse Prevention with Multiethnic Youth* (pp. 147-165). Sage Publications: Newbury Park, CA.

Fitzpatrick, K. M. (1997). Fighting among America's youth: A risk and protective factors approach. *Journal of Health and Social Behavior,* 38:131-148.

Flewelling, R. L., Ennett, S. T., Rachal, J. V. and Theisen, A. C. (1993). *National Household Survey on Drug Abuse: Race/Ethnicity, Socioeconomic Status, and Drug Abuse, 1991* (DHHS Publication No. SMA 93-2062). Substance Abuse and Mental Health Services Administration: Rockville, MD.

Gabriel, R. M., Hopson, T., Haskins, M. and Powell, K. E. (1996). Building relationships and resilience in the prevention of youth violence. *American Journal of Preventive Medicine,* 12:48-55.

Gabriel, R. M. and Larson, L. (1997). *Ethnic identity and violence prevention among African American youth: Measurement challenges and empirical results.* Presented at the Third National Conference on Family and Community Violence Prevention, October 12-14: New Orleans, LA.

Garmezy, N. (1985). Stress-resistant children: The search for protective factors. In J. E. Stevenson (Ed.), Recent research in developmental psychopathology. *Journal of Child Psychology and Psychiatry,* 4:213-233.

Garmezy, N., Masten, A. S. and Tellegen, A. (1984). The study of stress and competence in children: A building block for developmental psychopathology. *Child Development,* 55:97-111.

Gary, L. E. and Berry, G. L. (1985). Predicting attitudes toward substance use in a Black community: Implications for prevention. *Community Mental Health Journal,* 21: 42-51.

Gay, G. (1985). Implications of selected models of ethnic identity development for educators. *Journal of Negro Education,* 54:43-55.

Gottfredson, M. R. and Hirschi, T. (1990). *A General Theory of Crime.* Stanford University Press: Stanford, CA.

Gouges, R. A. (1986). The effects of prejudice and stress on the academic performance of Black Americans. In U. Merssen (Ed.), *The School Achievement of Minority Child: New Perspectives* (pp. 145-58). Erlbaum: Mahwah, NJ.

Hawkins, J. D. (1995). Controlling crime before it happens: Risk-focused prevention. *National Institute of Justice Journal,* August:10-18.

Hawkins, J. D., Catalano, R. F. and Miller, J.Y . (1992). Risk and protective factors for alcohol and other drug problems in adolescence and early adulthood: Implications for substance abuse preventions. *Psychological Bulletin,* 112:64-105.

Hawkins, J. D. and Weis, J. G. (1985). The social development model: An integrated approach to delinquency prevention. *Journal of Primary Prevention*, 6:73-97.

Hays, R. D. and Ellickson, P. L. (1996). Associations between drug use and deviant behavior in teenagers. *Addictive Behaviors*, 21:291-302.

Helms, J. E. (1980). An overview of black racial identity theory. In J. E. Helms (Ed.), *Black and White Racial Identity: Theory, Research, and Practice* (pp. 9-32). Greenwood Press: New York, Westport, Connecticut, London.

Helms, J. (1984). Toward a theoretical explanation of the effects of race on counseling: A black and white model. *Counseling Psychologist*, 12(3-4):153-165.

Herd, D. (1989). The epidemiology of drinking patterns and alcohol-related problems among U.S. blacks. In D. L. Spiegler, D. A. Tate, S. S. Aitken and C. M. Christian (Eds.), *Alcohol Use among U.S. Ethnic Minorities* (NIAAA Research Monograph No. 18, DHHS Publication No. ADM 89-1435, pp. 3-50). National Institute on Alcohol Abuse and Alcoholism: Rockville, MD.

Herd, D. (1993). An analysis of alcohol-related problems in black and white women drinkers. *Addiction Research*, 1:181-198.

Hirshi, T. (1969). *Causes of Delinquency*. University of California Press: Berkeley, CA.

Hutnik, N. (1991). *Ethnic Minority Identity. A Social Psychological Perspective*. Clarendon Press: Oxford.

Institute of Medicine (IOM), Committee on Prevention of Mental Disorders (1994). *Reducing Risks for Mental Disorders: Frontiers for Preventive Intervention Research*. In P. J. Mrazek and R. J. Haggerty (Eds.), National Academy Press: Washington, D.C.

Irwin, C. and Millstein, S. (1986). Biopsychosocial correlates of risk-taking behaviors during adolescence. *Journal of Adolescent Health Care*, 7:825-965.

Jackson, B. (1975). Black identity development. *Journal of Educational Diversity*, 2:19-25.

Jessor, R. and Jessor, S. (1977). *Problem Behavior and Psychological Development: A Longitudinal Study of Youth*. Academic Press: New York.

Kandel, D. B. (1992). The social demography of drug use. *The Milbank Quarterly*, 69:365-414.

Kaplan, H. B. and Peck, B. M. (1992). Self-rejection, coping style, and mode of deviant response. *Social Science Quarterly*, 73:903-919.

Kazdin, A. E. (1993). Adolescent mental health. Prevention and treatment programs. *American Journal of Psychology*, 48(2):127-141.

Malcolm, X. (1965). *Autobiography of Malcolm X*. Golden Press: New York.

Marcia, J. (1966). Development and validation of ego-identity status. *Journal of Personality and Social Psychology*, 3:551-558.

Marcia, J. E. (1980). Identity in adolescence. In J. Adelson (Ed.), *Handbook of Adolescent Psychology* (pp. 159-187). John Wiley: New York.

Markides, K. S., Krause, N. and Mendes de Leon, C. F. (1988). Acculturation and alcohol consumption among Mexican-Americans. *American Journal of Public Health*, 78:1178-1181.

Moritsugu, J. and Sue, S. (1983). Minority status as a stressor. In R. Felner, L. Jason, J. Moritsugu and S. Farber (Eds.), *Preventive Psychology: Theory, Research and Practice* (pp. 3-10). Pergamon Press: Elmsford, NY.

Newcomb, M. D. (1995). Drug use etiology among ethnic minority adolescents. *Drug Abuse Prevention with Multiethnic Youth* (pp. 105-29). Sage Publications: Thousand Oaks, CA.

Newcomb, M. D. and Felix-Ortiz, M. (1992). Multiple protective and risk factors for drug use and abuse: Cross-sectional and prospective findings. *Journal of Personality and Social Psychology*, 63:280-296.

Noack, H. (1988). The role of socio-structural factors in health behavior. In R. Anderson (Ed.), *Health Behavior Research and Health Promotion*. Oxford University Press: Oxford.

Oetting, E. R. (1993). Orthogonal cultural identification: Theoretical links between cultural identification and substance use. In M. R. De La Rosa and J. R. Adrados (Eds.), *Drug Abuse among Minority Youth: Advances in Research and Methodology* (pp. 32-56). NIDA Research Monograph 130.

Oetting, E. R. and Beauvais, F. (1991). Orthogonal cultural identification theory: The cultural identification of minority adolescents. *The International Journal of the Addictions*, 25:655-685.

Office of Applied Studies (1993). *National Household Survey on Drug Abuse: Main Findings 1991*. (DHHS Publication No. SMA 93-1980). Substance Abuse and Mental Health Services Administration: Rockville, MD.

Ogbu, J. U. (1983). Schooling the inner city. *Society*, 21, 1 (147), Nov-Dec, 75-79.

Osgood, D. W. (1995). *Drugs, Alcohol, and Adolescent Violence* (pp. 1-59). Institute of Behavioral Science, Regents of the University of Colorado: Colorado.

Osgood, D. W., Johnston, L. D., O'Malley, P. M. and Bachman, J. G. (1988). The generality of deviance in late adolescence and early adulthood. *American Sociological Review*, 53:81-93.

Parham, T. and Helms, J. E. (1985a). Attitudes of racial identity and self-esteem of Black students: An exploratory investigation. *Journal of College Student Personnel*, 26(2):143-147.

Parham, T. and Helms, J. (1985b). Relation of racial identity attitudes to self-actualization and affective states of Black students. *Journal of Counseling Psychology*, 32:431-440.

Parker, R. N. and McDowell, D. (1986). Constructing an index of officially recorded crime: The use of confirmatory factor analysis. *Journal of Quantitative Criminology*, 2: 237-250.

Phinney, J. S. (1989). Stages of ethnic identity development in minority group adolescents. *Journal of Early Adolescence*, 9:34-49.

Phinney, J. S. (1990). Ethnic identity in adolescents and adults: Review of research. *Psychological Bulletin*, 108:499-514.

Phinney, J. S. (1992). The multi-group ethnic identity measure: A new scale for use with diverse groups. *Journal of Adolescent Research*, 7:156-176.

Resnick, M. D., Bearman, P. S., Blum, R. W., Bauman, K. E., Harris, K. M., Jones, J., Tabor, J., Beuhring, T., Sieving, R. E., Shew, M., Ireland, M., Bearinger, L. H. and Udry, J.R. (1997). Protecting adolescents from harm. Findings from the National Longitudinal Study on adolescent health. *Journal of Medical Association*, 278: 823-832.

Richters, J., and Weintraub, S. (1990). Beyond diathesis: Toward an understanding of high-risk environments. In J. Rolf, A. S. Masten, D. Cicchetti, K. H. Nuechterlein and S. Weintraub (Eds.), *Risk and Protective Factors in the Development of Psychopathology*. Cambridge University Press: New York.

Ringwalt, C. L., Graham, L., Paschall, M. J., Browne, D. and Flewelling, R. L. (1996). Supporting adolescents with guidance and employment (SAGE). *American Journal of Preventive Medicine*, 12:31-38.

Rosenberg, M. and Finley, M. (1991). *Violence in America.* Oxford University Press: Oxford.

Rotheram-Borus, M. J. (1990). Adolescents' reference group choices, self-esteem, and adjustment. *Journal of Personality and Social Psychology*, 59:1075-1081.

Rutter, M. (1985). Resilience in the face of adversity: Protective factors and resistance to psychiatric disorder. *British Journal of Psychiatry*, 147:598-611.

Rutter, M. (1987). Psychosocial resilience and protective mechanisms. *American Journal of Orthopsychiatry*, 57:316-331.

Scheir, L. M., Botvin, G. J., Diz, T. and Ifill-Williams, M. (1977). Ethnic identity as a moderator of psychosocial risk and adolescent alcohol and marijuana use: Concurrent and longitudinal analyses. *Journal of Child and Adolescent Substance Abuse*, 6:21-47.

Sclar, E. D. (1980). Community economic structure and community well-being. A look behind the statistics. *International Journal of Health Services*, 10:563-579.

Singleton, E. G., Harrell, J. P. and Kelly, L. M. (1986). Differentials in the impact of maternal cigarette smoking during pregnancy on fetal development and mortality: Concerns for Black psychologists. *Journal of Black Psychology*, 12(2):71-83.

Smith, C., Lizotte, A.J., Thornberry, T. P. and Korhn, M. D. (1995). Resilient youth: Identifying factors that prevent high-risk youth from engaging in delinquency and drug use. *Current Perspectives on Aging and the Life Cycle*, 4:217-247.

Snyder, J., and Patterson, G. (1987). Family interaction and delinquent behavior. In H. C. Quay (Ed.), *Handbook of Juvenile Delinquency* (pp. 216-43). Wiley and Sons: New York.

Stacy, A. W., Newcomb, M. D. and Bentler, P. M. (1992). Interactive and higher-order effects of social influences no drug use. *Journal of Health and Social Behavior*, 33:226-241.

Steinberg, L. (1996). *Beyond the Classroom: Why School Reform has Failed and What Parents Need to Do* (pp. 62-77). Simon and Schuster: New York.

Taylor, J., Henderson, D. and Jackson, B. (1991). A holistic model for understanding and predicting depressive symptoms in African-American women. *Journal of Community Psychology*, 19(4):306-320.

Thomas, C. W., Ed. (1971). *Boys No More. A Black Psychologist's View of Community.* Glencoe: Beverly Hills, CA.

Thomas, C. W. (1987). Pride and purpose as antidotes to Black homicidal violence. *Journal of the National Medical Association*, 79:155-160.

Trimble, J. E. (1995). Toward an understanding of ethnicity and ethnic identity and their relationship with drug use research. In G. J. Botvin, S. Schinke and M. A. Orlandi (Eds.), *Drug Abuse Prevention with Multiethnic Youth* (pp. 3-27). Sage Publications: Thousand Oaks, CA.

Wallace, J. M. and Bachman, J. G. (1991). Explaining racial/ethnic differences in adolescent drug use: The impact of background and lifestyle. *Social Problems*, 38: 333-357.

Warfield-Coppock, N. (1992). *Afrocentric Theory and Applications: Vol. II. Advances in the Adolescent Rites of Passage.* Baobab Associates, Inc: Washington, D.C.

Weinreich, P. (1983). Emerging from threatened identities. In G. Breakwell (Ed.), *Threatened Identities*. Wiley: New York.

Weinstein, N. D. (1993). Some criteria for evaluating risk messages. *Risk Analysis,* 13(1): 103-114.

Welte, J. W. and Barnes, G. M. (1987). Youthful smoking: Patterns and relationships to alcohol and other drug use. *Journal of Adolescence,* 10:327-340.

Werner, E. E. (1984). Resilient children. *Young Children,* 40:68-72.

Werner, E. and Smith, R. (1992). *Overcoming the Odds: High Risk Children from Birth to Adolescence.* Cornell University Press: Ithaca, NY.

Whaley, A. L. (1992). A culturally sensitive approach to the prevention of interpersonal violence among urban black youth. *Journal of the National Medical Association,* 84:585-588.

White, C. and Burke, P. (1987). Ethnic role identity among Black and White college students: An interactionist approach. *Sociological Perspectives,* 30:310-331.

White, H., Labourie, E. and Bates, M. (1985). The relationship between sensation seeking and delinquency: A longitudinal analysis. *Journal of Research in Crime and Delinquency,* 22:197-211.

Zuckerman, M. (1979). *Sensation Seeking: Beyond the Optimal Level of Arousal.* Lawrence Erlbaum: Mahwah, NJ.

Zuckerman, M. (1983). *Biological basis of sensation seeking, impulsivity, and anxiety.* Lawrence Erlbaum: Mahwah, NJ.

PART II

Cultural Issues in Substance Abuse Prevention

CHAPTER 6

A State of the Art Review of Latinos and Substance Abuse

Melvin Delgado

The impact of alcohol, tobacco, and other drug abuse (ATOD) in the Latino community is well acknowledged in the professional and popular literature. There is increased concern of having the alcohol industry target Latinos for mass campaigns (Maxwell and Jacobson, 1989). There are few Latino families and communities in the United States that have not been impacted by drugs of various kinds. ATOD, in turn, has had a disproportionate impact on the youth of the community, seriously limiting the potential of this age-group to exercise current and future leadership within the community. The impact of ATOD, as a result, must go far beyond dollars and measured in human terms—by the lives lost, incarcerated, and wasted human potential.

ATOD has historically been viewed from a public health perspective with a focus on primary, secondary, and tertiary prevention (Coombs and Ziedonis, 1995). However, ATOD can also be viewed from a community organizing perspective. The problem of drug abuse can serve to mobilize communities to come together in search of common goals, as a means of empowerment, capacity enhancement, and control over their environment. However, for these lofty goals to be accomplished, the basic premise in viewing Latino communities must shift from a deficit to an asset perspective. Namely, a shift in paradigms is necessary that allows practitioners, be they organizers or prevention specialists (practitioners, researchers, etc.), to rethink common perceptions of Latino communities. A deficit-based paradigm must be discarded and a strengths-based paradigm embraced. In short, Latino communities must be viewed as having strengths, indigenous resources, etc., before addressing problems/needs such as substance abuse.

Strengths-based practice offers potential for reaching undervalued communities in the United States (Saleebey, 1992). This perspective, unlike the more commonly used deficits approach, identifies, mobilizes, and builds upon existing indigenous resources in the development of community solutions to community concerns (Delgado, 1995). A strengths-based paradigm lends itself to primary prevention and community organizing; a deficits approach, which is predicated on individuals, families, and communities being the source of problems and solutions being possible only if derived from and directed by external sources, does not lend itself to prevention, community capacity enhancement, and organizing (Delgado, 1997; McKnight and Kretzmann, 1990).

This chapter will provide a state of the art review of the professional literature, present a paradigm that stresses Latino strengths, and highlight practice-based examples of innovative prevention initiatives that have potential for use with community organizing strategies in urban-based Latino communities across the United States. The chapter will consist of six sections: (1) Overview of Approaches Toward Substance Abuse Prevention; (2) Challenges in Defining The Problem (focus on data gathering limitations and definitions of Latinos); (3) Extent of Use and Abuse of Alcohol, Tobacco, and Other Drug Abuse (data will be presented with a focus on urban areas and trends based on federal sources); (4) Innovative Intervention Strategies (case examples and illustrations on the most promising approaches); (5) Principles for Organizing and Prevention: Partnerships in Community Service (a series of key principles and considerations will be provided); and (6) Implications for Practice and Research.

OVERVIEW OF APPROACHES TOWARD SUBSTANCE ABUSE PREVENTION

Botvin (1995, pp. 29-30) does an excellent job of summarizing the components of successful prevention programs:

> Based on existing knowledge, it is clear that the most effective prevention strategy would be one that has multiple components, uses program providers and delivery channels that efficiently reach the target population, and provides ongoing intervention throughout the critical period for the initiation of drug use.

There are five general approaches toward preventing the onset of substance abuse. Most prevention initiatives utilize all or a combination of the following components: (1) information dissemination on the risks associated with drug use and abuse (widely considered of little value in preventing substance abuse); (2) psychosocial risk factors (increase awareness of the role of social factors in promoting drug use); (3) changing attitudes, beliefs, and normative expectations (individual or mass media campaigns focused on realistically addressing substance abuse); (4) resistance skills (training youth to deal with peer and media pressures to use drugs); and (5) personal and social skills (enhancing skills in order to promote competence and thereby reducing motivation to experiment and use drugs). The latter two approaches are widely considered to hold the greatest promise for achieving substance abuse prevention based upon available data. These two approaches, in turn, need to be specifically tailored to incorporate factors related to Latino communities and culture.

CHALLENGES IN DEFINING THE PROBLEM OF SUBSTANCE ABUSE

Assessing the extent of substance abuse among Latinos, as it will be noted in great detail, is very difficult as a result of a number of methodological and classification problems that have not changed dramatically over the past two decades (Humm-Delgado and Delgado, 1983; Rodriguez-Andrew, 1998). These limitations can be classified into the following categories: (1) reliance on arrest and treatment data (communities of color are signaled out); (2) type of drug frequently focused on by enforcement and treatment programs (White, non-Latinos, and middle class drug users can purchase drugs through legal means or illegal means that minimize exposure to law enforcement); (3) under counting by U.S. Census Bureau serves to reduce the total number of Latinos, and serves to increase the relative of reported substance abusers within the total population); and (4) statistics and reported studies have only recently separated Latinos from other groups of color, making historical comparisons and trend assessment difficult, if not impossible.

EXTENT OF USE AND ABUSE OF ALCOHOL, TOBACCO, AND OTHER DRUG ABUSE

The use and abuse of substance abuse is complex in nature and greatly influenced by a variety of factors. Substance use and abuse among Latinos must be viewed from a multidimensional perspective, taking into account a series of variables and noting how they interact, in order to develop a more accurate picture of substance abuse.

De La Rosa's (1998) analysis of the 1993 National Household Survey on Drug Abuse illustrates the complexity of making generations about Latino use of ATOD:

> Analysis of data from the 1993 NHSDA on the prevalence of past-month alcohol, heavy alcohol, marijuana, cocaine, and cigarette use among Hispanics by age, sex, and specific Hispanic sub-groups . . . indicates that persons of Central American ancestry had the lowest prevalence of past-month

use for these drugs across age and sex groupings. Among persons belonging to the other Hispanic sub-groups . . . Puerto Ricans had the highest prevalence of past-month cocaine use (1.5 percent, compared with 1.3 for all Hispanics) and cigarette use (28.8 percent compared with 22.4 percent for all Hispanics), and both Puerto Ricans and persons of South American ancestry had the highest prevalence of past-month marijuana use (5.3 percent, compared to 4.3 for all Hispanics). For past-month alcohol use, persons of South American ancestry had the highest prevalence rates (57.3 percent, compared with 46.0 percent for all Hispanics), and persons of Mexican ancestry reported the highest prevalence of past-month heavy alcohol use (6.9 percent compared with 5.5 percent for all Hispanics).

When age, residence (urban/rural, education), socioeconomic class, and length of residence in this country are taken into account, a complex picture emerges with implications for prevention, treatment, and community organizing.

Latino Subgroup

The 1990s have witnessed a dramatic increase in ATOD and a shift in the conceptual underpinnings for both understanding and intervening in the field (Cunningman, 1994, p. ix):

During the 1990s this community emphasis has evolved into the expanding awareness that communities are composed of groups representing multiple ethnicities and cultures. This shift from a service delivery model to a community development model . . . requires the field of AOD utilizes a framework and methodologies that integrate multi-cultures throughout all aspects of knowledge and skill development.

This shift has also made the field prevention much more complimentary to community organizing, both sharing a community base and a focus on undervalued groups. The Latino community is no longer restricted to three primary groups (Cubans, Mexicans, and Puerto Ricans). Recent demographic trends, particularly related to immigration, indicate that the Latino community is becoming more diverse (Castex, 1994). Few areas of the country have Latino communities consisting of just one group. Many areas have increased numbers of Central and South American groups who are recent arrivals to the United States. This increased diversity will prove very challenging to the fields of prevention and organizing, since such efforts must address historical distrust of various Latino subgroups that can be traced back several centuries.

Drug of choice will generally vary according to Latino sub-group. Puerto Ricans generally have the highest use of marijuana (5.3%), Mexican-Americans and Puerto Ricans are tied for use of cocaine (1.5%). Mexicans have the highest rate of heavy alcohol use (6.9%). In turning to cigarettes, Puerto Ricans have the highest percentage with 28.8 percent (National Household Survey on Drug Abuse, 1993).

Type of Drug Use

Substance abuse prevention requires practitioners and researchers to address drug-specific concerns. Campaigns that lump all drugs together are too generic to succeed in preventing use. Consequently, it is necessary for substance abuse programs to develop strategies and messages that are locality-based, with specific reference to local issues and concerns, not too dissimilar from community organizing campaigns.

Heavy alcohol use over the past month is the most prevalent form of abuse with 5.5 percent of all Latinos falling into this category. Marijuana use was indicated by 4.3 percent, followed by cocaine with 1.3 percent (no data were available on heroin use); use of cigarettes was mentioned by 22.4 percent (National Household Survey on Drug Abuse, 1993).

Urban/Rural

Unfortunately, rural areas of the United States have not been studied to the same degree as urban areas (Paz, 1998). Latinos are the most urbanized ethnic group in the United States with 92 percent compared to only 73 percent for non-Latinos (National Hispanic Leadership Agenda, 1996). In fact, there were nine cities in the United States with Latino populations numbering at least 500,000 (Morales and Bonilla, 1993): (1) Los Angeles (4.8 million); (2) New York (2.8 million); (3) Miami (1 million); (4) San Francisco (970,000); (5) Chicago (893,000); (6) Houston (772,000); (7) San Antonio (620,000); (8) Dallas (519,000); and (9) San Diego (511,000).

The large proportion of Latinos in urban areas results in a disproportionate amount of research focused on cities such as Los Angeles, Miami, and New York. As a result, relatively little is known about substance abuse among Latinos residing in small urban areas of the country. Ecological factors related to residing in large urban areas may not allow translation of research results to smaller urban areas.

Gender

There are some clear differences between males and females when studying drugs, although the gaps are closing (Colon, 1998; Mora, 1998). Prevalence rates among Latinas ranged from 5.8 percent (cigarettes) for women of Central American ancestry to 25.5 percent (cigarettes) for Puerto Ricans. Heavy alcohol use ranged from .3 percent for Central American women to 1.7 percent for Mexicans. Marijuana accounted for 2.9 percent with Puerto Rican (4.0) having the highest percentage and Central Americans the lowest (.8 percent). Cocaine accounted for 1.1 percent among Cubans and .2 percent for South Americans (National Household Survey on Drug Abuse, 1993).

Age

The research is quite strong in suggesting that the earlier an individual starts to use gateway drugs, the higher the likelihood that he/she will graduate to more powerful drugs. The twelve to seventeen age group was generally the second highest abusing group with the eighteen to twenty-five being the highest. This pattern can be seen with all drugs except use of alcohol (26 to 34 being highest) (National Household Survey on Drug Abuse, 1993).

INNOVATIVE INTERVENTION STRATEGIES

There is no question that the complexities faced by Latino communities in maximizing their potential for contributions in this society have increased in difficulty the last thirty years. Major structural changes in the economy, combined with dramatic demographic shifts in population characteristics, political climate, and social problems (i.e., HIV/AIDS), requires the development of bold and innovative strategies for empowering Latino communities.

There are a number of promising approaches toward substance abuse prevention that have applicability to other social problems. The work by Delgado and colleagues (Delgado, 1998e; Delgado and Barton, 1998; Delgado and Santiago, 1998) has focused primarily on Latinos, but is also applicable to other communities of color. An urban ecology perspective builds upon community assets, which are often overlooked or minimized. These assets can be represented in the form of murals, gardens, community-initiated playgrounds, and sculptures, bringing communities together in search of common goals.

These goals, in turn, generally encompass the following: (1) taking control over vacant lots, a source of criminal activity, and beautifying them through murals, gardens, etc.; (2) the stress on participation and development of indigenous leadership; (3) the focus on intergenerational activities whenever possible as a means of uniting various groups within a community; (4) a focus on mentoring, teaching, and learning for all participants; and (5) a stress on cultural pride and heritage as a cornerstone of any community-wide activity be it prevention or community organizing focused.

Murals represent a picture of what a community considers to be important. Unfortunately, the subject of murals has not been addressed in sufficient depth from a social science, prevention, and community organizing perspective. Murals have cultural meaning and influence on the internal audience, namely the community (Treguer, 1992). It would be simplistic to think that murals can be easily classified into categories (Holscher, 1976, p. 25):

One is impressed by the heterogeneity of the mural styles, subjects, and locations. The typical mural does not exist. There are too many of them, depicting numerous ideas and themes, painted in literally hundreds of different places, to allow us to form an unsophisticated conclusion about the reasons for their existence.

Drescher and Garcia's (1978) study of Latino murals (primarily based in Los Angeles) was done from an artistic and social (historical, political, and economic) perspective. Treguer (1992), in turn, considers murals as a cultural-based form of self- expression for communities that have few unregulated outlets for their public voices. Pounds (1996) notes that: "Murals express more than ethnic pride. It's about people expressing what their own issues are." Last, Holscher (1976-77), one of the few social scientists to study this phenomenon, has identified the socio-political value murals play in undervalued communities.

Delgado and Barton (1998) identified six themes related to content of Latino murals and one related to location: (1) symbols of ethnic and racial pride; (2) religious symbols; (3) issues related to social and economic justice; (4) decorative; (5) homages to national and local heroes; (6) memorials commissioned by local residents; and (7) location of murals (limited, targeted, and maximum audience exposure). These themes, in turn, provide a wealth of information about a community and the issues they consider to be salient.

Mural painting is an excellent means for involving community, primarily youth, in activities that can be considered prevention as well as organizing in nature. Delgado and Barton (1998), in addition, listed eleven knowledge and skill areas that are developed and enhanced for youth and their communities through mural painting: (1) research (undertaking library research on use of cultural and historical content); (2) negotiation (skill developed that can be transferred to other arenas); (3) safety consciousness and following rules (greater awareness of the importance of listening and creation of an accident-free mind-set); (4) team work (an ability and willingness to work together in pursuit of a common goal); (5) exposure to starting and completing a project (planning and implementation skills); (6) work habits (importance of attendance and punctuality); (7) communication skills (verbal and written); (8) knowledge of math and chemistry; (9) working across generations (enlisting the support and input of adults); (10) budgeting and scheduling (an in depth understanding of finances and planning); and (11) making a contribution to the community (youths are resources and assets that are often overlooked by adults).

Victory Gardens have a rich and important history in the United States, particularly their contributions during World War II. Gardens, however, have increased in popularity in recent years, with an estimated 300 to 500 cities in the United States having non-profit organizations devoted to urban gardening (Hamilton, 1996). Gardens, if viewed sociologically and politically, have taken on social development goals beyond the growing of food (Hill, 1996, p. 1): "People are more concerned about the environment. . . . We focus on low-income communities. Gardens have become a tool to help develop people." Urban gardens, as a result, have evolved into social interventions over the past three decades (Miller, 1995, C8):

> The initial appeal of urban gardens used to be a simple desire for home-grown vegetables. Now, it seems however, community gardens are becoming a way to improve relationships and neighborhoods. During the 1992 riots in South Central Los Angeles, the seven community gardens there escaped the barrage of damage. It is this attitude that has made the popularity of community gardens grow in recent years.

The presence of urban gardens has been widely credited with preventing or reducing drug abuse and crime. Gardens, in some initiatives, have specifically been developed as a means of preventing crime related to drug abuse. Vacant lots have been transformed into community-meeting grounds, making it difficult for drug dealers to conduct business. Further, the success of their gardens has inspired community residents to undertake other social problems through community organizing.

PRINCIPLES FOR ORGANIZING AND PREVENTION–PARTNERSHIPS IN COMMUNITY SERVICES

Substance abuse prevention lends itself to community organizing and development approaches. The goals of these two approaches generally compliment, if not overlap. A set of five principles can be identified that facilitate the integration of organizing into prevention, and prevention into organizing. These principles, in turn, will guide practitioners and organizations in developing more culture-specific, and thereby competent, approaches toward Latino communities throughout all regions of the United States.

Strengths (assets) must form the cornerstone of an intervention initiative.

Gordon provides a definition of resilience that is also applicable to a strengths perspective, and has profound implications for substance abuse prevention among Latino youths (1996, p. 63):

> Resilience [strengths] is a multifaceted phenomenon that encompasses environmental and personal factors. Comprehensively, resilience is the ability to thrive, mature, and increase competence in the face of adverse circumstances or obstacles. The obstacles may be severe and infrequent or chronic and consistent.

Substance abuse prevention for Latinos, as a result, must systematically utilize personal and environmental assets as a cornerstone of community-focused activities. A systematic effort necessitates the comprehensive mapping of community (indigenous resources).

The mapping of community assets is a necessary step whether the organization is interested in prevention or organizing. Latino community assets, however, may take on "unconventional" forms and necessitate a strengths perspective and open-mind—in short, assets may be manifested in many shapes and sizes, none of which may be "typical."

The professional literature has recently reported efforts at mapping Latino community assets as part of substance abuse prevention (Delgado, 1995). A Latino community mapping of assets was undertaken in Holyoke, Massachusetts, a city of approximately 44,000, located 100 miles west of Boston. The Latino community consisted primarily of Puerto Ricans.

The goals of mapping community assets are generally multifaceted and can encompass both prevention, organizing, and program development, like that those of the Holyoke study (Delgado, 1995, p. 117):

(1) provide a detailed description and location of Puerto Rican natural support systems . . . ; (2) provide youth with a resiliency perspective on the community; (3) raise the consciousness of human service organizations/providers concerning positive aspects of the Puerto Rican community; and (4) serve as a basis for a resource directory specifically focused on community assets.

Latino community assets can be integrated into prevention initiatives. Development of community gardens, for example, can play an instrumental role in substance abuse and crime prevention if vacant lots can be conceptualized as assets rather than deficits. Open spaces within high crime areas of a city can often be areas where individuals who are involved in criminal activities can congregate. Thus, converting these spaces into gardens represents an effort on the part of the community to exercise control, an important aspect of both prevention and organizing (Hill, 1996, p. 1), "The reason we purchased that lot was that there were a lot of drug dealers and prostitutes hanging out. It was county owned. We didn't have a lot of ways of monitoring it . . . But if we purchased it, then only certain people could use it."

Carrier (1997) makes a similar observation when stating:

Keeping her street safe was what Anna Baez hoped for her North Baker [Denver] community's new mini-garden planted by 100 volunteers. "I feel more comfortable because of fruits and vegetables," she said (p. B-05).

The examples described above illustrate how community gardening can serve as a substance abuse prevention and intervention, as well as organizing a community to take over activities within its boundaries.

Prevention, like organizing, must begin with what the community believes to be its priority for change.

Any form of intervention and organizing must be premised on a sound understanding of what the Latino community considers to be of paramount importance. If drugs are not considered to be of significant importance, then it will be difficult, if not impossible, to mobilize residents to address this social problem. Prevention, like organizing, must have the community address problems that are specific, can have immediate results, and be successful in achieving stated goals. Substance abuse, as a result, must be systematically broken down into components that are user-specific, such as age, gender, and drug-specific, such as tobacco, cocaine, etc. This specificity, in turn, allows for targeting of prevention and organizing efforts.

The likelihood that community-based prevention and organizing efforts start with what the Latino community considers its priority is increased when involving residents throughout all facets of a project. No project can achieve success without active and meaningful participation of Latino residents. This involvement can start with the formation of an advisory committee, hiring residents, contracting with local-based institutions, and development of information gathering methods that systematically tap all segments of the community.

Substance abuse, in turn, must be conceptualized as an enemy of the community, stressing the role of external forces. Drugs, regardless of the potential harm to the community, are brought into the community. Organizing would be much easier if the target of the change is outside of the community in the form of unresponsive government officials, slum landlords, a repressive police force, etc. Once success is achieved, then efforts can turn to internal players in the drug business.

Community-targeted efforts at prevention and change must be based upon community capacity enhancement goals.

Any initiatives at preventing substance abuse and organizing Latinos must endeavor to utilize local community resources and enhance resident capacities in the process. According to Aguirre-Molina and Parra (1995, p. 153):

> Community development is the ultimate goal of [substance abuse] prevention strategies employed to reduce risk factors and address the variables that contribute to their occurrence. *Community development*, as defined here, is

the process of involving the community in the identification and reinforcement of those aspects of everyday life, culture, and political activity that are conducive to health [italics added].

One project based in Dallas, Texas, specifically focused on community development as the central goal of substance abuse prevention (Colby and Rice, 1994, p. 147):

> Using community change strategies based on a bottom-up model, the NMP [Neighborhood Mentors Project] fosters inclusion and partnership by establishing a coalition of key power-based community institutions and empowered neighborhood residents.

In essence, the concepts of development and empowerment are not exclusively within the domain of community organizing; they, too, can be found in the substance abuse prevention field.

Capacity enhancement strategies necessitate in-depth knowledge of local issues, particularly when targeting youth (McLaughlin, 1993, p. 66):

> Effective leaders use local knowledge and credibility to craft programs and resources that provide the connective tissue between estranged, cynical inner-city youth and the broader social institutions essential to their productive futures and positive conceptions of self. The connective tissue is spun from personal knowledge of youngsters and their setting and from knowledge of social, political, and economic resources in the larger community. These effective leaders act as brokers, catalysts, and coaches, making the contacts and linkages necessary to enlarge the opportunities available to youth and providing confidence necessary to access.

Delgado (1997) stresses the importance of community-targeted initiatives identifying, recruiting, and training Latino youths for leadership positions in prevention and community organizing efforts. Youths represent a vast untapped resource within the Latino community and are often overlooked in the staffing of initiatives targeting the community. In addition, investment of resources into the preparation of Latino youths for leadership roles also represents an investment in the future of the community. In short, youths are an untapped indigenous resource for prevention and organizing efforts. However, Delgado (1997, p. 110) issues an important caution concerning the necessary steps before this goal can be realized: ". . . the development of Latino youth leaders can be accomplished only after they have developed a positive identity, including ethnic pride."

Cultural pride enhancement activities must form an integral part of any prevention and organizing initiatives.

Self-concept has recently been researched as a key factor in preventing substance abuse among Latinos (Gordon, 1996). A critical factor in self-concept is ethnic pride. McLaughlin (1993) stresses the importance of cultural-pride related activities for organizations targeting youth and succeed in achieving their goals:

> Many adults in these settings stressed the importance of alliance with some well-grounded cultural history as a component of general self-esteem and social competence. Youth workers understood the importance of cultural awareness and pride and of youths' development of a positive sense of this aspect of their identity. Within the broader community context, there is often little with which to ascribe value or pride to African American or Latino youth (p. 60).

Substance abuse prevention programs targeting Latinos must have a cultural component as a significant part of any initiative (Delgado, 1997; Hernandez and Lucero, 1996). This component necessitates youth developing greater awareness of their cultural heritage and developing pride in who they are. Cultural pride activities often encompass study of history, arts and dance, and the role of political oppression in shaping historical events such as migration. Painting of murals can play a role in helping youth express their cultural pride; murals, in turn, can convey to the internal and external communities a deepening sense of pride.

Substance abuse prevention and community organizing must encompass a comprehensive approach that serves to unite social problems.

Unfortunately, social scientists, politicians, and service providers of various kinds, have a tendency to compartmentalize social problems into "neat" boxes. This process of reductionism undermines efforts at addressing Latino community problems from a comprehensive perspective. Youth serving organizations must take a broader perspective on Latino youths and their needs, thus avoiding common traps concerning single-focused interventions (McLaughlin, 1993, p. 55):

> The needs of inner-city youth do not come in neat bundles or tidy problem definitions. Just as the identities of youth are embedded in the character and resources of the communities, neighborhoods, and families, so are their needs enmeshed and interrelated. Inner-city organizations that connect youth with larger society, promote a positive sense of purpose and personhood, and provide the resources that youngsters need to reach adulthood are not single-issue, single-purpose institutions . . . These organizations, in short, serve as

"family" for youth, meeting their needs and promoting their growth much in the inclusive way a family would.

There are numerous possibilities for prevention specialists and organizers to connect social problems together in the hopes of more efficiently addressing them within a community context. Very often we cannot separate crime, drugs, under or unemployment, sexual activities, and other risky behavior. This connectedness becomes very apparent when examined within a community and family context. Thus, a comprehensive approach increases the likelihood that limited outside community funding can have a maximum impact.

Comprehensive interventions must, in turn, be intergenerational and gender welcoming in nature as a means of uniting an entire community and not just one sector. As a result, these initiatives must systematically build in positions of leadership that take into account age as well as gender considerations. Leadership positions that rest solely on Latino adult males undermine significant sectors of the Latino community.

Latinas, too, for example, have leadership abilities and potentials and must not be systematically ruled out of prevention and community organizing campaigns. Lazzari, Ford, and Haughey's (1996) study of Latinas actively engaged in promoting social change in the community, listed numerous activities they were a significant part of that fall within typical prevention and organizing initiatives—promoting environmental changes to improve circumstances for Latino residents, creating, providing, and maintaining social services within the community, promoting self-esteem (cultural pride), and encouraging and sustaining individual and collective approaches to change. These Latinas could easily undertake and maintain community-based initiatives if provided with the same support that Latino males receive from the community.

IMPLICATIONS FOR PRACTICE AND RESEARCH

The content covered in this chapter raises important implications for practice and research in the field of substance abuse research with Latinos. This section of the chapter will highlight a variety of ways for initiating substance abuse prevention in urban-based Latino communities.

The perspective on open spaces addressed in this chapter must not be lost by both practitioners and researchers. The subject of open spaces within urban communities has not received the attention it deserves within the scholarly literature. Open spaces have usually been the focus of architects. However, open spaces have important roles to play in substance abuse prevention programming and activities. Open spaces represent excellent opportunities for creative community-based programming since these areas often play a pivotal role in drug transactions and the crime often associated with them. Most urban communities with high concentrations of Latinos tend to be low-income and socially marginal. Thus, these communities have high percentages of abandoned or razed buildings, and buildings destroyed by fires and their remains left standing—representing both safety and blights on the community. In circumstances where an empty lot is the result, they become a dumping ground for garbage, abandoned cars, etc., and a site for criminal-related activities.

Empowering communities to use these spaces as playgrounds and gardens, for example, not only serves to reduce an area used for drug activities, it also serves as a setting for increasing community participation. Youth, a prime target of any prevention effort, can be enlisted to develop lots for the benefit of the community. Murals and sculptures designed by youth can also be placed within community gardens and playgrounds, serving to enhance the positive messages being sent to the internal and external community. In essence, open spaces must be reclaimed for the benefit of a community. Failure to use these spaces will often relegate them to drug and criminal activity, making the impact of any prevention programming limited.

In the area of research, much can be done to expand the role of the community in designing and implementing studies related to substance abuse. The creation of an advisory committee, in addition to hiring local residents to serve as field interviewers, can enhance a research effort. An advisory committee can play an important role in helping researchers create questions that have meaning for both the community and practitioners in the field. In addition, the committee can assist researchers in defining the target area, getting research subjects, working research questions, enlisting the cooperation of the community, interpreting findings, and determining who should get copies of reports. Advisory committee members should be compensated for their time and effort. Community involvement through advisory committee participation, in turn, provides researchers with an opportunity to enhance the capacities of participants.

CONCLUSION

The impact of substance abuse in Latino communities has varied across the United States. However, although varied, few communities and families have escaped its devastating impact. The youthfulness of the Latino community increases the importance of society viewing substance abuse prevention as a high priority. As noted in this chapter, there are a number of promising approaches toward substance abuse prevention that not only seek to prevent the onset of use, but also serve to enhance community capacity in the process.

Enhancement of community capacity serves to involve, empower, and help identify strengths in the Latino community. These concepts are no different from those applied in community organizing, where a community must first believe in their capability to bring about social change and redress social injustices. Consequently, there is a natural alliance between prevention and community organizing.

REFERENCES

Aguirre-Molina, M. and Parra, P. A. (1995). Latino youth and families as active participants in planning change: A community-university partnership. In R. E. Zambrana (Ed.), *Understanding Latino Families: Scholarship, Policy, and Practice* (pp. 130-153). Sage Publications: Thousand Oaks, CA.

Botvin, G. J. (1995). Principles of prevention. In R. H. Coombs and D. Ziedonis (Eds.), *Handbook on Drug Abuse Prevention* (pp. 19-44). Allyn & Bacon: Boston, MA.

Carrier, J. (1997). Gardeners, rich and poor, sink roots across Denver. *Denver Post,* B-05.

Castex, G. M. (1994). Providing services to Hispanic/Latino populations. *Social Work,* 39:288-96.

Colby, I. and Rice, A. (1994). A community development approach to substance abuse prevention. *Journal of Applied Social Sciences,* 18:147-56.

Colon, E. (1998). Alcohol use among Latino males: Implications for the development of culturally competent prevention and treatment services. *Alcoholism Treatment Quarterly,* 16:147-161.

Coombs, R. H. and Ziedonis, D., Eds. (1995). *Handbook on Drug Abuse Prevention.* Allyn & Bacon: Boston, MA.

Cunningham, M. S. (1994). Foreword. In J. U. Gordon (Ed.), *Managing Multiculturalism in Substance Abuse Services* (pp. vii-ix). Sage Publications: Thousand Oaks, CA.

De La Rosa, M. (1998). Prevalence and consequences of alcohol, cigarette, and drug use among Hispanics. *Alcoholism Treatment Quarterly,* 16:21-54.

Delgado, M. (1998a). *Social services in Latino communities: Research and strategies.* Haworth Press: New York.

Delgado, M. (Ed.). (1998b). *Alcohol use/abuse among Latinos: Issues and examples of culturally competent services.* Haworth Press: New York.

Delgado, M. (1998c). *Social work practice in non-traditional urban settings.* Oxford University Press: New York.

Delgado, M. (in press d). Involvement of Puerto Rican and other Latinos in ATOD research. *Drugs & Society.*

Delgado, M. (1998e). Community social work practice in an urban context: A capacity enhancement perspective. Oxford University Press: New York.

Delgado, M. (1995). Community asset assessment and substance abuse prevention: A case study involving the Puerto Rican community. *Journal of Child and Adolescent Substance Abuse,* 4:57-77.

Delgado, M. (1996). Community asset assessments by Latino youths. *Social Work in Education,* 18:169-78.

Delgado, M. (1997). Strengths-based practice with Puerto Rican adolescents: Lessons from a substance abuse prevention project. *Social Work in Education,* 19:101-112.

Delgado, M. and Barton, K. (in press). Murals in Latino communities: Social indicators of community strengths. *Social Work,* 43:346-356.

Delgado, M. and Santiago, J. (1998). HIV/AIDS in a Puerto Rican/Dominican community: A collaborative project with a botanical shop. *Social Work.,* 43:183-186.

Drescher, T. and Garcia, R. (1978). Recent Raza murals in the U.S. *Radical America*, 12:14-31.

Gordon, K. (1996). Resilient Hispanic youths' self-concept and motivational patterns. *Hispanic Journal of Behavioral Sciences*, 18:63-73.

Hamilton, N. (December 23, 1996). Building neighborhoods with community gardens. *The Des Moines Register*:11.

Hernandez, L. P. and Lucero, E. (1996). DAYS La familia community drug and alcohol prevention program: Family centered model for working with inner-city Hispanic families. *Journal of Primary Prevention*, 16:255-272.

Hill, M. (July 3, 1996). D. M.'s inner city turning green. *The Des Moines Register*:1.

Holscher, L. M. (1976). Artists & murals in East Los Angeles and Boyle Heights: A sociological observation. *Humboldt Journal of Social Relations*, 3:25-29.

Holscher, L. M. (1976-77). Tiene arte valor afuera del barrio (Art has value outside of the community): The murals of East Los Angeles and Boyle Heights. *Journal of Ethnic Studies*, 4:42-52.

Humm-Delgado, D. and Delgado, M. (1983). Hispanic adolescents and substance abuse: Issues for the 1980s. *Child and Youth Services*, 6:71-87.

Lazzari, M. M., Ford, H. R. and Haughey, K. J. (1996). Making a difference: Women of action in the community. *Social Work*, 41:197-205.

Maxwell, B. and Jacobson, M. (1989). *Marketing Disease to Hispanics: The Selling of Alcohol, Tobacco, and Junk Foods*. Center for Science in the Public Interest: Washington, D.C.

McKnight, J. L. and Kretzmann, J. P. (1990). *Mapping Community Capacity*. Northwestern University, Center for Urban Affairs and Policy Research: Evanston, IL.

McLaughlin, M. W. (1993). Embedded identities: Enabling balance in urban contexts. In S. B. Heath and M. W. McLaughlin (Eds.), *Identity & Inner-City Youth: Beyond Ethnicity and Gender* (pp. 36-68). Teachers College Press: New York.

Miller, A. (July 11, 1995). A little patch of Eden blooms in the D.C. sun; Community gardens grow food, friendships. *The Washington Times*:C8, Policy.

Mora, J. (1998). The treatment of alcohol dependency among Latinas: A feminist, cultural and community perspective. *Alcoholism Treatment Quarterly*, 16:163-177.

Morales, R. and Bonilla, F. (1993). Restructuring and the new inequality. In R. Morales and F. Bonilla (Eds.), *Latinos in a Changing U.S. Economy* (pp. 1-27). Sage Publications: Newbury Park, CA.

National Household Survey on Drug Abuse: (1991-1993). Substance Abuse and Mental Health Administration: Rockville, MD.

National Hispanic Leadership Agenda. (1996). *1996 policy summary*. Washington, D.C.

Paz, J. (1998). The drug free workplace in rural Arizona. *Alcoholism Treatment Quarterly*, 16:133-145.

Pounds, J. (1996). Personal communication.

Rodriguez-Andrew, S. (1998). Alcohol use and abuse among Latinos: Issues and examples of culturally competent services. *Alcoholism Treatment Quarterly*, 16:55-70.

Saleebey, D. S., Ed. (1992). *The Strengths Perspective in Social Work Practice*. Longman Publishers: New York.

Treguer, A. (1992). The Chicanos—muralists with a message. *U.N.E.S.C.O. Courier*, 45, 22-24.

CHAPTER 7

Substance Abuse Prevention in African-American Communities

Lawrence S. Brown, Jr. and Stanley John

Even as we near the end of the last decade of the twentieth century, substance abuse continues to have a significant impact on the social fabric, the economic landscape, and the public health of all Americans. For Americans of African descent, the effects are even more profound. For this reason, it is critical that society supports efforts to understand the fundamental mechanisms that underlie substance abuse and to develop effective substance abuse prevention programs. These intervention efforts must be built upon a sound scientific base and the experience of previous successful prevention efforts. The purpose of this chapter is to explore substance abuse issues relevant to Americans of African descent and to discuss the barriers to substance abuse prevention in many African-American communities.

Before proceeding, one question deserves immediate attention. How does one accurately and adequately describe this very important population of Americans? African Americans represent diverse multicultural subpopulations. There are African Americans who are descendants of African slaves and who were born in the United States. There are African Americans who are descendants of African slaves of the Caribbean and who migrated to the United States. There are African Americans who were born in Africa and migrated to the United States. Each of these subcultures has unique characteristics, which easily differentiate one group from another. Such characteristics reflect aspects of their colonizing mother country and include dialect, traditional dress and festivities, and religion. The geographic distribution of African-American subcultures varies considerably. For example, in New York City, African Americans of Caribbean origin are concentrated in some Brooklyn neighborhoods. On the other hand, African

Americans of American birth are more predominant in the Bushwick/Brownsville areas of Brooklyn, and African Americans of recent migration from Africa are localized predominately in the Harlem neighborhood of Manhattan (John, et. al., 1995).

SUBSTANCE USE AND PREVALENCE

According to the National Household Survey on Drug Abuse, as of 1996, thirteen million persons twelve years and older currently use an illicit drug. This information demonstrated that there was no significant change since 1995 and has been rather stable since 1992. As in previous years, marijuana was the most commonly used illicit drug as 54 percent of those who responded admitted to the use of this substance.

This same survey, conducted by the Substance Abuse and Mental Health Services Administration, indicated that White Americans comprised a larger portion of current illicit drug users. However, African-American males between twelve and thirty-five years of age were much more likely to be users of an illicit substance compared to their White counterparts. Indeed, 6.1 percent of Whites admitted to the use of an illicit substance as compared to 7.5 percent of Blacks. This is particularly the case for cocaine use. African-American and Latino women were more likely than White women to have used crack cocaine, a form of cocaine which many believe to be especially virulent (National Institute on Drug Abuse, 1988a). On the other hand, data from the National High School Senior Survey (National Institute on Drug Abuse, 1988b) indicated that the rate of drug use among African-American high school seniors was lower for all drugs, except heroin and marijuana. An equal percentage of African Americans and Whites between the age of twelve and seventeen had used an illicit drug in their lifetime, in the past year, or past month (National Institute on Drug Abuse, 1995).

The patterns of substance abuse among both African-American males and females entering substance abuse treatment programs are much different than patterns seen in other groups. Nearly 45 percent of African-American women and 30 percent of African-American men entering treatment reported crack (smoked cocaine) as the primary drug of abuse. These rates are much higher than rates among Puerto Rican females (5%) and males (about 2%). The exchange of sex for drugs, especially crack cocaine, has greatly increased the risk of HIV transmission among African American women (Amuleru-Marshall, 1995).

Substance abuse among African Americans has received considerable attention (Amuleru-Marshall, 1991; Brown, 1981; Brown, 1993; Brown and Alterman, 1992; Johnson and Nishi, 1976; Maddox and Borinski, 1964; Musto, 1973; Novotny, et. al. 1988; Robins and Murphy, 1967; Tucker, 1985). Large-scale surveys provide an intriguing picture of substance among African Americans. However, drug use surveys have many limitations that may disproportionately affect African Americans.

First, many of these surveys miss populations at risk for illegal substance use. These populations include the homeless, high school dropouts, and imprisoned persons. Because a significant percent of these hidden populations are comprised of African Americans, the true picture of substance abuse among African Americans is unclear. The National Household survey, like other data sets, has sparse data on poverty. This is a significant limitation to efforts to separate effects of income from proxy and potentially confounding variables of employment, place of residence, and education. These surveys rarely use multivariate analyses due to sample size and funding limitations and there is rare encouragement for secondary analysis.

All of the surveys, except for the Drug Use Forecasting System (DUF), rely on self-reporting. As indicated by comparisons of self-reports and urinalysis results from DUF data, drug use tends to be underreported. This is of particular importance because these surveys deal with a stigmatized and patently illegal behavior. Consequently, the validity of the results is always an issue of discussion. Just as important is the question of whether there are cultural differences in the validity of the self-reported results. It is certainly possible that African Americans may differ from other populations in their receptivity to responding to questions of this sort.

Finally, because surveys focus on the use of psychoactive substances, there is limited usefulness for clinicians, who care for patients with a substance abuse disorder. Clinicians focus their efforts on persons who meet clinical definitions of abuse or dependence. Consequently, surveys of substance use are not necessarily predictive of the consequences likely to occur as a result of use or the costs to society for the use of illegal substances.

CONSEQUENCES OF SUBSTANCE ABUSE

African Americans sustain a disproportionately higher rate of the consequences of consuming illicit drugs and alcohol. Drug abuse-related emergency department cases reported to the Drug Abuse Warning Network (DAWN) consistently demonstrated an overrepresentation of African Americans (NIDA, 1990; Rouse, 1989). Between 1994 and 1995, Blacks had a 13 percent increase in drug/alcohol-related emergency room visits, while Whites experienced a 11 percent increase. Of the 460,910 emergency room visits in 1993, Blacks comprised 28 percent of the visits with cocaine followed by alcohol as the reasons for these visits. In comparison, alcohol followed by cocaine, were the most frequent reasons for emergency room visits for Whites.

Drug-related deaths reported by medical examiners are another component of DAWN for which African Americans are represented at a higher rate than

Hispanics or Whites. Of the 8,541 drug-related deaths in 1993, Blacks were over-represented and comprised 30 percent of the deaths. For Blacks, cocaine, opiates, and alcohol (from greatest to least) were the most common causes of substance-related deaths. For Whites, opiates, alcohol, and cocaine (from greatest to least) were the most common causes of substance-related deaths.

The acquired immunodeficiency syndrome (AIDS) and human immuno-deficiency virus (HIV) infection represent other ways in which psychoactive drug use can kill. The literature is replete with citations of the association between HIV/AIDS and injecting drug use among African Americans (Brown, et. al., 1988; Brown and Primm, 1990; Coates, et. al., 1988). Although AIDS cases among African Americans are distributed among all AIDS exposure categories, AIDS case reports associated with injecting drug use and heterosexual contact increased in 1993 (Centers for Disease Control and Prevention, 1993). More than 50 percent of the cumulative AIDS cases associated with heterosexual contact have been related to sex with an injecting drug user. Taken together, these two facts underscore the pivotal role injection drug use plays in HIV infection and AIDS in the United States. This information also explains why African Americans now comprise the largest percent and number of new AIDS cases.

It is also evident that the use of alcohol and other psychoactive substances through non-injecting routes of administration may put users at risk of HIV infection (Auerbach, et. al., 1994; Bolton, et. al., 1992; Leigh and Stall, 1993; Miller, et. al., 1990; National Commission on AIDS, 1991). Unfortunately, African Americans are also at higher risk for these behaviors as well.

Additionally, higher rates of cirrhosis and esophageal cancer among African Americans are attributed to alcohol consumption (Herd, 1989; National Institute on Alcohol Abuse and Alcoholism, 1990). Finally, the social and economic dislocations associated with substance abuse are evident in African-American communities and have been discussed previously (see the excellent review by Bell, 1990).

In summary, our knowledge about the epidemiology of substance abuse among African Americans can be characterized in the following way. Because the reliability of self-reported information from African Americans is unknown and because many African-American communities may be underrepresented in national surveys of drug use but over-represented in indices of substance abuse-related consequences, the findings from surveys of drug and alcohol use should be viewed as suggestive, at best.

CULTURAL ISSUES SURROUNDING SUBSTANCE ABUSE

Current prevention strategies flow from theories that share an attempt to explain some of the determinants of human behavior. The importance of drug-using behaviors makes it especially important to understand factors in the individual and the environment that influence these very intense and intimate behaviors. Much more information is available about the psychological and sociological than the neurobiological basis of drug-using behaviors.

Some social scientists have argued that behavior change is more likely through use of social networks to modify social norms. Advocates of this approach argue that individual behaviors are more efficiently changed through this mechanism as individuals are linked to neighborhoods and communities. These social scientists further argue that sociogenetic perspectives have a greater propensity for reflecting cultural sensitivities as well as gender dynamics.

Psychological and other social science perspectives have been useful, but their limitations are significant. Many currently used models assume that drug use behaviors are regulated by individually formulated action plans, immune to the impulsivity of sexual encounters or cues in the environment associated with drug abuse. Additionally, the major models do not reflect contextual personal and socio-cultural variables, such as gender, race/ethnicity, culture, and class. Finally, most models focus on the individual, without consideration of other levels of interest such as the community. The relevance of these theoretical issues to African Americans has been reviewed by a host of investigators (Mays, 1989; Mays and Cochran, 1988; Schilling, et. al., 1989; Thomas and Quinn, 1991; Thompson-Fullilove, et. al., 1990).

As in many cultures, the use of some psychoactive substances, especially alcohol, is often deeply linked to beliefs about individual responsibility and the importance of family and kinship networks. Every culture has evolved its own beliefs and behaviors for understanding and coping with the pain of illness and death, including some of the life-threatening complications of substance abuse, such as cirrhosis and AIDS.

Substance abuse-related interventions in African-American communities, organized and administered by governmental and even some private agencies are often viewed as part of the "white establishment." These programs have to overcome a century-long legacy of mistrust of public health programs. It was not until the late 1980s that public health efforts sought approaches that involved the Black community as partners rather than as subjects of inquiry and experiment (Jenkins, et. al., 1993), and federal agencies increased funding for prevention and treatment. However, since 1992, much of the funding has evaporated, reflecting public concerns about a weakening economy and dwindling support for health and social services and exacerbating mistrust in the African-American community. And while the current American economy is far from the perception of weakness, societal interests in public health programs, in general, and substance abuse programs, in particular, remain unpopular targets for public support.

There are many other major barriers to overcome in developing substance abuse prevention efforts among African Americans. Because of a host of other serious health and social problems facing the community, many African

Americans regard prevention—whether substance abuse-related or otherwise—as a luxury. Because of the long-term, pervasive impact of discrimination and racism, many African Americans have a sense that their future is predetermined. Many believe they have no control over their fate (Cummings, 1969; Jenkins, et. al., 1993), a chilling barrier to any type of prevention effort, especially one targeting a potentially fatal consequence. Failure to involve African-American community leaders, especially religious leaders, in planning prevention efforts and failure to understand the role of religious practices and beliefs in the community are faults of many prevention programs targeting African Americans. This may, in part, explain community resistance to siting of drug abuse treatment programs and to controversial approaches such as needle exchange.

Some prevention programs lack the understanding of the weak sociopolitical networks of some African-American communities (De La Cancela, 1989). Many more prevention programs fail to appreciate the traditional, gender-differentiated power roles (Thompson-Fullilove, et. al., 1990) among African Americans. These programs do not include an understanding of the economic and psychological dependence of many African-American women on their male counterparts (Cochran and Mays, 1993; Worth, 1989) and the lack of eligible African-American men compared with the numbers of African-American women (Mays and Cochran, 1988). For many African-American women the threat of physical and sexual abuse (Wyatt, 1985) is very real.

Investigators at the Drug Abuse Research Center at the University of California at Los Angeles (UCLA) have uncovered a number of additional factors with some relevance to substance abuse prevention. In a sample of 122 African-American arrestees in the Los Angeles area, Longshore, et. al. (1997) demonstrated that the key determinant of desire for help was interpersonal problem recognition. These investigators also showed that conventional moral beliefs and expected benefit of drug treatment were also associated with the desire for help. However, treatment motivation, as opposed to desire for help, was only associated with problem recognition and perceived treatment benefit (Longshore, et. al., 1998). These researchers noted that this association was especially strong among study subjects who endorsed Africentric values (Grills and Longshore, 1996).

In another publication involving this same study population, Longshore and Grills (1998) reported that drug problem recognition was most closely linked to conventional moral beliefs and neighborhood drug/alcohol problems. Collectively, these reports suggest that while the strengths of the association may vary, the desire for help, the motivation for drug abuse treatment, and drug problem recognition among some African Americans are linked to neighborhood drug/alcohol problems and conventional moral beliefs.

Admittedly, these studies certainly have their limitations. First, because they were conducted among African-American arrestees, it is difficult to generalize to other African-American populations in other geographical locations. Second, some may argue that the findings are at best relevant to populations who are already drug users and may have little benefit to interventions among African Americans who are not current drug users. With respect to the first issue, the investigators admit that there is critical need to replicate their investigations in other African-American communities. As for the second limitation, it is true that drug abuse interventions involving current drug users may meet the strict public health definition of primary prevention. However, some variables associated with drug initiation also influence continued drug use. Additionally, to the extent that initiation of drug use is associated with exposure to current drug users, effective interventions among current drug users may be viewed as primary prevention of drug use among persons who are not current users. Taken together with well-known and previously described medical, social, and economic complications of alcohol and drug abuse, any interventions that halt continued drug use among current drug users have unequivocal public health benefits. Finally, the UCLA studies, as a group, are among the first to demonstrate that Africentric values have an influence on the motivation for drug abuse treatment. The question that remains is what is the extent to which Africentric values influence consumption of substance abuse prevention and desirable outcomes to these same interventions.

Because of these issues, some have suggested a dramatically different approach since previous approaches lack the potential to uncover significant differences among racial and ethnic populations. As Gordon (1985) stipulates, "the search for universals has inhibited rather than enhanced the encirclement of social science knowledge." The resources necessary to pursue a more culturally sensitive, relevant, and competent direction may be substantial, given the ethnic and racial diversity of the United States.

The inclusion of an Africentric approach, recognizing the burdens experienced by and the strengths of African Americans, has been recommended for substance abuse-related interventions targeting African Americans. Advocates contend that this approach will offer the best prospects for improving current prevention programs and for ensuring that the next generation of prevention programs is more receptive to the wide range of issues relevant to Americans of African descent.

The Africentric (or Afrocentric) approach has been defined by Amuleru-Marshall (1992), Rowe and Grills (1993), and Grills and Longshore (1996) as theory and practice rooted in the cultural image. Africentrism is based on the seven principles or the *Nguzo Saba*. These include:

1. *Umoja* (Unity)—to strive for and maintain unity in the family, community, nation, and race;
2. *Kujichagulia* (Self-determination)—to define ourselves, name ourselves, create for ourselves, and speak for ourselves instead of being defined, named, created for, and spoken for by others;

3. *Ujima* (Collective work and responsibility)—to build and maintain our community together and make our sisters' and brothers' problems our problems and to solve them together;

4. *Ujamaa* (Cooperative economics)—to build and maintain our own stores, shops, and other businesses and to profit from them together;

5. *Nia* (Purpose)—to make our collective vocation the building and developing of our community to restore our people to their traditional greatness;

6. *Kuumba* (Creativity)—to do always as much as we can, in the way we can, to leave our community more beautiful and beneficial than we inherited it; and

7. *Imani* (Faith)—to believe with all our heart in our people, our parents, our teachers, and the righteousness and victory of our struggle.

Advocates contend that this approach has the interest of African people with reaffirming life experiences, history, values, and traditions as the foundation for analyzing, interpreting, and transforming individual and collective reality. Expressing a high level of agreement, many African-American social scientists have identified certain cultural attributes as indigenous to the African life experience (Dixon, 1976; Kambon, 1992; Myers, 1988; Nobles, 1991). Communalism or collectivism, cooperation and interdependence, spirituality, eldership, and intergenerational connectedness are among the components of an Afrocentric world view. (For a comprehensive discussion of these ideas, see Ani, 1994.)

As advocates further contend, these themes provide a framework from which prevention messages can be developed. The notion that the individual is subservient to the collective offers alternative approaches to conventional appeals to individual interests. It also provides an opportunity to shift attention away from individual rights and to the well-being of the collective. Similarly, cooperation and interdependence emphasize responsibility to others and do not pit an individual's interests against those of others. One's life obligates one to those who have gone before and those who follow. Finally, an emphasis on the nature of human existence as fundamentally spiritual has implications for primary, secondary, and tertiary interventions, including bereavement and the preparation for dying. Despite all of its virtues, advocates must admit that there is a paucity of published reports evaluating interventions using an Africentric approach. This is primarily because this approach has not enjoyed the financial support of other more traditional methods.

Fortunately, there are a few published studies among African Americans testing substance abuse interventions that include Africentric principles and that deserve discussion. In a sample of 222 African-American drug users, Longshore, Grills, and Annon (in press), randomly assigned some subjects to either the experimental condition of an Engagement Project or a control condition of referral based on a comprehensive needs assessment. The Engagement Project is a culturally-congruent, one-time intervention of a meal, a video about African-American accomplishments, and focused dyadic counseling (involving the client, a peer, and a counselor), using the technique of motivational interviewing and based on Africentric principles. Using a multi-item questionnaire containing six domains (involvement, counselor rapport, motivation, participation, disclosure, and preparation), these investigators reported that subjects assigned to the Engagement Project scored significantly higher on the involvement, motivation, participation, disclosure, and preparation domains. The researchers admit that they cannot predict whether their findings will be sustained over time or which components of the Engagement Project were responsible for the beneficial effects. In addition, it is not clear from where their African-American drug using subjects were recruited, so it is difficult to determine the extent to which the findings can be generalized. Furthermore, since the researchers did not provide any information on the length of the Engagement Project or the control condition, it might be said that length of the Engagement Project and not its components were responsible for its effects. Nonetheless, the study offers additional evidence that an Africentric drug abuse intervention can be beneficial among African-American drug users.

Perhaps because of the limitations of the above study, the investigators pursued their research with a larger sample (364 African-American drug users not in treatment) and evaluated the effects after a year using the same type of Africentric intervention (personal communications). Self-reported drug use at the one-year follow-up period was the criterion measure. Unadjusted drug use rates after one year was greater for the subjects randomly assigned to the control condition than among those assigned to the experimental condition. This study also contained some of the limitations of their prior study, especially as it pertains to the ability to generalize to other populations of African Americans and to determine which components of the intervention were responsible for the observed effects. Additionally, it is not clear whether the researchers assessed any of the subjects for other factors that might explain their findings. For example, the experimental subjects might have enrolled in drug abuse treatment to a greater extent or length as compared to the control subjects. Even so, this study extended the range of areas in which cultural congruence can enhance the effectiveness of interventions.

EVALUATION OF EXISTING PREVENTION EFFORTS

Only a small fraction of substance abuse programs contain evaluation components and an even smaller number of these evaluation efforts have found their way to publication. Lack of funding is certainly a significant problem in the evaluation of prevention efforts. Unfortunately, this is not the only limitation.

Many prevention programs fail to fully describe the population targeted and the context in which the targeted population is engaged. The size of the population and the lack of diversity in the targeted population often limit the extent to which one can extrapolate the results to other populations. There is also often inadequate information about the manner in which the targeted population is selected; there is often no comparative population.

The choice of outcome measures and bias in the ascertainment of outcome measures are additional problems. Most prevention programs only focus on short-term or individual outcomes when long-term outcomes and the use of the community as the unit of outcome measure are particularly more potent and more meaningful. While self-reported changes in behaviors are potentially valuable, reliance on self-reported change in behaviors has its limitations, especially for stigmatized behaviors.

Prevention programs also must clarify whether the efforts are targeted at primary prevention (before persons become drug users), secondary prevention (preventing complications of drug use), and/or tertiary prevention (reducing the mortality rate of drug abuse associated medical complications).

Just as important in understanding prevention programs is an appreciation of the actual intervention utilized. Unfortunately, few published reports of prevention programs provide an adequate description of the intervention(s) used or any concurrent phenomenon that may influence the impact of the intervention.

CONCLUSIONS

Substance abuse continues to be an issue of critical concern for Americans of African descent. Epidemiological data demonstrate that alcohol, tobacco, and use of illegal drugs is appreciable among African Americans. African Americans sustain a disproportionately greater range and level of consequences associated with substance abuse, yet little information is available about the extent to which these epidemiological sources represent use, abuse, or dependence on alcohol and illicit drugs among African Americans. Thus, it is necessary to commit an adequate level of resources to determine the extent to which currently used national surveys represent the magnitude of alcohol and illicit drug use, abuse, and dependence in African-American communities. It is just as important to assess the utility of epidemiological techniques in gathering the same types of data across various racial and ethnic populations. And it is crucial to encourage secondary analyses to separate race/ethnicity from markers of poverty and chronic economic underdevelopment.

Substance abuse among African Americans represents a pivotal pathway for a vast array of social and medical sequelae, including HIV infection and AIDS. Therefore, a better understanding is crucial of the relationships between African-American substance abuse and the medical, social, and economic consequences of substance abuse. The importance of this information for developing and evaluating prevention programs for African Americans is unquestionable.

There is a need to know the limitations of currently available data on the prevalence of substance abuse among African Americans. Without this information, the substrate of data underlying prevention efforts will remain limited. The life threatening implications of substance abuse make it untenable to postpone prevention efforts until adequate information is available to guide substance abuse-related interventions.

Some signs of hope are on the horizon. Some prevention efforts rely on sociogenetic perspectives (as suggested by the work of Grills and colleagues, 1996), as opposed to more individualistic psychological approaches. The use of peers or outreach workers is an example of prevention efforts based on social networks. Whether this approach will enhance the effectiveness of prevention programs with African Americans remains to be seen. Including gender and cultural issues, removing socioeconomic barriers that challenge participation in prevention efforts, and recognizing the legacy of discrimination will strengthen the likelihood that prevention efforts will be effective with African Americans.

REFERENCES

Amuleru-Marshall, O. (1991). African Americans. In J. Kinney (Ed.), *Clinical Manual of Substance Abuse,* Mosby-Year Books: St. Louis, MO.

Amuleru-Marshall, O. (1992). Nurturing the black adolescent male: culture, ethnicity and race. In L. W. Abramczyk and J. W. Ross (Eds.), *Nurturing the Black Adolescent Male in the Family Context: A Public Health Responsibility,* University of South Carolina College of Social Work: Columbia, SC.

Amuleru-Marshall, O. (1995). Introduction. In O. Amuleru-Marshall (Ed.), *Substance Abuse Treatment in the Era of AIDS* (pp. 1-16), Volume II.

Ani, M. Yurugu (1994). *An African-Centered Critique of European Cultural Thought and Behavior.* African World Press, Inc.: Trenton, NJ.

Auerbach, J. D., Wypijewska, C., and Brodie, H. K. H., Eds. (1994). *AIDS and Behavior: An Integrated Approach.* National Research Council, National Academy Press: Washington, D.C.

Bell, P. (1990). *Chemical Dependency and the African American, Counseling Strategies and Community Issues.* Hazelden Foundation: Center City, MN.

Bolton, R., Vincke, J. and Mak, R. (1992). Alcohol and risky sex in search of an elusive connection. *Medical Anthropology,* 14:323-363.

Brown, L. S. (1981). Substance abuse and America, historical perspective on the federal response to a social phenomenon. *Journal of the National Medical Association,* 73:497-505.

Brown, L. S. (1993). Alcohol abuse prevention in African-American communities. *Journal of the National Medical Association,* 85:665-673.

Brown, L. S. and Alterman, A. I. (1992). African Americans. In J. G. Lowinson, P. Ruiz and R. B. B. Millman (Eds.), *Substance Abuse: A Comprehensive Textbook* (pp. 861-867). 2nd ed. Williams and Wilkins: Baltimore, MD.

Brown, L. S., Murphy, D. L. and Primm, B. J. (1988). The acquired immunodeficiency syndrome: Do drug dependence and ethnicity share a common pathway. In L. Harris (Ed.), *Problems of Drug Dependence 1987. Proceedings of the 49th Annual Scientific Meeting. Committee on Problems of Drug Dependence* (pp. 188-94). NIDA Research Monograph 81, DHHS Publication No. (ADM) 888-1564.

Brown, L. S. and Primm, B. J. (1998). Intravenous drug abuse and AIDS in minorities. *AIDS and Public Policy,* 3:5-15.

Centers for Disease Control and Prevention (1993). *HIV/AIDS Surveillance Report.* US Department of Health and Human Services, Center for Disease Control and Prevention: Washington, D.C.

Coates, T. J., Des Jarlais, D. C., Miller, H. G., Moses, L E., Turner, C. F. and Worth, D. (1988). The AIDS epidemic in the second decade. In H.G. Miller, C. F. Turner and L. E. Moses (Eds.), *AIDS: The Second Decade* (pp. 38-80). National Research Council, National Academy Press: Washington, D.C.

Cochran, S. D. and Mays, V. M. (1993). Applying social psychological models for predicting HIV-related sexual risk behaviors among African Americans. *Journal of Black Psychology* 19:142-154.

Cummings, S. (1969). Family socialization and fatalism among black adolescents. *Journal of Social Issues,* 25:13-27.

De La Cancela, V. (1992). Minority AIDS prevention: Moving beyond cultural perspectives towards sociopolitical empowerment. *AIDS Education and Prevention,* 1:141-153.

Dixon, V. (1976). Worldviews and research methodology. In L. King, V. Dixon and W. W. Nobles (Eds.), *African Philosophy: Assumptions and Paradigms for Research on Black Persons.* Fanon Center Publication, Charles Drew Postgraduate Medical School: Los Angeles, CA.

Gordon, E. W. (1985). Social science: Knowledge production and minority experience. *Journal of Negro Education,* 54:117-133.

Grills, C. and Longshore, D. (1996). Africentrism: Psychometric analyses of a self-report measure. *Journal of Black Psychology,* 22:86-106.

Herd, D. (1989). The epidemiology of drinking patterns and alcohol-related problems among US blacks. In *The Epidemiology of Alcohol Use and Abuse among US Minorities* (pp. 12-21). U.S. Government Printing Office, DHHS Publication No. (ADM) 8-1402: Washington, D.C.

Jenkins, B., Lamar, V. L. and Thompson-Crumble, J. (1993). AIDS among African Americans: A social epidemic. *Journal of Black Psychology,* 19(2):108-122.

John, S., Brown, L. S., Jr. and Primm, B. J. (1997). African Americans: Epidemiologic, prevention, and treatment issues. In J. H. Lowinson, P. Ruiz, R. B. Millman and J. G. Langrod (Eds.), *Substance Abuse: A Comprehensive Textbook* (pp. 699-705). 3rd ed. Williams and Wilkins.

Johnson, B. J. and Nishi, J. M. (1976). Myths and realities of drug use by minorities. In P. Iiyama, J. M. Nishi and B. D. Johnson (Eds.), *Drug Use and Abuse among US Minorities.* Praeger Publications.

Kambon, K. K. K. (1992). *The African Personality in America: An African-Centered Framework*. Nubian Nation Publications: Tallahassee, FL.

Leigh, B. and Stall, R. (1993). Substance use and risky sexual behavior for exposure to HIV: Issues in methodology, interpretation and prevention. *American Psychologist*, October: 1035-1045.

Longshore, D., Grills, C., Anglin, M. D. and Annon, K. (1997). Desire for help among African American drug-users. *Journal of Drug Issues*, 27(4):755-770.

Longshore, D., Grills, C., Anglin, M. D. and Annon, K. (1998). Treatment motivation among African American drug-using arrestees. *Journal of Black Psychology*, 24: 126-144.

Longshore, D., Grills, C. and Annon, K. (in press). Effects of a culturally congruent intervention on cognitive factors relevant to drug use recovery. *Substance Use and Misuse*.

Longshore, D., Grills, C., Annon, K. and Grady, R. (1998). Promoting recovery from drug abuse: An Africentric intervention. *Journal of Black Studies*, 28(3):319-333.

Maddox, G. and Borinski, E. (1964). Drinking behavior in Negro collegians. *Quarterly Journal of Studies of Alcohol*, 25:651-668.

Mays, V. M. (1989). AIDS prevention in Black populations: Methods of a safer kind. In V. M. Mays, G. Albee and S. Schneider (Eds.), *Primary Prevention of AIDS* (pp. 264-279). Newbury Park, CA.

Mays, V. M. and Cochran, S. D. (1988). Issues in the perception of AIDS risk reduction activities by Black and Hispanic/Latina women. *American Psychologist*, 43: 949-957.

Miller, H. G., Turner, C. F. and Moses, L. E. (1990). *AIDS: The Second Decade*. National Research Council, National Academy Press: Washington, D.C.

Myers, L. J. (1988). *Understanding an Afrocentric World View: Introduction to an Optimal Psychology*. Kendall/Hunt Publishing Co.: Dubuque, IA.

National Commission on AIDS. (1991) *Report: The Twin Epidemics of Substance Abuse and HIV*. National Commission on AIDS: Washington, D.C.

National Institute on Drug Abuse (1988a). *National Household Survey on Drug Abuse: Main Findings 1985*. DHHS Publication No. (ADM) 88-1586. Superintendent of Documents, U.S. Government Printing Office: Washington, D.C.

National Institute on Drug Abuse (1988b). *Illicit Drug Use, Smoking and Drinking by America's High School Students, College Students, and Young Adults (1975-1987)*. DHHS Publication No. (ADM) 89-1602. Superintendent of Documents, U.S. Government Printing Office: Washington, D.C.

National Institute on Alcohol Abuse and Alcoholism (1990). *Seventh Special Report to the US Congress on Alcohol and Health*. U.S. Government Printing Office, DHHS Publication No. (ADM) 281-880002: Rockville, MD.

National Institute on Drug Abuse (1990). Substance abuse among blacks in the U.S. *NIDA Capsules*, February.

National Institute on Drug Abuse (1995). Drug use among racial/ethnic minorities. NIH Publication No. 95-3888.

Nobles, W. W. (1991). African philosophy: Foundations for black psychology. In R. L. Jones (Ed.), *Black Psychology*, 3rd ed. Cobb & Henry Publishers: Berkeley, CA.

184 / SUBSTANCE ABUSE PREVENTION

Novotny, T. E, Warner, K. E., Kendrick, J. S. and Remington, P. L. (1988). Smoking by Blacks and Whites: Socioeconomic and demographic differences. *American Journal of Public Health*, 78:1187-1189.

Robins, L. N. and Murphy, G. E. (1967). Drug use in a normal population of young Negro men. *American Journal of Public Health*, 57:1580-1596.

Rouse, B. (1989). *Drug Abuse Among Racial/Ethnic Minorities: A Special Report*. National Institute on Drug Abuse: Rockville, MD.

Rowe, D. and Grills, C. (1993). African-centered drug treatment: An alternative conceptual paradigm for drug counseling with African American clients. *Journal of Psychoactive Drugs*, 25(1):21-33.

Schilling, R. F., Schninke, S. P., Nichols, S. E., Zayas, L. H., Miller, S. O., Orlandi, M. A. and Botvin, G.J. (1989). Developing strategies for AIDS prevention research with Black and Hispanic drug users. *Public Health Reports*, 104:2-11.

Thomas, S. and Quinn S. (1991). The Tuskegee syphilis study, 1932 to 1972: Implications for HIV education and AIDS risk education programs in the black community. *American Journal of Public Health*, 81:1498-1505.

Thompson-Fullilove, M., Fullilove, R. E., Haynes, K. and Gross, S. (1990). Black women and AIDS prevention: A view towards understanding the gender rules. *Journal of Sex Research*, 27:47-64.

Tucker, M. B. (1985). US ethnic minorities and drug abuse: An assessment of the science and practice. *International Journal of Addiction*, 20:1021-1047.

Worth, D. (1989). Sexual decision making and AIDS: Why condom promotion among vulnerable women is likely to fail. *Studies in Family Planning*, 20:297-307.

Wyatt, G. D. (1985). The sexual abuse of Afro-American and White American women in childhood. *Child Abuse and Neglect*, 9:507-519.

CHAPTER 8

The Complexities of Diversity: Substance Abuse Among Asian Americans

Saskia Karen Subramanian and
David Takeuchi*

The abuse of and dependence upon alcohol and other legal and illegal substances is a pervasive social and economic problem in the United States. The National Comorbidity Study (NCS), a large-scale investigation of over 8,000 survey respondents between the ages of fifteen to fifty-five, estimated that about one in four residents in the United States had experienced some substance abuse or dependence disorder in their lifetime; 11 percent had the disorder within the twelve months prior to the interview. Males had at least double the risk for having a substance abuse problem than females. The lifetime and current prevalence rates for males were 35 percent and 16 percent compared to 18 percent and 7 percent for females. As expected, alcohol abuse was the most prevalent substance abuse problem. Though men had higher rates than women for alcohol and drug problems, the prevalence pattern for both were quite similar (e.g., alcohol problems were higher than drug problems). While individuals use and abuse substances, the consequences that accrue because of their addiction and dependence has an imposing presence over close relationships and society in general. For example, the social and economic costs of substance abuse is estimated at $150 billion a year (Zane and Kim, 1994).

*The authors gratefully acknowledge the research assistance of Mary Hurst.

Alcohol and other drug (AOD) abuse has become conspicuous across different demographic groups (e.g., socioeconomic status, race, and ethnicity, etc.). It is hardly surprising, then, that research on the prevention and treatment of AOD has increased substantially in recent decades. Discrepancies exist, however, in the amount of research conducted on different ethnic groups. For the most part, empirical investigations on AODs has focused primarily on White and African-American populations. More specifically, the proportion of investigations focusing on Asian Americans has not matched the growth rate of this group.

The population surge of Asian Americans over the past three decades must be taken within context of the overall demographic transformations that the United States has undergone. Immigration accounts for a large part of the demographic change in the United States. Because of various immigration laws and policies over the past two decades, more than ten million people have come to the United States—an increase that matches the rise in the immigrant population in the early part of this century. Of course, this figure does not consider the magnitude of undocumented migrants, which could increase this figure by about two million (Muller, 1993). Approximately four out of five immigrants have settled in large urban areas such as Los Angeles, Boston, San Francisco, New York, Miami, and Washington D.C. (Portes and Rumbaut, 1990). A major difference between the rise in the immigrant population in the early 1900s and the current increase is the countries from which immigrants have come. In the early part of the 1900s, most of the immigrants moved from Europe and Canada; the recent immigrants have come primarily from Asia and Latin America. Muller (1993) notes that these patterns have led to a change in the racial composition of the United States unseen since the late seventeenth century when Black slaves became part of the labor force in the south.

As a result of immigration patterns, Asian Americans have become a visible presence in the United States, especially in major urban areas. In 1980, the population of Asian Americans exceeded 3.7 million, easily doubling the 1.5 million figure in 1970. By 1990 the population nearly doubled again by exceeding 7.1 million. It is estimated that by the end of the twenty-first century, Asian/Pacific Islanders will constitute about 12 percent of the US population, while Blacks will represent nearly 15 percent and Hispanics will constitute 23 percent (Bouvier and Gardner, 1986). Over half (56%) of Asian/Pacific Islanders live in the West. The ethnic groups that comprise this category are quite diverse in terms of cultural background, country of origin, and circumstances for coming to the United States. For example, more than twenty ethnic groups, speaking one of more than thirty different languages, are included in the Asian-American category (O'Hare and Felt, 1991). The three largest Asian-American ethnic groups are Chinese, Japanese, and Filipino. Koreans and Southeast Asians (e.g., Vietnamese, Cambodians, Laotians) also comprise a significant proportion of the Asian-American population. The three largest groups among Pacific Islanders are Native Hawaiians, Samoans, and Chamorros (Guamanians) (Asian Week, 1991).

Given these demographic changes, there is little question that Asian Americans and immigrants are increasingly comprising a rather substantial segment of society. However, relatively little is known about this population with regard to the types and prevalence of social problems that Asian communities face, including the extensiveness of AOD abuse. Even with data that are available, not much effort has been expended in attempting to understand the underlying structures and causes. All too frequently when considering social problems such as substance abuse, we find ourselves reporting statistics rather than examining the social forces that cause vulnerability and risk among certain populations. Furthermore, prevention and treatment programs designed to address AOD abuse often lack socio-cultural components that clearly address the needs of minority populations. This chapter endeavors to bridge practice with theory by: discussing substance abuse patterns in Asian groups through a review of current representative research on substance abuse that does include Asians, as well as the few studies that have explored abuse within Asian subpopulations; examining the social forces that seem to increase risk for certain Asian subgroups; considering how an understanding of abuse patterns and socio-cultural factors can help to inform prevention strategies; and, suggesting some future directions for research in this area. Zane and Kim (1994) and Kuramoto (1997) provide more exhaustive reviews of the specific studies and their findings; our modest contribution is to identify some key themes in previous investigations and to indicate some potential directions for future research in order to advance a new generation of studies on substance abuse in Asian-American communities.

PREVIOUS RESEARCH

Most studies maintain that Asian Americans have lower rates of substance use and abuse than do Whites and African Americans. For example, in a study comparing the drinking patterns of Asian and White college students, Asians drank less, abstained more frequently, and reported fewer drinking problems than Whites (O'Hare, 1995). Data from the High School Seniors Survey indicate that Asian-American students had the lowest use of marijuana—less than half that of Whites—and matched African Americans in having the lowest annual usage of cigarettes and alcohol (Johnston, O'Malley, and Bachman, 1991). A composite analysis of fifty-three U.S. surveys collecting data on alcohol, tobacco, and other drug use by youth between 1985 and 1991 reported that "Blacks and Asians typically are the lowest using groups" (Pollard, 1993).

However, a few studies indicate that Asian Americans may, in fact, have far higher rates of usage than previously believed—in some cases paralleling their White counterparts. Kim and colleagues (1992) assert, with regard to heavy drinking, that Asian-American youth are comparable to White youth. Lifetime prevalence studies of adolescents—over the age period of twelve to eighteen—

show that Blacks and Asians "catch up" to their White peers in terms of alcohol experimentation (Pollard, 1993). A county-wide study in North Carolina revealed that Asian/Pacific Islanders used barbiturates, cocaine, and amphetamines at rates equaling or surpassing non-Asians in the sample (Kim, McLeod, and Shantzis, 1992). The use of illicit drugs among Asian students exceeded that of African Americans and Hispanics in a west coast study that also determined that Asians tended to initiate substance abuse through illicit drugs, later followed by tobacco and alcohol consumption (Ellickson, Hayes, and Bell, 1992).

A small body of research has investigated substance abuse patterns across ethnic subgroups within the Asian population. One such study (McLaughlin, et al., 1987) found that "there is not a consistently clear pattern of predictors of alcohol and other drug use among Asian Americans. That is to say, all Asian Americans are not alike in their patterns of alcohol and other drug use or in their attributes that appear to be predictive of substance use." Studies on the drinking patterns of Chinese, Japanese, Korean, and Filipino respondents (Chi, Lubben, and Kitano, 1989; Kitano and Chi, 1985) illustrate wide variance across different Asian groups in percent of heavy drinkers, with Japanese having the highest percentage and Chinese having the lowest. The 1991 California Student Substance Abuse Survey, which sampled students from approximately fifty high schools across the state, determined, for cigarette and alcohol consumption, that Pacific Islanders reported the highest usage rates, followed by Koreans, Filipinos, Japanese, Southeast Asians, and Chinese. Similar patterns were seen in an analysis of illegal drug use, with the exception of Southeast Asians, who ranked first in use of cocaine and high in their use of amphetamines (Kuramoto, 1997).

That there is variation in rates and patterns of usage indicates that a variety of socio-cultural forces moderate the extent to which various Asian subgroups are at risk of AOD abuse. While not exhaustive, the following section discusses some factors that should be considered with regard to Asian populations' risk propensity.

Acculturation and Social Isolation

While arguments persist over whether the rates of AOD use among Asian Americans are lower or higher than other comparison groups, some investigators have moved beyond the examination of prevalence into understanding the social and cultural factors that may explain ethnic differences. Because immigrants comprise a large proportion of the Asian-American ethnic category, a key construct in examining the heterogeneity within and between the group and others is acculturation. Acculturation represents changes in cultural attitudes, values, and behaviors that are the result of the interaction between two distinct cultures (Berry, Trimble, and Olmedo, 1986). The focus of acculturation has been on how minority or immigrant groups relate to the dominant (or host) society (Phinney, 1990). The term "acculturation" appears prominently in the social science literature to explain the social and psychological adaptation of immigrants and groups who live apart from the mainstream society (e.g., American Indians who live on reservations). Acculturation began as a promising construct because researchers speculated that the adaptation of immigrants to a new society created many adjustment problems.

Empirical results about acculturation and AOD is mixed. With regard to Asian populations, however, the polar extremes of acculturation both impact likelihood of substance use. On the one end of the spectrum, there is evidence that "Asians' use of alcohol and other substances appears to increase with entry into mainstream American life" (Austin and Pollard, 1993; Austin, Prendergast, and Lee, 1989; D'Avanzo, Frye, and Froman, 1994; see also Johnson and Nagoshi, 1990; Kuramoto, 1997; Sue, Zane, and Ito, 1979). While this is generally thought to be a result of the attenuation of traditional norms disapproving of drug and alcohol use, it is also likely that highly acculturated Asians who have internalized Western goals and expectations, but are constrained from significant attainment due to institutional barriers, will engage in withdrawal behaviors such as retreatism. Described by Merton (1968) as a modality by which individuals reconcile high aspirations with constrained cultural means, retreatism through the use of drugs and alcohol represents a release mechanism for acculturated individuals who are frustrated by social limitations entrenched in discrimination.

On the other end of the acculturation spectrum, however, the abuse of substances is also more prevalent for socially isolated immigrants with low levels of acculturation (Austin, Prendergast, and Lee, 1989; Cheung, 1993; D'Avanzo, Frye, and Froman, 1994; Yee and Thu, 1987). Migration to the United States profoundly affects the basic construct of social life for immigrants, particularly in the cases of older individuals. Many emigrate with the belief that they will be afforded greater economic opportunities; however, unanticipated to some, the transition from the relatively homogenous culture of their homeland to one characterized by great complexity and heterogeneity effectively engenders a sense of dislocation, isolation, and normlessness. Tonnies (1887, 1963) defined the former society as one supporting "gemeinshaft" relations (community oriented, intimate) as opposed to the "gesellschaft" interactions (impersonal, heterogeneous, formal) found in the city. The alienation felt by some immigrants can have profound negative impacts and result in a range of behaviors, including the use and abuse of substances to mitigate loneliness and anomie.

Mental Illness

In the general population, "substance abusers exhibit higher rates of psychiatric symptoms than nonclinical populations" (Kendall, Sherman, and Bigelow, 1995). There is some indication that drugs and alcohol may be used for self-medication by Asians who are experiencing psychiatric symptoms but who do not seek help for a variety of reasons (McLaughlin, et al., 1987), including fear of "losing face" in the community and reluctance to use services where only English is spoken (Bui and Takeuchi, 1992). While many studies have shown that Asians tend to be underrepresented in psychiatric clinics and hospitals (Bui and Takeuchi, 1992; Cheung and Snowden, 1990; Sue, 1994; Sue, et al., 1991), other research has found that Asians score higher on some measures of psychiatric disturbance than do their White counterparts (Crystal, 1989; see also Sue, 1994). If indeed Asians are more reluctant to enter into psychiatric treatment despite symptoms, they may be alternatively coping through the use of alcohol, street drugs, and/or prescription drugs. Refugee populations may be at greatest risk for such behaviors given the level of trauma experienced before immigration to the United States as well as the difficulty of managing the stresses of living in a new country (Austin, Prendergast, and Lee, 1989; Yee and Thu, 1987; Zane and Kim, 1994); one survey indicated that Southeast Asian refugees needed mental health services at a rate of 11.7 percent, with Cambodians requiring such services at a rate of 34 percent (Cheung and Snowden, 1990).

Stigma and a "Conspiracy of Silence"

A major impediment in accurately identifying substance abuse in Asian populations is the unwillingness of abusers, and often too of their family members, to acknowledge that a problem exists (Austin, Prendergast, and Lee, 1989): "because drug abuse and dependency are considered to be a serious breach of behavior within most of these groups, acknowledging this problem often leads to a significant loss of face for both the individuals in question and their families . . . consequently, both the family and the community itself may avoid or deny the behaviors in question at an intensity beyond the levels of denial usually associated with substance abuse" (Ja and Aoki, 1993). Denial, in fact, was cited as a significant obstacle to seeking treatment by key informants (Hatanaka, et. al., 1991, summarized in Kuramoto, 1997) from six Asian populations: Chinese, Japanese, Korean, Pacific Islander, Filipino, and Southeast Asians.

Immigrant Youth and Loss of Social Control

Studies have shown that, in general, Asian youth are less likely to engage in substance abuse due to peer pressure than are other youth (Austin and Pollard, 1993, pp. 27, 39; Austin, Prendergast, and Lee, 1989). Parental disapproval, on the other hand, strongly influences decisions to abstain or moderate substance use (Johnson and Nagoshi, 1990). As such, the family can represent an important locus of behavior modification for Asian children. The process of immigration, however, can greatly diminish familial ties and concurrent social control. Those youth who come to America with their families may find that their parents and other household adults are forced to work multiple jobs and/or long hours, effectively forcing offspring to be "latchkey children" with little supervision. Similar social dislocation can be experienced by children sent to the United States whose families remain in their homeland: housed with strangers or distant relatives, these youth may also experience elevated risk for substance abuse as parental influence is absent.

The "Model Minority"

Typically, Asians living in America are considered a "model minority": their "apparently successful efforts at assimilation, achieved with a minimum of discomfort to the dominant culture," coupled with the stereotypical traits assigned to them such as intelligence, willingness to sacrifice and work hard, and trustworthiness, has led Asians to be viewed as "an exemplary group of . . . citizens" (Crystal, 1989). Unfortunately, this depiction of Asians as a model minority has served to obscure not only substance abuse issues for this group, but also has minimized other social problems such as poverty and unemployment. Reports of median family incomes by race, for example, have depicted Asians as more successful than Whites, while in fact Asian households tend to have more workers per household. Additionally, while poverty rates tend to be low for Asians, the Asian poor are disproportionately represented by female-headed families and the elderly. Immigrants, portrayed by the mass media as embodying the American dream through rags-to-riches stories, often continue to experience significant economic hardship after several years in the United States: for Indochinese refugees arriving in the 1980s, for example, 55 percent of the households relied on public assistance and 32 percent were below the poverty level after more than four years in the United States (Gould, 1988).

The net result of the model minority myth is that it has effectively disenfranchised Asian immigrants and Asian Americans from forms of social welfare and attention that would otherwise ameliorate certain conditions. Specifically with regard to substance abuse prevention programming, this stereotype has reinforced perceptions of Asians as not being at risk for AOD abuse and has resulted in a striking absence of initiatives and services directed toward Asians. Presumably, then, high-risk Asians are even more disadvantaged than their White counterparts in that few treatment and prevention resources are allocated to these populations.

PREVENTION CONSIDERATIONS

As previously discussed, Asians may be unwilling to seek treatment for AOD addictions. The emphasis on shame in Asian culture, which at the extreme can inhibit treatment seeking altogether, needs to be addressed in dealing with potential AOD abuse in this population. Some clinicians feel that, because of their desire to minimize shameful situations, Asian clients prefer short-term treatment oriented toward problem solving (Berg and Miller, 1992). Additionally, those who do enter into treatment programs may only be willing to do so for a short time (Berg and Miller, 1992); one program in San Francisco noted that "[m]ost Asian patients . . . did not complete their treatment episodes" (Perez-Arce, Carr, and Sorensen, 1993). Short term or incomplete substance abuse treatment, however, may do very little of consequence. As such, it can be imagined that prevention initiatives may represent a more functional social service for Asian populations.

There are, however, few prevention and treatment initiatives directed specifically toward Asian populations. A 1986 analysis of 143 prevention programs revealed that only 4 percent of the program effects dealt with minorities (Austin and Pollard, 1993, p. 34). Additionally, although it is generally agreed by experts in the field that drug prevention programs should include "family, background variables, cultural and ethnic values" (Maddahian, Newcomb, and Bentler, 1988), there is little consensus as to how this should be accomplished. Ideally, research should inform prevention initiatives in order to maximize their effectiveness within target populations. While AOD research on Asian populations is far from extensive, previous studies do indicate that certain Asian subpopulations may be at greater risk for substance abuse; hence, it may be helpful in designing and implementing prevention initiatives to directly address some of the issues associated with increased risk.

For example, although some professionals in the field believe that ethnic minority clients are unconcerned about the ethnic origin of social service providers (Berg and Jaya, 1993) and indeed maintain that clients may prefer to meet with someone outside of their community in order to preserve privacy, there is a great deal of evidence that culturally appropriate outreach and service provision makes a difference to Asian populations. A number of studies have shown that services where only English is spoken are underutilized by Asian Americans who do not speak English as a first language (Bui and Takeuchi, 1992; Sue, et al., 1991). Additionally, "in an evaluation of ethnic minority staffing, Wu and Windle (1980) found that a minority staff presence predicted minority utilization" (Cheung and Snowden, 1990). Employing a strategy that utilizes ethnically similar staff as well as culturally sensitive curricula that reinforce norms and values specific to the Asian subgroup being targeted should yield greater responsiveness on the part of the clients.

Another issue lies in the accurate identification and appropriate treatment of mental illness for certain Asian groups. It is assumed that refugees may be most at risk for psychopathology due to their experiences both prior to emigration as well as to the difficulty of adjusting to life in the United States; given that mental health services are poorly utilized by Asian groups and that there is some indication that Asians suffering from psychopathology may be self-medicating with AOD, much greater outreach must be made to recent immigrant populations. Strengthening informal support networks can be of great value in this effort: "workers should utilize . . . churches, ethnic clubs, and family associations as well as community leaders, such as priests, doctors, indigenous healers, and elders, in their work with

Asian clients" (Crystal, 1989). Research on the fallacy of the "model minority" suggests that this stereotype needs to be addressed. This strategy has two benefits. First, the acknowledgment that Asian clients face significant social and economic hardships, as do other minority populations, helps clients to identify substance abuse in part as a function of institutional stressors less than of personal weakness. This externalization may potentially diminish some of the denial and closeting associated with AOD abuse and allows for enhanced dialogue about substance abuse in the community. Second, publicizing data contradicting the model minority stereotype more widely may well help to turn public attention—and potentially some funding—to this much neglected area of research, prevention, and treatment.

Finally, there is some evidence that creating strong primary group associations for latchkey and parachute children may be effective in stemming AOD abuse. A study by Bankston (1995) on the effects of strong community ties in diminishing substance abuse practices found that community entrenchment and social integration can provide social control and support for young Asians and counterbalance risk. Asian children who do not have the benefit of parental or close familial interaction need to have other positive primary group associations. This can be accomplished through concerted efforts on the parts of schools and communities to provide mentoring, after-school supervision, and extracurricular activities run by respected community leaders and role models. There is evidence that "outreach programming targeted for Asian-American student populations may result in increased utilization rates for their dealing with . . . substance abuse concerns" (Solberg, et al., 1994). As such, greater effort should be made in the realm of school and community outreach.

FUTURE RESEARCH DIRECTIONS

Initial findings from research on Asian populations indicate that Asian AOD abuse is a far more complex issue than had been previously thought and worthy of careful study and consideration by researchers and policy makers alike. Based on existing studies, it seems likely that some Asian-American ethnic groups do have lower rates of use and abuse of some substances. This statement seems to contradict what we might expect of an ethnic minority group in the United States. Furthermore, the historical record suggests that Asian immigrants have not been strangers to the use of various substances. For example, some early Chinese settlers to the United States were addicted to opium (Ja and Aoki, 1993). The Narcotic Act of 1914 essentially eradicated opium use in America until its resurrection by Indochinese refugees in recent years (Westermeyer, et al., 1991). In addition, the strains of being an ethnic minority in the United States and, in the case of immigrants, the stressors they undergo to negotiate life in a new country may provide the context for using AOD to cope with everyday and episodic problems. Despite these conditions of life, if some Asian-American ethnic groups are less likely to use and abuse AOD, what truly accounts for this pattern? Past research, as noted above, offers us glimpses of the underlying causes, but it is clear that there remain ample avenues for research.

One possible research direction may lie in understanding community contexts in a more systematic manner than has been done in the past. Recently, Sampson, Raudenbush, and Earls (1997) conducted a study of 8782 residents of 343 neighborhoods in Chicago. The focus of their study was to identify the correlates of violent activities that occur in neighborhoods, and they tested the hypothesis that community level variables, in particular social cohesion and trust among neighbors, would have an independent effect over and beyond individual level variables (e.g., gender, marital status, homeownership, ethnicity, mobility patterns, age, and socioeconomic status). The investigators found that social cohesion was negatively associated with perceived violence in the neighborhood, victimization, and number of homicides committed in the neighborhood.

Some available evidence, as detailed in previous sections, suggests that social cohesion and social relationships in general may account for the low level of AOD use in Asian American communities (e.g., Bankston III, 1995; Johnson and Nagoshi, 1990). While these isolated studies provide important findings, it is clear that more can be done to identify the community factors that facilitate or constrain dysfunctional behaviors including AOD use and abuse. Moreover, it is important to develop a better understanding about how Asian-American communities differ or are similar to other types of communities in notions of social cohesion, trust, values, and other dimensions of social relationships. Much speculation has been made about the role of Asian constructs in shaping social relationships (e.g., "loss of face," "utang la loob," "amae"), but too few investigations have examined these constructs beyond individual relationships to how they shape broader community ties.

Related to issues involving community contexts and variations among communities is the consideration of other dependent variables beyond AOD. If Asian Americans in "high-risk" situations do not use or abuse AOD, do these "high-risk" situations lead to other types of problems? This research direction argues for the examination of multiple variables to better understand the social consequences of distress. Studies, for example, that focus exclusively on AOD at the expense of omitting other forms of individual problems (e.g., family violence, low self-esteem) may draw erroneous conclusions about how "vulnerable" or "resilient" some groups are when confronted with high-risk social conditions. An example of this point can be taken from literature on stress. Aneshensel, Rutter, and Lachenbruch (1991) take as a common finding that men and women have different rates of depression, which has eventually led to the conclusion that women are more vulnerable to stress than men. In analyses of the Epidemiological Catchment Area (ECA) data, the investigators find that stress is associated with depression for women and substance use among men. If only depression had been used as the outcome variable, the results would have supported the traditional explanation that women are more vulnerable than men. However, by including several outcomes, Aneshensel's analyses demonstrate that men and women are equally vulnerable to stress, but express their distress in very different ways. Aneshensel and her colleagues provide an excellent example of the different conclusions that can be drawn when single and multiple indicators of health are used.

Our final suggested area of research is in the area of response bias in reporting AOD use in survey research. A number of studies describe the unwillingness of abusers, and of their family members, to acknowledge that AOD problems may exist (see, for example, Austin, Prendergast, and Lee, 1989; Ja and Aoki, 1993; and Hatanaka, et. al., 1991, summarized in Kuramoto, 1997). Accordingly, more methodological studies are needed to identify (1) how cultural factors influence reports on AOD abuse, and (2) how questions about use/abuse might be asked in culturally appropriate ways that improve reporting. These types of studies will lend greater credibility when examining prevalence estimates across different ethnic groups.

CONCLUSION

Asian Americans have been included in few large scale AOD studies. When Asian Americans are considered, most data indicate that, as a population, this group has significantly lower rates of alcohol and other drug (AOD) abuse. More recently, however, social scientists have begun to acknowledge that the designation of Asian populations as low-risk for AOD abuse may be problematic for a number of reasons. The encompassing of many diverse and distinct populations under the broad category of "Asian," for example, potentially downplays the need for prevention and treatment initiatives that might be vitally important to certain subsets of the Asian population at greater risk for AOD abuse. Additionally, there is some indication that substance abuse among Asian populations may be greatly underreported as families mask drug and alcohol problems in order to avoid stigma. Because substance abuse is seen as little of a problem among Asian groups, few treatment and prevention resources are allocated to these populations to the detriment of those in need. Overall, Asian substance abuse is slowly being recognized as an underresearched and poorly understood phenomena in the United States.

Even if we were to conclude that AOD abuse is statistically less prevalent among Asian Americans and immigrants, substance abusers within this population are in far greater danger of not receiving the treatment services that they need because of the paucity of services dedicated to this group. Thus, the "needs of the few"—the at-risk Asian populations—are being sacrificed to the "needs of the many," but potentially at great social cost long term, particularly given the recent and projected population increases for Asian people.

Although the studies on Asian AOD abuse to date are extremely useful and often illuminating, there is no question that researchers, policy makers, and clinicians alike are still floundering in the proverbial dark when it comes to fully understanding the socio-cultural factors underlying the patterns of usage both within specific Asian populations as well as in contrast to White and other minority groups. More systematic research is warranted in this area as is the creation of linkages between data, social theory, and program interventions.

REFERENCES

Aneshensel, C., Rutter, C. and Lachenbruch, P. A. (1991). Social structure, stress and mental health: Competing conceptual and analytic models. *American Sociological Review*, 56:166-178.

Asian Week (1991). *Asians in America: 1990 Census Classification by States*. Asian Week: San Francisco.

Austin, G. and Pollard, J. A. (1993). *Substance Abuse and Ethnicity: Recent Research Findings*. Western Regional Center for Drug-Free Schools and Communities: Southwest Regional Laboratory: Portland, OR.

Austin, G., Prendergast, M. and Lee, H. (1989). *Substance Abuse Among Asian American Youth*. Western Regional Center for Drug-Free Schools and Communities: Portland, OR.

Bankston III, C. L. (1995). Vietnamese ethnicity and adolescent substance abuse: Evidence for a community level approach. *Deviant Behavior*, 16:59-80.

Berg, I. K. and Jaya, A. (1993). Different and same: Family therapy with Asian-American families. *Journal of Marital and Family Therapy*, 19(1):31-38.

Berg, I. K. and Miller, S. D. (1992). Working with Asian American clients: One person at a time. *Families in Society: The Journal of Contemporary Human Services*, June: 356-363.

Berry, J. W., Trimble, J. E. and Olmedo, E. L. (1986). Assessment of acculturation. In W.J. Lonner and J.W. Berry (Eds.), *US Field Methods in Cross-Cultural Research. Cross-Cultural Research and Methodology Series, Vol. 8*. Sage Publications: Beverly Hills, CA.

Bouvier, L. F. and Gardner, R. W. (1986). Immigration to the US: The unfinished story. *Population Bulletin*, 41(November):27.

Bui, K. V. and Takeuchi, D. (1992). Ethnic minority adolescents and the use of community mental health care services. *American Journal of Community Psychology*, 20(4): 403-417.

Cheung, Y. W. (1993). Beyond liver and culture: A review of theories and research in drinking among Chinese in North America. *The International Journal of the Addictions*, 28(14):1497-1513.

Cheung, F. and Snowden, L. (1990). Community mental health and ethnic minority populations. *Community Mental Health Journal*, 26(3):277-291.

Chi, I., Lubben, J. and Kitano, H. (1989). Differences in drinking behavior among three Asian American groups. *Journal of Studies on Alcohol*, 50:15-23.

Crystal, D. (1989). Asian Americans and the myth of the model minority. *Social Casework*, 70(7):405-413.

D'Avanzo, C., Frye, B. and Froman, R. (1994). Culture, stress, and substance use in Cambodian refugee women. *Journal of Studies on Alcohol*, 55(4):420-426.

Ellickson, P., Hayes, R. and Bell, R. (1992). Stepping through the drug use sequence. *Journal of Abnormal Psychology*, 101(3):441-451.

Gould, K. (1988). Asian and Pacific Islanders: Myth and reality. *Social Work*, 33(2): 142-147.

Ja, D. Y. and Aoki, B. (1993). Substance abuse treatment: Cultural barriers in the Asian American community. *Journal of Psychoactive Drugs*, 25(1):61-70.

Johnson, R. C. and Nagoshi, C. T. (1990). Asians, Asian-Americans, and alcohol. *Journal of Psychoactive Drugs*, 22(1):45-52.

Johnston, L., O'Malley, P. and Bachman, J. (1991). *Drug Use among American High School Seniors, College Students, and Young Adults: 1975-1990*. NIDA: Rockville, MD.

Kendall, J., Sherman, M. and Bigelow, G. (1995). Psychiatric symptoms in polysubstance abusers: Relationship to race, sex, and age. *Addictive Behaviors*, 20(5):685-690.

Kim, S., McLeod, J., Rader, D. and Johnston, G. (1992). An evaluation of a prototype school-based peer counseling program. *Journal of Drug Education*, 22(1):420-426.

Kim, S., McLeod, J. and Shantzis, C. (1992). Cultural competence for evaluators working with Asian American communities. In M. Orlandi (Ed.), *Cultural Competence for Evaluators*. Center for Substance Abuse Prevention: Rockville, MD.

Kitano, H. and Chi, I. (1985). Asian Americans and alcohol: The Chinese, Japanese, Koreans, and Filipinos in Los Angeles. In D. Spiegler, D. Tate, S. Aitken and C. Christian (Eds.), *Alcohol Use among Ethnic Minorities*. National Institute on Alcohol Abuse and Alcoholism: Rockville, MD.

Kuramoto, F. H. (1997). Asian Americans. In J. Philleo, F. L. Brisbane and L. Epstein (Eds.), *Cultural Competence in Substance Abuse Prevention*. NASW Press: Washington, D.C.

Maddahian, E., Newcomb, M. D. and Bentler, P. M. (1988). Adolescent drug use and intention to use drugs: Concurrent and longitudinal analyses of four ethnic groups. *Addictive Behaviors*, 13:191-195.

McLaughlin, D., Raymond, J., Murakami, S. R. and Goebert, D. (1987). Drug use among Asian Americans in Hawaii. *Journal of Psychoactive Drugs*, 19(1):85-94.

Merton, R. K. (1968). *Social Theory and Social Structure*. Free Press: New York.

Muller, T. (1993). *Immigrants and the American City*. Population Reference Bureau: Washington, D.C.

O'Hare, T. (1995). Differences in Asian and White drinking: Consumption level, drinking contexts, and expectancies. *Addictive Behaviors*, 20(2):261-266.

O'Hare, W. and Felt, J. (1991). *Asian Americans: America's Fastest Growing Minority Group*. Population Reference Bureau: Washington, D.C.

Perez-Arce, P., Carr, K. and Sorensen, J. (1993). Cultural issues in an outpatient program for stimulant abusers. *Journal of Psychoactive Drugs*, 25(1):35-44.

Phinney, J. S. (1990). Ethnic identity in adolescents and adults: Review of research. *Psychological Bulletin*, 108(3):499-514.

Pollard, J. A. (1993). *An Integration of Survey Findings Regarding Substance Use for Minority Youth: 1985-1991.* Southwest Regional Education Laboratory: Los Alamitos, CA.

Portes, A. and Rumbaut, R. (1990). *Immigrant America: A Portrait.* University of California Press: Berkeley, CA.

Sampson, R., Raudenbush, S. and Earls, F. E. (1997). Neighborhoods and violent crime: A multilevel study of collective efficacy. *Science,* 277:918-924.

Solberg, V. S., Ritsma, S., Davis, B. J., Tata, S. P. and Jolly, A. (1994). Asian American students' severity of problems and willingness to seek help from university counseling centers: Role of previous counseling experience, gender, and ethnicity. *Journal of Counseling Psychology,* 41(3):275-279.

Sue, S. (1994). Mental health. In N. Zane, D. Takeuchi and K. Young (Eds.), *Confronting Critical Health Issues of Asian and Pacific Islander Americans.* Sage Publications: Thousand Oaks, CA.

Sue, S., Fujino, D., Hu, L., Takeuchi, D. and Zane, N. (1991). Community mental health services for ethnic minority groups: A test of the cultural responsiveness hypothesis. *Journal of Consulting and Clinical Psychology,* 59(4):533-540.

Sue, S., Zane, N. and Ito, J. (1979). Alcohol drinking patterns among Asian and Caucasian Americans. *Journal of Cross-Cultural Psychology,* 10:41-56.

Tonnies, F. (1887, 1963). *Community and Society.* Harper: New York.

Westermeyer, J., Lyfoung, T., Westermeyer, M. and Neider, J. (1991). Opium addiction among Indochinese refugees in the United States: Characteristics of addicts and their opium use. *American Journal of Drug Alcohol Abuse,* 17(3):267-277.

Wu, I-H. and Windle, C. W. (1980). Ethnic specificity in the relative minority use and staffing of community mental health centers. *Community Mental Health Journal,* 16:156-168.

Yee, B. and Thu, N. D. (1987). Correlates of drug use and abuse among Indochinese refugees: Mental health implications. *Journal of Psychoactive Drugs,* 19(1):77-83.

Zane, N. and Kim, J. H. (1994). Substance use and abuse. In N. Zane, D. Takeuchi and K. Young (Eds.), *Confronting Critical Health Issues of Asian and Pacific Islander Americans.* Sage Publications: Thousand Oaks, CA.

CHAPTER 9

Psychosocial Factors Influencing Substance Abuse in Black Women and Latinas

Kathy Sanders-Phillips

The magnitude of substance abuse among Black women and Latinas and the significant health risks for these women and their children confirm that drug abuse among ethnic minority women is a significant public health problem (Carr, 1975; National Pregnancy and Health Survey, 1996). Currently, more than 4.4 million women in the United States use illicit drugs and women constitute more than 37 percent of the illicit drug using population (Mathias, 1995). Women who abuse drugs also engage in other risk behaviors and tend to have other health problems including complications of pregnancy, poor nutrition, and increased exposure to AIDS (Curtiss, Lenz, and Frei, 1993). Existing data indicate that Black women and Latinas are disproportionately impacted by substance abuse and illicit drug use is higher among Black women than White women or Latinas (Leigh, 1994).

The purpose of this chapter is twofold. First, based on existing literature, factors influencing substance use and abuse in women in general and Black women and Latinas in particular will be examined with emphasis on the social, psychological, and cultural factors influencing these behaviors. Factors specifically related to alcohol, tobacco, and illegal drug use will be identified. Second, approaches to substance abuse prevention for Black women and Latinas are reviewed and effective strategies for preventing and/or decreasing substance use in these populations are discussed.

PSYCHOSOCIAL FACTORS INFLUENCING ALCOHOL AND TOBACCO USE IN WOMEN

There is considerable evidence that psychosocial variables such as stressful life events, psychological status, social support, ethnic identity, and quality of interactions with the health care system influence health and risk behaviors in women more than men (Bullough, 1972; Cohen, et al., 1982; Cohen, et al., 1991; Gottlieb and Green, 1984; Hibbard, 1985; Makuc, Fried, and Kleinman, 1989; Morris, Hatch, and Chipman, 1966; Rakowski, 1988; Seeman and Evans, 1962; Seeman and Seeman, 1983; Shumaker and Hill, 1991). Although causal relationships between these variables have not been established, exposure to stressful life events and lack of social support may be specifically related to the initiation and maintenance of risk behaviors in women. Stressful life events such as exposure to violence may result in feelings of powerlessness and alienation which are related to perceptions of poor health status and decreased health promotion behaviors (Sanders-Phillips, 1996). Higher levels of depression are also related to fewer health promotion behaviors, as are experiences of racial discrimination (Bullough, 1972; Cohen, et al., 1982; Cohen, et al., 1991; Hibbard, 1985; Leftwich and Collins, 1994; Morris, Hatch, and Chipman, 1966; Seeman and Evans, 1962; Seeman and Seeman, 1983). Perceptions of the health care system and quality of interactions with health care staff also impact level of healthy behaviors and compliance with treatment among women. Women who report poorer relationships with health care staff and medical institutions tend to engage in less healthy behaviors (Freimuth and Mettzger, 1990; Harrison and Harrison, 1971; James, et al., 1984; Makuc, Fried, and Kleinman, 1989; Perez-Stable, 1987; Webb, 1984). Thus, ecological variables such as a women's exposure to violence and other stressors and the nature of her interactions with the larger social and health care system may be important determinants of health and risk behaviors.

Research on factors related to alcohol and tobacco use among women provide additional support for gender differences in risk and health behaviors and suggest that factors influencing the use of alcohol and tobacco in women are similar to those influencing other health and risk behaviors. For example, there is a well-documented relationship between stressful life events and women's use of tobacco and alcohol. Stressful life events are related to smoking initiation, cessation, and alcohol use for women (Gottlieb and Green, 1984). Gottlieb and Green (1984) concluded that relationships between stress, alcohol consumption, and smoking in women may be strong enough to justify sex-specific norms for smoking and drinking as coping mechanisms for stress.

Social support, as measured by church attendance and marital status, is related to lower levels of smoking and consumption of alcohol in women. Social network influences, including the availability of substances, modeling of their use, and attitudes toward their use, are correlates of substance abuse in women (Ferguson, Lennox, and Lettieri, 1976; Gottlieb, 1982). Women's substance use, particularly alcohol use, is also related to parental substance abuse and the quality of family relationships (Beckman, 1975; Ensminger, Brown, and Kallam, 1982; Swinson, 1980). Demographic characteristics such as older age and full time employment are also related to higher alcohol consumption in women but, unlike men, older age in women is not related to smoking cessation (Gottlieb and Green, 1984). Definitions of gender roles also influences alcohol consumption in women. Problem drinking is highest among women with untraditional gender role identities (Wilsnack, Klassen, and Wright, 1985).

Mental health status is also a predictor of women's smoking and drinking behavior. A history of marital conflict and depression is associated with higher levels of drinking and smoking (Cohen, et al., 1991; Lex, 1991). Among women with depression, the odds of smoking are 90 percent greater and the odds of moderate or heavy drinking are 120 percent greater compared to women without a history of depression (Cohen, et al., 1991). Marital conflict was related to an increased probability of smoking only among women who were not working full time, which supports the conclusion that relationships between stress and risk behaviors may be more significant for women of lower income. The findings also confirmed that mental health factors may be better predictors of health behaviors for women than men, particularly for substance abuse (Lex, 1991).

While relationships between stressful life events, depression, smoking, and drinking have also been found for ethnic minority women, the sources of stress related to substance use and factors related to depression in ethnic minority women may differ, social norms and support for smoking may vary within groups of ethnic minority women, and factors such as racial discrimination and level of acculturation may significantly impact depression as well as smoking and drinking behaviors.

Among Black women, education is negatively related to age of smoking onset, amount smoked, and perceived difficulties in quitting (Manfredi, Lacey, Warnecke, and Buis, 1992). It is positively related to plans to quit, beliefs that smoking is related to lung cancer and serious health problems, and knowledge of where to go for help. Black women with more education are also more likely to live in environments that support smoking cessation and have fewer smokers. Education and level of acculturation are also important predictors of smoking behavior in Latinas, but the nature of the relationships differ. More acculturated Latinas tend to smoke in greater numbers than women with lower levels of acculturation and those with less education (Marin, Marin, and Perez-Stable, 1989) and Mexican-American women have been found to smoke at higher levels than Mexican immigrant women (Zambrana, Hernandez, Dunkel-Schetter, and Scrimshaw, 1991). Level of acculturation has also been shown to influence attitudes, norms, and expectancies about smoking in Latino groups (Marin, Marin, Otero-Sabogal, Sabogal, and Perez-Stable, 1989).

Higher acculturation and education in Latinas are also positively related to alcohol consumption, as are older age and employment; however, drinking patterns among Latinas are not related to length of residence in the United States (Black and Markides, 1993; Caetano and Mora, 1988). These findings support previous reports that risk behaviors such as smoking and alcohol consumption tend to increase as Latinos become more acculturated (Marcus and Crane, 1985; Marcus, Herman-Shipley, Crane, and Enstrom, 1986); however, Zambrana, et al. (1991) found few differences in the consumption of alcohol between Mexican-American women and recent Mexican immigrants. Low income in Latinas is also an important predictor of alcohol consumption with poor Latinas consuming more drinks per occasion and more likely to be drinkers than higher income Latinas (Black and Markides, 1993).

In a study of factors related to alcohol consumption in Black women, Taylor, Henderson, and Jackson (1991) found that stressful life events such as exposure to violence and internalized racism accounted for a significant proportion of the variance in alcohol consumption. Internalized racism was defined as the degree to which Black women internalized negative racial stereotypes from the dominant society. Higher levels of internalized racism were associated with higher consumption of alcohol. Greater involvement in religious activities was related to higher alcohol consumption, depression, and internalized racism. These findings are consistent with previous reports that increased religious involvement is associated with higher depression among Blacks experiencing chronic economic strain (Brown, Gary, Greene, and Milburn, 1992).

Singleton, et al. (1986) have also reported that smoking among Black women is related to psychosocial stress and experiences of racism. They also note that smoking in Black women may be related to gender role difficulties including problems of assertion, independence, rebellion, or identification in relationships with males. This conclusion is supported by findings indicating that women who quit smoking are more likely to be married, have the support of their spouses, and are employed (United States Public Health Service, 1980). Conversely, Black women, who are more likely to be single and live in environments of high stress, are less likely to quit smoking than Whites (Singleton, et al., 1986).

Studies of depression in Black and Latino women indicate that negative life events, internalized racism, and social support are significant predictors of depression. Negative life events including exposure to violence, internalized racism, and social support predict depression in Black women but stressful life events have a greater effect on depression than social support (Taylor, Henderson, and Jackson, 1991). Although social support was inversely related to depressive symptoms, it was unrelated to alcohol consumption. Several investigators have shown that acculturative stress is related to depression in Latinos (Golding and Burnam, 1990; Ring and Marquis, 1991; Salgado de Snyder, 1987; Vega, Kolody, Valle, and Hough, 1986; Williams and Berry, 1991). Similar to Black women, experiences of racial discrimination contribute to higher rates of acculturative stress and depression in Latinas (Salgado de Snyder, 1987). Among Latino professional women, marital conflict and racial discrimination are significant predictors of depression (Amaro, Russo, and Johnson, 1987).

The above studies document relationships between stressful life events, depression, alcohol consumption, and tobacco use in women and suggest that racial discrimination, exposure to violence, and lack of social support may precipitate acculturative stress and depression, particularly in Black women and Latinas. These findings are consistent with Ferrence's (1988) observation that women's risk behaviors are related to social status and interactions outside the home and Krieger's (1990) finding that experiences of racism affect health outcomes.

These results also underscore the importance of psychological and social variables to the use and abuse of tobacco and alcohol in women and support previous findings that psychological and social factors are significant predictors of risk behaviors among all women and subgroups of ethnic minority women. It is also clear that ethnic differences exist in the sources of stress related to health behaviors and in the factors that precipitate stress and depression.

FACTORS INFLUENCING ILLEGAL DRUG USE IN WOMEN

Much previous research on factors related to drug abuse has been conducted with males (Hser, Anglin, and Booth, 1987). Therefore, less data is available on factors related to illegal drug abuse in women (Hser, Anglin, and Booth, 1987). It has been reported that more White women (35%) and Black women (33%) report using illicit drugs at some point in their lives than Latinas (25%) and current use of any illicit drug is higher among Black women than White women or Latinas (Leigh, 1994).

Patterns of drug use and factors related to drug use differ for men and women (Lex, 1991). Women who use illegal drugs, both during pregnancy and at other points in their lives, tend to be multiple drug users who use a number of drugs concurrently; report somewhat higher levels of drugs used but less money spent on drugs; are more likely to be living with a drug dependent partner; are likely to show symptoms of depression and isolation; and report more family and job pressures (Carr, 1975; Frank, et al., 1988; Lex, 1991; Singer, Arendt, and Minnes, 1993; Singer, Farkas, and Kleigman, 1992; Streissguth, et al., 1991). Girls are also more likely to become polydrug users or to self-medicate for depression than boys (Booth, Castro, and Anglin, 1991). Women's initiation into drug use and their progression through the addiction cycle is significantly influenced by their male partner (Hser, Anglin, and Booth, 1987).

In comparison to women who do not report use of illegal drugs, drug using women are more likely to be single, separated, or divorced; have less than a high school education; use alcohol and tobacco in addition to illegal drugs; and have fewer sources of social support (Beckwith, 1987; Singer, Arendt, and Minnes, 1993; Streissguth et al, 1991). Trauma, especially exposure to violence, may be a particularly important predictor of women's illegal drug use. Pregnant victims of abuse were more likely to use alcohol, marijuana, and cocaine than non victims and women who experienced maternal battering admitted more alcohol and cocaine use than non-battered women (Singer, Arendt, and Minnes, 1993). In addition to histories of childhood physical and sexual abuse, women drug abusers are more likely to be physically and sexually abused during the time of their drug use and exposed to stigmatization from the public and peers (Fullilove, Lown, and Fullilove, 1992).

A study of personality characteristics of male and female cocaine and alcohol abusers indicated that women cocaine abusers were more likely to have an Axis I DSM-III-R diagnosis in addition to substance abuse (Johnson, Tobin, and Cellucci, 1992). Depression was the most common disorder in women, while only men reported antisocial personality characteristics. Gender differences in depression persisted over time and women showed slower recovery from depression regardless of sociodemographic characteristics (Griffin, Weiss, Mirin, and Lange, 1989). These findings suggest that previous reports of higher rates of antisocial behaviors in cocaine users may have been confounded by collapsing data from male and female samples.

Women who abuse illegal drugs also experience a wide range of health problems. As indicated, marijuana, alcohol, and cigarette use are almost three times higher in drug abusing women as compared to non-drug-abusing samples from similar racial and social class groups (Frank, et al., 1988; Singer, Song, Warshawsky, and Kliegman, 1991). Poor prenatal care is also common among drug using pregnant women (Singer, Song, Warshawsky, and Kliegman, 1991). Women who use cocaine during pregnancy also tend to weigh less during pregnancy and at delivery which may be related to anorexia and poor maternal nutrition (Frank, et al., 1988; Singer, Song, Warshawsky, and Kliegman, 1991). Drug using women are also more likely to have a high prevalence of health problems including sexually transmitted diseases, anemia, and dental disease (Curtiss, Lenz, and Frei, 1993). Medical problems such as heart disease, surgical conditions, and breast disease are higher (Curtiss, et al., 1993) and their use of drugs, and possible involvement in prostitution, increase risk for HIV exposure and AIDS (Fullilove, Fullilove, Bowser, and Gross, 1990). Current statistics indicate that approximately 67 percent of AIDS cases among women are drug related (1993 National Household Survey, 1994).

Since many of the previous studies of women using illegal drugs have utilized samples from public urban hospitals serving predominantly low-income, ethnic minority populations, relatively few comparison studies of drug use in women have been conducted. Over reporting of ethnic minority drug abusing women to public health and/or social service agencies has also biased previous samples (Chasnoff, Landress, and Barrett, 1990). Thus, studies of ethnic differences among women drug abusers are limited. Zambrana, Hernandez, Dunkel-Schetter, and Scrimshaw (1991) examined ethnic differences in alcohol, cigarette, and illegal drug use in Mexican-American, Mexican immigrant, and African-American women. Consumption of alcohol and use of marijuana, cocaine, PCP, heroin, and over the counter medications were highest in Black women. Use of illegal drugs was low in the Mexican American and immigrant groups; however, Mexican immigrant women were slightly more likely to report using illegal drugs. There was also a trend for more Black women to be smokers and Mexican-American women were more likely to be smokers than Mexican immigrant women. Women who used alcohol, illegal drugs, or cigarettes during pregnancy were older, more likely to report negative life events, less likely to be living with the baby's father, and less likely to have planned the pregnancy.

The relationship between a planned pregnancy and drug use in the Zambrana, et al. (1991) study is interesting in light of previous data that a planned pregnancy is highly correlated with healthier behaviors, more positive health attitudes, greater involvement in prenatal care, and higher levels of self-care practices to protect the health of the baby (Cramer, 1987). Conversely, failure to plan pregnancy is associated with depression, alienation, and powerlessness (Groat and Neal, 1967) which, as indicated, are related to poorer health behaviors in women.

De La Rosa, Khalsa, and Rouse (1990) reported that prevalence of drug use differs among Hispanic subgroups and degree of acculturation influenced rates of drug use in Hispanic populations. Puerto Ricans and Mexican Americans who were born in the United States and whose primary language was English were most vulnerable to the use of illegal drugs. Greater drug use in these groups may be related to higher rates of poverty, limited school and employment opportunities, and racial discrimination (De La Rosa, Khalsa, and Rouse, 1990). Drug use among younger Hispanics is associated with acculturative stress, particularly loss of identification with the Hispanic culture. Lower levels of ethnic identity are also related to an increased risk of illegal drug use among Blacks (Ringwalt and Paschall, 1995).

Several studies have documented gender and ethnic differences in the initiation, addiction, and treatment phases of narcotic drug use and male-female differences in drug use behavior are more pronounced among Latinos than for other ethnic or cultural groups. For example, shorter times from initiation to addiction have been noted for Latinas and Latinas were more likely than other groups to use heroin (Anglin, Hser, and McGlothlin, 1987). Both illegal and prescription drug use may serve as forms of self-medication to cope with the stresses of acculturation in Latinas (Booth, Castro, and Anglin, 1991). Latina drug abusers also have lower self-esteem, lower self-efficacy, and more risk behaviors than Black women drug users (Grella, Annon, and Anglin, 1995).

Compared to White female narcotic users, Latinas are less likely to be employed and more likely to receive welfare or disability payments. Latinas are also more likely to come from single parent, low-income households and report family dysfunction. These circumstances, combined with lower education and a cultural milieu which disapproves of drug use in women and women working outside of the home, encourage greater dependence on an addicted partner and/or on welfare and disability payments (Anglin, Booth, Ryan, and Hser, 1988) and suggest that Latinas who use drugs are significantly influenced by cultural gender norms (Booth, Castro, and Anglin, 1991). Cultural differences in expectations regarding women and their roles may also contribute to drug dependent Latinas becoming marginal persons: marginal to the larger White society and marginal within the Latino community (Anglin, Booth, Ryan, and Hser, 1988). Anglin, Hser, and Booth (1987) have concluded that sex role conflicts, restricted job opportunities, and other marginal attributes influence all women addicts, but their impact may be more severe on Latinas.

Response to drug treatment also differs by gender and ethnicity. Perceived need for treatment is higher among women drug abusers, but, women are more likely to seek treatment based on crisis events rather than degree of drug dependence (Longshore, Hsieh, and Anglin, 1993). Black and Latino drug users are less likely to report having been in drug treatment; Latino drug users are most likely to report that they do not seek treatment because they do not need it; and Blacks are more likely to hold unfavorable views of treatment (Longshore, Hsieh, Anglin, and Annon, 1992). Both Blacks and Latinos may refuse treatment because they may view it as a form of oppression that is associated with racism (Longshore, et al., 1993). Latinas may cite pregnancy as a reason for seeking drug treatment, but report that treatment programs do not help (Anglin, Hser, and Booth, 1987).

Finally, social and environmental risk factors occurring at the community level appear to be important correlates of patterns of drug use. Community norms regarding alcohol and drug use influence perceptions of the prevalence of drug use and acceptance of drug use (Fitzpatrick and Gerard, 1993). In a study conducted by Lillie-Blanton, et al. (1993), the availability of drugs, community contacts with police, premature death rates, mechanisms for coping with life stressors, distribution of wealth, and access to social resources were related to residents' drug use patterns. Ethnic differences in illegal drug use did not persist after accounting for differences in these factors.

The findings on factors related to drug use for women and ethnic minority subgroups are important for several reasons. First, there is consistency in the factors related to alcohol, tobacco, and illegal substance abuse among women. Psychological, ecological, and interpersonal variables are salient factors related to these risk behaviors in women and relationships between these variables and risk behaviors are pronounced in Black women and Latinas. Second, drug use is associated with involvement in other unhealthy behaviors although it is not clear whether other unhealthy behaviors precede, accompany, or succeed drug addiction. Physical disability and poor health are cited as primary reasons for discontinuing drug use for many women (Longshore, et al., 1993). Third, in some drug abusing women, pregnancy is a time of greater motivation to engage in healthier behaviors, decreased drug use, and improved self-care practices. Fourth, for ethnic minority women, factors related to drug use are complex; however, it appears that ethnic minority women are more likely to be exposed to the factors related to unhealthy lifestyle behaviors, alcohol and tobacco use, and illegal drug use; that psychological status and functioning may be more marginal in these groups; and issues related to ethnic identity and acculturation may influence drug abuse behavior. Lastly, trauma and depression have been identified as etiologic factors in women's drug abuse. It has been suggested that women drug users experience a cycle of initiating drug use to relieve symptoms of depression or trauma, experiencing trauma in their efforts to secure drugs, and relieving the new trauma by continuing drug use (Fullilove, Lown, and Fullilove, 1992).

IMPLICATIONS FOR THE PREVENTION OF SUBSTANCE ABUSE IN BLACK WOMEN AND LATINAS

This review of factors related to the use of alcohol, tobacco, and illegal drugs suggests that involvement in these risk behaviors is associated with a complex array of individual, psychosocial, and environmental factors. Therefore, substance abuse prevention programs for women must acknowledge and address the multiple determinants of these behaviors.

The findings regarding women's use of alcohol, tobacco, and illegal drugs are consistent with an ecological conceptualization of health and risk behaviors and suggest an ecological approach to prevention. An ecological approach focuses on the environmental, cultural, and social correlates of health behaviors, acknowledges the individual factors that contribute to health behaviors, and utilizes social networks to effect behavior change. In an ecological framework, effective prevention programs must identify and address the social, cultural, psychological, and economic factors that influence women's substance use as well as the cultural and community factors that maintain health and risk behaviors (Stokols, 1992).

Based on previous prevention studies utilizing this approach, several conclusions can be reached about successful prevention programs for women. For example, cognitive approaches to health behavior change, in the absence of attention to psychological, social, and cultural determinants of health behaviors, may be ineffective in promoting behavior change (Israel, 1982, 1985; Lacey, 1992; Lacey, Manfredi, and Warnecke, 1991; Schorr, 1990; Thomas, 1990). Self-efficacy is an important predictor of health behavior change in women; cooperative learning methods may be most effective in promoting behavior change; and knowledge is a relatively poor predictor of behavior change (Amezucua, McAlister, Ramirez, and Espinoza, 1990; Hargreaves, Baquet, and Gamshadzahi, 1989; Schaefer, Falciglia, and Collins, 1990; Vega, et al., 1988). Successful programs should be based in the community and utilize naturally occurring social networks. Low income, socially isolated women may profit most from programs that address their immediate needs for companionship and mutual support and provide them with methods of self-improvement (Lacey, 1992). In light of relationships between exposure to violence and health behaviors in women (Sanders-Phillips, 1994a, 1994b, 1996) and data that low income ethnic minority women are more likely to experience traumatic events such as violence (Bell and Jenkins, 1991), prevention programs for women must acknowledge the impact of trauma and/or exposure to violence on risk behaviors.

Lay health advisors have been used successfully in prevention programs to promote health behavior change in women, especially ethnic minority women, and address the social and cultural barriers to healthy behaviors (Amezucua, et al., 1990; Hargreaves, et al., 1989). The effectiveness of lay health advisors in overcoming the cultural and social barriers to healthy behaviors, in recruiting women to health promotion interventions, and in increasing health promotion behaviors in women has been well documented (Brownstein, Cheal, Ackerman, Bassford, Campos-Outcalt, 1992; Levine, Becker, and Bone, 1992; Salber, 1979; Warnecke, Graham, Mosher, Montgomery, and Schotz, 1975; Warnecke, Graham, Mosher, and Montgomery, 1976). The importance of using lay health advisors who are similar to the target population and who conduct interventions in programs where there is a shared sense of identity has also been stressed (Israel, 1982, 1985; Warnecke, et al., 1975). The success of prevention programs for women that focus on increasing ethnic identity and pride as a mechanism for changing health behaviors (DiClemente and Wingood, 1995) also supports the use of indigenous community workers and underscores the importance of addressing issues related to ethnicity.

Indigenous, lay health advisors operating in close-knit social networks may exert a greater social influence than those functioning in loosely-knit programs that lack a common identity or purpose (Gottlieb, 1981; Israel, 1985). The use of lay health advisors in health promotion and/or intervention programs is also consistent with findings that women tend to turn to informal support systems and other women for health advice and information (Leutz, 1976; Neighbors and Jackson, 1984; Schaefer, et al., 1990; Warnecke, et al., 1976). Among low income, Black women, the use of lay health advisors is related to lower levels of depression and healthier behaviors (Cohen, et al., 1991; Gottlieb and Green, 1987; Rhodes, Ebert, and Fisher, 1992; Taylor, Henderson, and Jackson, 1991). Lay health advisors may also provide the social support for women that is necessary for health behavior change (Israel, 1985). Social support offered by lay health advisors may reduce stress, increase coping skills (Gottlieb, 1981; Hirsch, 1981; Salber, 1979), and increase self-efficacy and perceived control over health (Hibbard, 1985).

Consistent with these findings, an ecological approach to the prevention of drug abuse and treatment of drug abusing women has been recommended by several investigators. Although relatively few drug abuse prevention programs for women have been developed and evaluated, successful programs of drug treatment for women have provided critical insights regarding potential strategies for drug abuse prevention for women. For example, Longshore, et al. (1993) have concluded that special efforts may be needed to engage women, particularly ethnic minority women, into programs. Special efforts may be especially important for clients who seek help because of family pressure, legal coercion, or other external motivators. Engagement of women can be facilitated by designing intake and referral services that are culturally specific and appropriate and providing staff who are ethnically compatible with the targeted group. Staff-client interactions may improve if staff are bilingual and trained to adopt interaction styles that are consistent with the cultural group being served. Closer ties should also be established between program staff and community caregivers in neighborhood health clinics, school programs, and/or churches. Lay counselors may be recruited and community-based resources should be utilized as adjuncts to the program (Longshore, et al., 1993).

The provision of trauma treatment services may also be an integral component of drug abuse prevention for women. Fullilove, et al. (1992) have suggested that peer support to address experiences of trauma may be a critical element in recovery for women addicts. A focus on self-affirmation and self efficacy in overcoming drug abuse problems may also need to be incorporated into drug prevention programs. Given the unique influence of a male partner on drug use patterns among women, prevention and intervention programs may also need to provide treatment for or solicit the support of male partners in the treatment of women (Anglin, Hser, and Booth, 1987). Finally, prevention and treatment programs for women may need to capitalize on the motivation of pregnancy to improve health for the well-being of the baby. In fact, pregnancy may be a critical point for substance abuse prevention and intervention for women.

Increased rates of disease and disability in drug abusing women also suggest that programs of prevention and intervention should provide comprehensive medical care and must address other risk behaviors in drug abusing women. These findings also suggest that substance abuse prevention should be an integral component of general health care for women. A more comprehensive approach to women's health that does not focus exclusively on substance abuse, but addresses the factors that promote unhealthy lifestyle behaviors including substance abuse, may result in better overall health outcomes and changes in substance abuse behavior in women.

Finally, substance abuse behaviors in women, particularly those of ethnic minority groups, must be understood and addressed in terms of both the personal characteristics that promote drug use as well as the community characteristics that contribute to drug use, regardless of individual characteristics (Lillie-Blanton, Anthony, and Schuster, 1993). An ecological approach suggests that interventions designed to prevent risk behaviors and promote healthy behavior may have to be implemented at the macrosocial, mesosocial, and microsocial levels (Taylor,

Henderson, and Jackson, 1991). At the microsystem level, the effects of life events, social support, depressive symptoms, and poor health on risk behaviors in women suggest the need for programs to enhance coping skills, to improve social management skills, and to encourage health promotion. At the mesosystem level, the roles of religious orientation, internalized racism, and socioeconomic status in promoting risk behaviors suggest the need for church-based support and intervention, cultural programs to replace negative racial stereotypes, and social/ vocational programs to improve educational and economic status. Macrosystem approaches should include public and cultural policies that support the microsystem and mesosystem interventions (e.g., public policies supporting job development, technical training, and employment). As McLeroy, et al. (1992) concluded, the goals of health education for all women should not only include changes in health-related behaviors and health status, but changes in the capacity of individuals, networks, organizations, communities, and political structures to address health problems.

REFERENCES

Amaro, H., Russo, N. F. and Johnson, J. (1987). Family and work predictors of psychological well-being among Hispanic women professionals. *Psychology of Women Quarterly*, 11:505-521.

Amezucua, C., McAlister, A., Ramirez, A. and Espinoza, R. (1990). A su salud: Health promotion in a Mexican-American border community. In N. Bracht (Ed.), *Health Promotion at the Community Level* (pp. 257-276). Sage Publications: Newbury Park, CA.

Anglin, M. D., Booth, M. W., Ryan, T. M. and Hser, Y. I. (1988). Chicano and Anglo addiction career patterns. In Special Issue, Ethnic differences in narcotics addiction. *The International Journal of the Addictions*, 23:1011-1027.

Anglin, M. D., Hser, Y. I. and Booth, M. W. (1987). Treatment. In Special Issue, Sex differences in addict careers. *American Journal of Drug and Alcohol Abuse*, 13:253-280.

Anglin, M. D., Hser, Y. I. and McGlothlin, W. H. (1987). Becoming Addicted. In Special Issue, Sex differences in addict careers. *American Journal of Alcohol Abuse*, 13:59-71.

Beckman, L. J. (1975). Women alcoholics: A review of social and psychological studies. *Journal of Studies on Alcohol*, 36:797-824.

Beckwith, J. B. (1987). Psychological functions of eating, drinking, and smoking in adult women. *Social Behavior and Personality*, 15:185-206.

Bell, C. and Jenkins, E. (1991). Traumatic stress and children. *Journal of Health Care for the Poor and Underserved*, 2:175-188.

Black, S. A. and Markides, K. S. (1993). Acculturation and alcohol consumption in Puerto Rican, Cuban-American, and Mexican-American Women in the United States. *American Journal of Public Health*, 83:890-893.

Booth, M. W., Castro, F. G. and Anglin, M. (1991). What do we know about Hispanic substance abuse? A review of the literature. In R. Click and J. Moore (Eds.), *Drugs in Hispanic Communities* (pp. 21-43). Rutgers University Press: New Brunswick, NJ.

Brown, D. R., Gary, L. E., Greene, A. D. and Milburn, N. G. (1992). Patterns of social affiliation as predictors of depressive symptoms among urban Blacks. *Journal of Health and Social Behavior*, 33:242-253.

Brownstein, J. N., Cheal, N., Ackerman, S. P., Bassford, T. L. and Campos-Outcalt, D. (1991). Breast and cervical cancer screening in minority populations: A model for using lay health educators. *Journal of Cancer Education*, 7:321-332.

Bullough, B. (1972). Poverty, ethnic identity and preventive health care. *Journal of Health and Social Behavior*, 13:347-359.

Caetano, R., and Mora, E. M. (1988). Acculturation and drinking among people of Mexican descent in Mexico and the United States. *Journal of Studies on Alcohol*, 49:462-471.

Carr, J. N. (1975). Drug patterns among drug-addicted mothers. *Pediatric Annals*, 4:65-77.

Chasnoff, I. J., Landress, H. J. and Barrett, M. E. (1990). The prevalence of illicit-drug use during pregnancy and discrepancies in mandatory reporting in Pinellas County, Florida. *The New England Journal of Medicine*, 322:1202-1206.

Cohen P., Struening E., Muhlin G., Genevie L., Kaplan S. and Peck H. (1982). Community stressors, mediating conditions and wellbeing in urban neighborhoods. *Journal of Community Psychology*, 10:377-391.

Cohen, S., Schwartz, J., Bromet, E. and Parkinson, D. (1991). Mental health, stress, and poor health behaviors in two community samples. *Preventive Medicine*, 20:306-315.

Cramer, J. C. (1987). Social factors and infant mortality: Identifying high-risk groups and proximate causes. *Demography*, 24:299-322.

Curtiss, M. A., Lenz, K. M. and Frei, N. R. (1993). Medical evaluation of African American women entering drug treatment. *Journal of Addictive Diseases*, 12:29-44.

De La Rosa, M. R., Khalsa, J. H. and Rouse, B. A. (1990). Hispanics and illicit drug use: A review of recent findings. *The International Journal of the Addictions*, 25:665-691.

DiClemente, R. and Wingood, G. (1995). A randomized controlled trial of an HIV sexual risk-reduction intervention for young African-American women. *Journal of the American Medical Association*, 274:1271-1276.

Ensminger, M. E., Brown, C. H. and Kallam, S. G. (1982). Sex differences in antecedents of substance use among adolescents. *Journal of Social Issues*, 38:25-42.

Ferguson, P., Lennox, T. and Lettieri, D., Eds. (1976). *Drugs and Family/peer Influence. Research Issues* (pp. 77-186). National Institute on Drug Abuse. DHEW Pub. No. (ADM) vol. 4.

Ferrence, R. G. (1988). Sex differences in cigarette smoking in Canada, 1900-1978: A reconstructed cohort study. *Canadian Journal of Public Health*, 79:160-165.

Fitzpatrick, M. L. and Gerard, K. (1993). Community attitudes toward drug use: The need to assess community norms. *The International Journal of the Addictions*, 28: 947-957.

Frank, D. A., Zuckerman, B. S., Amaro, H., Aboagye, K., Baucher, H., Cabral, H., Fried, L., Hinson, R., Kayne, H., Levenson, S., Parker, S., Reece, H. and Vinci, R. (1988). Cocaine use during pregnancy: Prevalence and correlates. *Pediatrics*, 82:888-895.

Freimuth, V. and Mettger, W. (1990). Is there a hard-to-reach audience? *Public Health Reports*, 105:232-238.

Fullilove, R. E., Fullilove, M. T., Bowser, B. and Gross, S. (1990). Crack users: The new AIDS risk group. *Cancer Detection and Prevention*, 14:363-368.

Fullilove, M. T., Lown, A. and Fullilove, R. E. (1992). Crack 'hos and skeezers': Traumatic experiences of women crack users. *The Journal of Sex Research*, 29:275-287.

Griffin, M. L., Weiss, R. D., Mirin, S. M. and Lange, U. (1989). A comparison of male and female cocaine abusers. *Archives of General Psychiatry*, 34:122-126.

Golding, J. and Burnam, A. (1990). Immigration, stress, and depressive symptoms in a Mexican-American community. *The Journal of Nervous and Mental Disease*, 178:161-171.

Gottlieb, B. H. (1981). Preventive interventions involving social networks and social support. In B. H. Gottlieb (Ed.), *Social Networks and Social Support*. Sage Publications: Beverly Hills, CA.

Gottlieb, N. H. (1982). The effects of peer and parental smoking and age on the smoking careers of college women: A sex-related phenomena. *Social Science and Medicine*, 16:595-600.

Gottlieb, N. and Green, L. (1984). Life events, social network, life-style, and health: An analysis of the 1979 national survey of personal health practices and consequences. *Health Education Quarterly*, 11:91-105.

Gottlieb, N. and Green, L. (1987). Ethnicity and lifestyle health risk: Some possible mechanisms. *American Journal of Health Promotion*, 2:37-51.

Grella, C. E., Annon, J. J. and Anglin, M. D. (1995). Ethnic differences in HIV risk behaviors, self-perceptions, and treatment outcomes among women in methadone maintenance treatment. *Journal of Psychoactive Drugs*, 27:421-433.

Groat, H. and Neal, A. (1967). Social psychological correlates of urban fertility. *American Sociological Review*, 32:945-949.

Hargreaves, M. K., Baquet, C. and Gamshadzahi, A. (1989) Diet, nutritional status and cancer risk in American Blacks. *Nutrition and Cancer*, 12:1-28.

Harrison, I. and Harrison, D. (1971). The Black family experience and health behavior. In C. Crawford (Ed.), *Health and the Family: A Medical-Sociological Analysis* (pp. 175-199). Macmillan: New York.

Hibbard, J. (1985). Social ties and health status: An examination of moderating factors. *Health Education Quarterly*, 12:23-34.

Hirsch, B. J. (1981) Social networks and the coping process: Creating personal communities. In B.H. Gottlieb (Ed.), *Social Networks and Social Support*. Sage Publications: Beverly Hills, CA.

Hser, Y. I., Anglin, M. D. and Booth, M. W. (1987). Sex differences in addict careers. 3. Addiction. *American Journal of Drug and Alcohol Abuse*, 13: 231-251.

Israel, B. A. (1982). Social networks and health status: Linking theory, roles and practice. *Patient Counseling and Health Education*, 4:65-77.

Israel, B. A. (1985). Social networks and social support: Implications for natural helper and community level interventions. *Health Education Quarterly*, 12:65-80.

James, S., Wagner, E., Strogatz, D., Bresford, S., Kleinbaum, D., Williams, C., Vutchin, L. and Ibraham, M. (1984). The Edgecombe county (NC) high blood pressure control program II: Barriers to the use of medical care among hypertensives. *The American Journal of Public Health*, 74:468-472.

Johnson, R. S., Tobin, J.W. and Cellucci, T. (1992). Personality characteristics of cocaine and alcohol abusers: More alike than different. *Addictive Behaviors*, 17:159-166.

Krieger, N. (1990). Racial and gender discrimination: Risk factors for high blood pressure. *Social Science and Medicine*, 30:1273-1281.

Lacey, L. (1992). Helping low-income minority women reduce cancer risk. *Oncology*, 7:22.

Lacey, L., Manfredi, C. and Warnecke, R. B. (1991). Use of lay health educators for smoking cessation in a hard-to-reach urban community. *Journal of Community Health*, 16:269-282.

Leftwich, M. J. T. and Collins, F. L. (1994). Parental smoking, depression, and child development: Persistent and unanswered questions. *Journal of Pediatric Psychology*, 19:557-570.

Leigh, W. (1994). *The Health Status of Women of Color*. Joint Center for Political and Economic Studies: Washington, D.C.

Leutz, W. (1976). The informal community caregiver: A link between the health care system and local residents. *American Journal of Orthopsychiatry*, 44:678-683.

Levine, D. M., Becker, D. M. and Bone, L. R. (1992). Narrowing the gap in health status of minority populations: A community-academic medical center partnership. *American Journal of Preventive Medicine*, 8:319-323.

Lex, B. W. (1991). Some gender differences in alcohol and polysubstance users. *Health Psychology*, 10:121-132.

Lillie-Blanton, M., Anthony, J. and Schuster, C. (1993). Probing the meaning of racial/ethnic group comparisons in crack cocaine smoking. *Journal of the American Medical Association*, 269:993-997.

Longshore, D., Hsieh, S. and Anglin, M. D. (1993). Ethnic differences in drug user's perceived need for treatment. *The International Journal of the Addictions*, 28:539-558.

Longshore, D., Hsieh, S., Anglin, M. D. and Annon, T.A. (1992). Ethnic patterns in drug abuse treatment utilization. *Journal of Mental Health Administration*, 19: 268-277.

Makuc, D. M., Fried, V. M. and Kleinman, J. (1989). National trends in the use of preventive health care by women. *American Journal of Public Health*, 79:21-26.

Manfredi, C., Lacey, L., Warnecke, R. and Buis, M. (1992). Smoking-related behavior, beliefs, and social environment of young Black women in subsidized public housing in Chicago. *American Journal of Public Health*, 82:267-272.

Marcus, A. and Crane, L. (1985). Smoking behavior among US Latinos: An emerging challenge for public health. *American Journal of Public Health*, 75:169-172.

Marcus, A., Herman-Shipley, N., Crane, L. and Enstrom, J. (1986). *Recent Trends in Cancer Incidence among U.S. Latinos*. Proceedings of the meeting of the American Public Health Association: Las Vegas, NV.

Marin, G., Marin, B. V. and Perez-Stable, E. (1989). Cigarette smoking among San Francisco Hispanics. *American Journal of Public Health*, 79:196-199.

Marin, G., Marin., B. V. O., Otero-Sabogal, R., Sabogal, F. and Perez-Stable, E. (1989). The role of acculturation in the attitudes, norms, and expectancies of Hispanic smokers. *Journal of Cross-Cultural Psychology*, 20:399-415.

Mathias, R. (1995). Filling the gender gap in drug abuse research. *NIDA Notes*, 10(1-5 whole volumes).

McLeroy, K. R., Steckler, A. B., Goodman, R. M. and Burdine, J. N. (1992). Health education research: Theory and practice-future directions. *Health Education Research Theory and Practice*, 7:1-8.

Morris, N., Hatch, M. and Chipman, S. (1966). Alienation as a deterrent to well-child supervision. *American Journal of Public Health*, 56:1874-1882.

National Pregnancy and Health Survey (1996). *Drug Abuse among Women Delivering Livebirths: 1992*. National Institute on Drug Abuse, U.S. Department of Health and Human Services. National Institutes of Health. NIH Publication No. 96-3819.

1993 National Household Survey on Drug Abuse (1994). NIDA National Pregnancy and Health Survey. Centers for Disease Control and Prevention. HIV/AIDS Surveillance Report, June.

Neighbors, H. W. and Jackson, J. S. (1984). The use of informal and formal help: Four patterns of illness behavior in the Black community. *American Journal of Community Psychology*, 12:629-644.

Perez-Stable, E. (1987). Issues in Latino health care—Medical staff conference. *The Western Journal of Medicine*, 146:213-218.

Rakowski, W. (1988). Predictors of health practices within age-sex groups: National survey of personal health practices and consequences, 1979. *Public Health Reports*, 103:376-386.

Rhodes, J. E, Ebert, L. and Fisher, K. (1992). Natural mentors: An overlooked resource in the social networks of young, African American mothers. *American Journal of Community Psychology*, 20:445-461.

Ring, J. and Marquis, P. (1991). Depression in a Latino immigrant medical population: An exploratory screening and diagnosis. *American Journal of Orthopsychiatry*, 61:298-302.

Ringwalt, C. and Paschall, M. (1995). *Ethnic Identity, Drug Use, and Violence among African-American Male Adolescents*. Paper presented at the meeting of the American Public Health Association: San Diego, CA.

Salber, E. (1979). The lay advisor as a community health resource. *Journal of Health Politics, Policy and Law*, 3:469-478.

Salgado de Snyder, V. N. (1987). Factors associated with acculturative stress and depressive symptomatology among married Mexican immigrant women. *Psychology of Women Quarterly*, 11:475-488.

Sanders-Phillips, K. (1994a). Health promotion behavior in low-income Black and Latino women. *Women and Health*, 21:71-83.

Sanders-Phillips, K. (1994b). Correlates of healthy eating habits in low-income Black women and Latinas. *Preventive Medicine*, 23:781-787.

Sanders-Phillips, K. (1996). The ecology of urban violence: Its relationship to health promotion behaviors in Black and Latino communities. *American Journal of Health Promotion*, 10:88-97.

Schaefer, N., Falciglia, G. and Collins, R. (1990). Adult African-American females learn cooperatively. *Journal of Nutrition Education*, 22:240D.

Schorr, L. B. (1990). Successful health programs for the poor and underserved. *Journal of Health Care for the Poor and Underserved*, 1:271-277.

Seeman, M. and Evans, J. (1962). Alienation and learning in a hospital setting. *American Sociological Review*, 27:772-782.

Seeman, M. and Seeman, T. (1983). Health behavior and personal autonomy: A longitudinal study of the sense of control in illness. *Journal of Health and Social Behavior*, 24:144-160.

Shumaker, S. A. and Hill, D. R. (1991). Gender differences in social support and physical health. *Health Psychology*, 10:102-111.

Singer, L., Arendt, R. and Minnes, S. (1993). Neurodevelopmental effects of cocaine. *Clinics in Perinatology*, 20:245-262.

Singer, L., Farkas, K. and Kleigman, R. (1992). Childhood medical and behavioral consequences of maternal cocaine use. *Journal of Pediatric Psychology*, 17:389-406.

Singer, L. T., Song, L., Warshawsky, L. and Kliegman, R. (1991). Maternal gravidity predicts prematurity in cocaine-exposed infants. *Pediatric Research*, 26:266A.

Singleton, E. G., Harrell, J. P. and Kelly, L. M. (1986). Acial differentials in the impact of maternal cigarette smoking during pregnancy on fetal development and mortality: Concerns for Black psychologists. *The Journal of Black Psychology*, 12:71-83.

Stokols, D. (1992). Establishing and maintaining healthy environments. *American Psychologist*, 47:6-22.

Streissguth, A. P., Grant, T. M., Barr, H. M., Brown, Z. A., Martin, J. C., Mayrock, D. E., Ramey, S. L. and Moore, L. (1991). Cocaine and the use of alcohol and other drugs during pregnancy. *American Journal of Obstetrics and Gynecology*, 164: 1239-1243.

Swinson, R. P. (1980). Sex differences in the inheritance of alcoholism. In O.J. Kalant (Ed.), *Alcohol and Drug Problems in Women: Research Advances in Alcohol and Drug Problems* (Chapter 5). Plenum Press: New York.

Taylor, J., Henderson, D. and Jackson, B. B. (1991). A holistic model for understanding and predicting depressive symptoms in African-American women. *Journal of Community Psychology*, 19:306-320.

Thomas, S. B. (1990). Community health advocacy for racial and ethnic minorities in the United States: Issues and challenges for health education. *Health Education Quarterly*, 17:13-19.

United States Public Health Service (1980). *The Health Consequences of Smoking for Women*. DHEW Publication No. 0-326-003. U.S. Government Printing Office: Washington, D.C.

Vega, W., Kolody, B., Valle, R. and Hough, R. (1986). Depressive symptoms and their correlates among immigrant Mexican women in the United States. *Social Science and Medicine*, 22:645-652.

Vega, W. A., Sallis, J. F., Patterson, T. L., Rupp, J. W., Morris, J. A. and Nader, P. R. (1988). Predictors of dietary change in Mexican American families participating in a health behavior change program. *American Journal of Preventive Medicine*, 4:194-199.

Warnecke, R. B., Graham, S., Mosher, W. and Montgomery, E. (1976). Health guides as influentials in Central Buffalo. *Journal of Health and Social Behavior*, 17:22-34.

Warnecke, R. B., Graham, S., Mosher, W., Montgomery, E. and Schotz, W. E. (1975). Contact with health guides and use of health services among Blacks in Buffalo. *Public Health Reports*, 90:213-222.

Webb, H. (1984). Community health centers: Providing care for urban Blacks. *Journal of the National Medical Association*, 76:1063-1067.

Williams, C. L. and Berry, J. W. (1991). Primary prevention of acculturative stress among refugees: Application of psychological theory and practice. *American Psychologist*, 46:632-641.

Wilsnak, R. W., Klassen, A. D. and Wright, S. I. (1985). Gender-role orientations and drinking among women in a U.S. national survey. In S. C. Wilsnak (Ed.), *Women and Alcohol: Health-Related Issues*. National Institute on Alcohol Abuse and Alcoholism, Division of Extramural Research: Rockville, MD.

Zambrana, R. E., Hernandez, M., Dunkel-Schetter, C. and Scrimshaw, S. C. M. (1991). Ethnic differences in the substance use patterns of low-income pregnant women. *Family and Community Health*, 13:1-11.

PART III

Policy and Community Issues in Substance Abuse Prevention

CHAPTER 10

Determinants of Effective School and Community Programs for Tobacco, Alcohol, and Drug Abuse Prevention: Cross-Cultural Considerations

C. Anderson Johnson

Over the last two decades there have been important scientific contributions, if only sporadic application, of knowledge about how to prevent tobacco, alcohol, and other drug abuse through school based interventions. Two recent research consensus statements have agreed that school based programming must contain certain basic elements in order to be effective (NIDA, 1997; Sussman and Johnson, 1996). These support the recommendations of an earlier NCI consensus statement (Glynn, 1989), CDC school smoking prevention guidelines (Centers for Disease Control, 1994), report on prevention of tobacco use in youth. It is no secret what works in schools to prevent tobacco use. *Yet a huge gap exists between what is known about prevention science and what is practiced in schools and the community.* The increase in cigarette smoking and other substance use over the last five years can be attributed largely to the failure of schools to apply these known prevention principles. Beginning next fall the Department of Education will require that school based drug abuse prevention programs, which generally subsume tobacco prevention programs, must contain certain empirically validated components in order to receive federal support (NPR, 1997).

We now know quite a lot about how to prevent smoking and other drug abuse through school programming. We know clearly that the acquisition of smoking is a social psychological process. Youth begin using other drugs because they see others using drugs, and they assume that smoking has social utility. Drug use may be seen as capacity expanding from the perspective of the adolescent, particularly in regard to social capacities. The perception of social utility is instilled, reinforced, and prompted to memory by imagery in the media and by fashion in the youth and young adult cultures to which youth aspire.

It is important to consider whether the determinants of drug use onset and progression and means for effective prevention hold uniformly across cultures and subcultures. I review briefly here the evidence relative to determinants of drug use and prevention in youth, both by international comparison and for specific subcultures within the United States. In considering factors that influence the onset of smoking, the focus here is on those that are readily amenable to school and community interventions. Genetic variation in addiction potential, mental health status, variation in individual cognitive abilities, psychological status, academic achievement, and general health and physical characteristics, while potentially important as risk factors, may not be readily amenable to school and community interventions. Perceptions, memory, cognitive attributions, group influences, and skill acquisition may, on the other hand, malleable through school and community interventions.

TRAJECTORY OF ONSET IN DRUG USE

In most cultures and subcultures the first notable upswing in drug use begins in the preadolescent and adolescent years, peaking in late adolescence to early adulthood. This varies somewhat by drug and culture. Among American Whites, tobacco and alcohol use tend to precede use of marijuana by two years or more. Onset of marijuana use relative to other drugs tends to occur earlier for Hispanic Americans. And use of all drugs tends to be considerably delayed for African Americans. Among some Asian populations, use of illicit drugs may sometimes anticipate later use of tobacco and alcohol. Onset of smoking in China occurs at a later age than in the United States, but a higher proportion of youthful smokers report regular, daily smoking than in the U.S. (National Prevalence Survey of Smoking Pattern, 1996). It is not clear the extent to which these differences are the result of the economic changes occurring in these cultures.

INFLUENCES ON DRUG USE IN YOUTH

Factors known to be associated with the onset of drug use in youth include environmental and social influences such as association with peers who use drugs, parents who use drugs, sensation-seeking and risk-taking tendencies, and drug availability. Intra-individual variables can also be important, including physiological responses (e.g., flushing response among many Asians) and perceptions of pleasure/displeasure associated with physiological changes. Escalation of drug use into addiction and dependence is influenced additionally by psychological factors, including emotional distress, poor school performance, absenteeism (Newcomb and Earlywine, 1996), and genetics. Even so, social and environmental variables continue to influence transitions into problematic use, and at least some programs that are effective in preventing onset of use have been found to prevent transitions to problematic levels of use as well (Chou, Montgomery, Pentz, et al., 1998).

There is remarkable consistency over ethnic and cultural groupings in the social, environmental, and intra-individual influences on drug use. Use by friends and parents is a consistently strong predictor for American Asians, Hispanics, Africans, and Whites, as well as youth in Northern Europe, Africa, and China. Risk-taking, curiosity, and sensation-seeking are consistent predictors across cultures, as is drug availability. And these findings tend to hold across substances, including tobacco, alcohol, and marijuana. Some factors may be particularly important influences for some cultures, including risk-taking, anger, and greater television exposure for African Americans; improved self-image and perceived adult approval for Hispanics; and socioeconomic status for Whites and African Americans, but not Hispanic Americans. Smoking increases dramatically in third world nations as they begin to emerge into affluent market economies. Often, increases in other drug use tend to follow shortly thereafter. This is clearly observed in Southeast Asia and China. A similar trend has been observed in Europe with economic development there, e.g., Spain and Greece. The same trend occurs for the youth of immigrant populations to the United States, i.e., smoking and other drug use tend to increase in succeeding generations.

PERCEIVED SOCIAL NORMS

The major influences on early tobacco, alcohol, and drug use are *social norms*. These include *perceptions about prevalence* of use in the society and perceptions of *social approval* for use. The perceived prevalence of use by friends, parents, and other peers (arguably in that order) all predict smoking onset. Perceptions of friends' use are probably the strongest and most robust influence on onset of tobacco and other substance abuse in youth. The typical youth at age of increased risk of smoking or drug use (ages 10 to 15) overestimates the number of peers who use most drugs, including tobacco, and this overestimation influences subsequent use. Figure 1 represents illustrative data from a longitudinal study of approximately 800 Los Angeles youth, measured first at eighth grade and again at ninth grade (Nezami, Johnson, and Chou, 1997). Perception of friends' use at grade eight was the strongest independent influence on marijuana use at grade nine. Perceived marijuana use among friends at grade eight predicted marijuana use at grade nine controlling for eighth grade use, parental use, perceived responses of friends and parents, and marijuana accessibility. Perception of parents' use

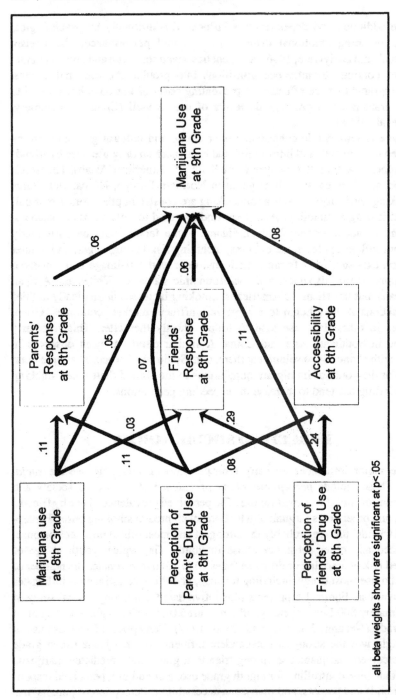

Figure 1. Prospective social and environmental risk factors for marijuana use.
Source: Nezami, Johnson, and Chou, 1997.

all beta weights shown are significant at p<.05

was also a strong independent influence on later use, when controlling for all the other variables, including perceptions of friends' use. We have found these same influences, friends' use, and parents' use to be strong predictors of smoking among youth in central (Wuhan) China (Chen, Johnson, Li, et al., in preparation).

Perceptions of social approval also influences tobacco and other drug use onset. Figure 1 shows that the perceived responses (approval/disapproval) of both friends and parents were independent influences on the later marijuana use of Los Angeles youth. The more approving friend and parental responses were expected to be, the more likely youth were to begin using marijuana, all other things held constant. We found that the same trends held for youth smoking in central China (Chen, Johnson, Li, et al., in preparation).

Exaggerated perceptions of use can create the expectation that use is desirable and has utility. It would not be surprising to find that greater use by friends and parents is seen as evidence of greater tolerance, and the attribution of social approval for use might mediate, or account for, some of the effect of perceived prevalence on subsequent use. This appears to have been the case in that the perceived responses of friends and parents mediated partially the effects of perceived prevalence for friends and parents, respectively. This can be seen by the beta weights of paths from perceived prevalence to perceived responses together with the beta weights of paths from responses to drug use. The mediated effect, like the direct prevalence effect, was stronger for friends than parents, but clearly independently significant for both.

The effects of perceived prevalence may be mediated in part by increased access to drugs or the perception of greater access, if friends, parents, and other peers smoke or use drugs. This can be seen in the significant paths from perceived friend and parent use to perceived accessibility, together with the significant path from accessibility to marijuana use. From the standpoint of prevention strategy, this mediation path differs from the others in having the potential for linkage with public policy. This kind of *environmental norm*, expectations about the occurrence of environments which provide easy or difficult access to tobacco, clearly has prevention implications that go beyond the classroom.

Both estimates of prevalence and perceptions of social approval, whether accurate or not, are amenable to classroom intervention. A whole new set of perceptions about prevalence of use and social disapproval can be generated through skillfully applied classroom exercises. Experimental trials have found that otherwise effective programs stripped of normative interventions were no longer effective in preventing tobacco and other drug use (Donaldson, Sussman, MacKinnon, et al., 1996; Hansen and Graham, 1991). And "effective" programs have been shown to be truly effective only for those for whom shifts in perceived norms actually occurred (MacKinnon, Johnson, Pentz, et al., 1991). There is evidence that some of the most popular school programs fail to work because they do not contain effective normative interventions (Hansen and McNeal, 1997).

There do not appear to be important differences in the effectiveness of these programs for different populations and ethnic groups. Programs that have focused on normative influences on drug use have been found to be equally effective in preventing cigarette, alcohol, and marijuana use among Asian-, African-, Hispanic-, and European-American youth (Graham, Johnson, Hansen, et al., 1990). The approach appears to be equally effective with largely White and mixed ethnic groupings in the classroom (Ellickson and Bell, 1990). And a general population "Life-Skills Training" program was just as effective as a culturally focused program for Hispanics and African Americans in reducing intentions to drink alcohol. However, there may be important differences in programs with regard to their community acceptability. For example, we found emphasis on peer leadership to be unacceptable in Alaskan Eskimo and Indian communities. Tuning programs to be more culturally sensitive may increase both their community acceptability and relevance to youth. One of the advantages of the class of programs shown to be effective for preventing drug use onset is that by design they are culturally responsive. They are designed to be sensitive to the prevailing cultural norms and influences in the populations they serve, which likely accounts for their generally universal effectiveness.

COMMUNITY NORMS

At the community level, policy interventions have been effective in reducing tobacco use. In California, location-specific smoking restrictions have been shown to lead to reduced smoking among workers (Pierce, et al., 1994). Pentz and colleagues (1997) found the lowest rates of youth smoking in schools with clearly articulated policies regarding smoking restrictions and requirements for prevention programming. No doubt some of the effect of policy enactment is mediated by restricted or difficult access, as when workers experience limited access to places to smoke at work, or students find few if any places at school where it is safe to smoke. This is an example of the mediation effect for environmental norms.

Much of the effect of policy enactment, however, may be mediated directly by perceived social norms. Policies that are strictly enforced convey the message that smoking is counter normative, i.e., not typically practiced or approved in the society. One view of public policy is that formal polices are nothing more than codification of already existing societal norms about which there is great consensus.

Whether by limiting access, providing for formal sanctions, or drawing attention to societal consensus, public policy is an important tool in the tobacco prevention arsenal. Rarely, however, is public policy implemented as part of a carefully thought out strategy in concert with school tobacco prevention programming. The public policy people do their own thing, and the education people rarely interact with tobacco control advocates or anyone else outside the school system (Rohrbach, et al., 1996). Shamefully, there are those in public policy advocacy, most egregiously some academics, who disdain educational approaches to prevention. And there are those in education who distrust policy advocates as espousing unrestrained invasion of government into the private lives of citizens. It has not been easy to get educators and public policy advocates together to plan for strategic policy that supports the objectives of school prevention programming, and for school curriculum that supports enlightened policy action. One potential exception has been the considerable effort in many California communities to involve youth in sting operations to expose and curtail illegal sales of tobacco to minors (Rogers, et al., 1995). Even these efforts have more often than not involved schools only informally and tangentially, if at all. In a limited number of schools, curricular activities have been directed at this very important public policy issue.

Rarely have public policy and school interventions been programmed to provide consistent messages that smoking is counter normative. Tobacco prevention components of the Midwestern Prevention Study (Johnson, Pentz, Weber, et al., 1990; Pentz, MacKinnon, Dwyer, et al., 1989), The Minnesota Heart Health Program (Perry, Klepp, Halper, et al., 1986), and the North Karelia (Finland) Project (Vartiainen, Pallonen, McAllister, and Puska, 1990) are examples of where public policy has been enacted and enforced at the same time and consistent with school based smoking education and prevention programs. The hostility between those in policy advocacy and those in public education has been notably absent in Finland. Prevention was always seen as a joint enterprise of policy decision makers, educators, the media, and lay leaders. The Minnesota and Midwestern Prevention Projects adopted similar models. Of the three, the Midwestern Project has been arguably the most school-centric, and the North Karelia Project the most effective in public policy enactment. But all three developed an integrated approach to public education, community involvement, and public policy enactment. It is notable that these three comprehensive community prevention programs have produced among the strongest and clearly longest lasting smoking prevention effects in the literature.

THE MEDIA AND NORMS

The influence of the media on societal norms and individual perceptions of norms can be enormous. Surveys have documented that the public perception of violent crime has risen steadily in recent years along with increased coverage of violence in the media, even in the face of substantial and consistent declines in the actual numbers of violent crimes. The media have been rightly criticized for over reporting sensational events, in politics as well as crime, often at the expense of public anxiety and distrust.

More to the point of public policy and societal norms, studies in Finland found that most of the increase in seat belt use occurred during media coverage of impending seat belt legislation and the ensuing public debate. Very little additional seat belt usage was detected after the seat belt law went into effect. In California, it appears that there was an acceleration in the decline in smoking in 1988 during the period of debate over Proposition 99 continuing through the end of 1988 prior to the tobacco tax's going into effect. These findings demonstrate the power of media coverage of public health and health policy issues to shape community norms and modify individual behavior.

There are potentially important cultural differences in media usage and influence. African Americans tend to watch television to a greater extent and get more of their health information from television than other ethnic groups. Hispanic, and perhaps other recently immigrated groups, show a tendency to consume radio programming to a greater extent.

It is almost as rare for school tobacco programs to be orchestrated with media programming as with policy action. Where it has happened, i.e., the North Karelia Project, the Minnesota Heart Health Program, and the Midwestern Prevention Program, the results have been notable.

ESTABLISHING COMMUNITY NORMS ABOUT THE PRACTICE OF PREVENTION IN OUR SCHOOLS

There needs to be established clear norms regarding the practice of prevention. Until now federal and state agencies have played a largely passive role, advisory at most, regarding school programming for prevention. This has to change. It is important that federal and state educational and tobacco control agencies adopt and enforce empirically based prevention program standards such as those suggested in the consensus statements issued by NIDA (1997), the Irvine Prevention Conference (Sussman and Johnson, 1996), NCI (Glynn, 1989), and CDC.

Of course the problem of quality standards in education is not unique to tobacco and drug abuse prevention. There is no lack of innovative ideas and experimentation in public education. All sorts of approaches have emerged for teaching math, reading, and the physical and social sciences. Once promulgated, unproved innovations in education then are modified, tweaked, and filtered in application at the local level, all with little or no standardized outcome assessment. It can be argued that the major problem with public education is that it encourages curricular diversity and experimentation, i.e., curricular pluralism, at the expense of enlightened discrimination in the interest of progress. There is no effective mechanism for establishing public norms about what is effective in curriculum, what the standards of practice should be, how to enforce practice standards, and how to monitor and assure progress in curricular outcomes. This is certainly true in regards to tobacco and drug abuse prevention curricula.

It is in the context of individual school autonomy and benign teacher neglect that the forces of prevention program marketing are played out. Programs and curricula are promoted, gain recognition, and eventually become fashionable in the same way that basketball shoes, VCR formats, and even cigarettes do, not through an appeal to reason and scientific validation, but through savvy marketing practices. These marketing practices appeal to emotion (in the case of drug abuse curricula, typically fear), and typically present products in slick and convenient packaging, all delivered through highly efficient distribution systems. Often the marketing of school prevention programs thrives on consumer ignorance, sometimes promoting it by suppressing or disparaging evidence contrary to program effectiveness, sometimes going to extreme ends to undermine the credibility of responsible researchers. In the world of marketing perhaps all is seen as fair.

What is needed is a social norm, an ethic about the practice of drug abuse prevention, one in which standards of program selection, implementation, community coordination, and evaluation are made very explicit and are reinforced unequivocally. The recent consensus statements of prevention expert panels, and the endorsement by key federal agencies are steps in the right direction. But they are not enough.

We cannot assume that teachers trained and experienced in didactic classroom instruction, can move easily into the role of facilitator and processor that research has shown to be necessary for effective program delivery (Rohrbach, et al., 1996). Fundamental changes in youths' perceptions of social norms, so necessary for prevention effectiveness, cannot be brought about by lecture and discipline alone, but require teaching through interactive modalities, including role playing, structured social comparison with peers and ideal role models, vicarious learning, and processes of group consensus.

Community norms about the practice of prevention, therefore, must include the expectation that: (1) teachers be selected for qualities compatible with effective drug prevention education, (2) teachers be thoroughly trained and periodically re-trained to teach and otherwise deliver prevention programming in a standardized and rigorously reinforced manner, and (3) quality assurance standards be established to assure not only that programs are implemented well, but that intended outcomes are achieved, i.e., effective reductions in tobacco and other substance use.

Any attention to community norms and their modification should be sensitive to cultural issues. Inner-city youth who are disproportionately African-American, Hispanic-American, and recent Asian-American immigrants may be more concerned with day-to-day survival and consumed by feelings of despair regarding long-term aspirations. Youth in China are in the midst of dramatic economic and

228 / SUBSTANCE ABUSE PREVENTION

social changes where Confucian and Marxist ideologies are being uprooted by Western and free-economy influences. Youth in Russia are also in the midst of dramatic economic and cultural changes that for the short-term at least are considerably for the worse for the majority. Normative change and normative conflict are fundamental considerations for school and community based prevention programming for much of the world, including our own urban settings.

In the end, norms must be addressed at all relevant levels, from the perceptions of youth, to the behavioral standards of cultures and subcultures, to environmental support for prevention, to community expectations about effective prevention programming. Researchers, educators, parents, and public policy decision makers should attend to the synergistic potential of school, media, community, and public policy programming to create and sustain consistent anti-tobacco norms. A multi-faceted approach to shaping norms provides the potential synergism that may provide for breakthroughs in tobacco and other drug abuse prevention.

REFERENCES

Chen, X., Johnson, C. A., Li, Y., and Unger, J. (in preparation). *Who Contributes More to Adolescent Smoking in China: Parents or Peers?* Results from a pilot study in Wuhan, China.

Chou, C. P., Montgomery, S., Pentz, M. A., Rohrbach, L. A., Johnson, C. A., Flay, B. R. and MacKinnon, D. P. (1998). Effects of a community-based prevention program on decreasing drug use in high risk adolescents. *American Journal of Public Health*, 88:944-948.

Donaldson, S. I., Sussman, S., MacKinnon, D. P., Severson, H. H., Glynn, T., Murray, D. M. and Stone, E. J. (1996). Drug use prevention programming: Do we know what content works? *American Behavioral Scientist*, 39(7):868-883.

Ellickson, P. and Bell, R. (1990). Drug prevention in junior high: A multi-site longitudinal test. *Science*, 247:1299-1305.

Glynn, T. (1989). Essential elements of school-based smoking prevention programs. *Journal of School Health*, 59:181-189.

Graham, J. W., Johnson, C. A., Hansen, W. B., Flay, B. R. and Gee, M. (1990). Drug use prevention programs, gender, and ethnicity: Evaluation of three seventh-grade Project SMART cohorts. *Preventive Medicine*, 19:305-313.

Hansen, W. B. and Graham, J. W. (1991). Preventing alcohol, marijuana, and cigarette use among adolescents: Peer pressure resistance training versus establishing conservative norms. *Preventive Medicine*, 20:414-430.

Hansen, W. B. and McNeal, R. B. (1997). How D.A.R.E. works: An examination of program effects on mediating variables. *Health Education and Behavior*, 24(2):165-176.

Johnson, C. A., Pentz, M. A., Weber, M. D., Dwyer, J. H., Baer, N., MacKinnon, D. P. and Hansen, W. B. (1990). Relative effectiveness of comprehensive community programming for drug abuse prevention with high-risk and low-risk adolescents. *Journal of Consulting and Clinical Psychology*, 8:447-456.

Johnson, C. A., Yan, L., Chen, X., Guo, Q., Unger, J. and Trinidad, D. (in preparation). Predictors of early smoking in Wuhan, China.

MacKinnon, D. P., Johnson, C. A., Pentz, M. A., Dwyer, J. H., Hansen, W. B., Flay, B. R. and Wang, E. Y. (1991). Mediating mechanisms in a school-based drug prevention program: First-year effects of the Midwestern Prevention Project. *Health Psychology*, 10:164-172.

National Prevalence Survey of Smoking Pattern (1996). In F. Lixin, H. Zhengjing, L. Futian, C. Aiping, K. Becker, Y. Jie, M. Enbo, T. Minxin, and L. Lauter (Eds.), *Smoking and Health in China*.

National Institute on Drug Abuse. (1997). *Monitoring the future study*. Rockville, MD: Author.

National Public Radio (broadcast), September 1997.

Newcomb, M. and Earleywine, M. (1996). Intrapersonal contributors to drug use. *American Behavioral Scientist*, 39(7):823-837.

Nezami, E., Johnson, C. A. and Chou, C. P. (1997). Direct and indirect or normative perception of marijuana use on future use among adolescents. Poster presented at the Society of Behavioral Medicine's 18th Annual Meeting, San Francisco, CA, April 16-19, 1997.

Pentz, M. A., MacKinnon, D. P., Dwyer, J. H., Wang, E. Y. I., Hansen, W. B., Flay, B. R. and Johnson, C. A. (1989). Longitudinal effects of The Midwestern Prevention Project (MPP) on regular and experimental smoking in adolescents. *Preventive Medicine*, 18:304-321.

Pentz, M. A., Sussman, S. and Newman, T. (1997). The conflict between least harm and no-use tobacco policy youth: Ethical and policy implications. *Addiction*, 92(9): 1165-1173.

Perry, C. L., Klepp, K. I., Halper, A., Hawkins, K. G. and Murray, D. M. (1986). A process evaluation study of peer leaders in health education. *Journal of School Health*, 56:62-67.

Pierce, J. P., Evans, N., Farkas, A. J., Cavin, S. W., Berry, C., Kramer, M., Kealey, S., Rosbrook, B., Choi, W. and Kaplan, R. M. (1994). *Tobacco Use in California: An Evaluation of the Tobacco Control Program 1989-1993*. University of California, San Diego: San Diego, CA.

Rogers, T., Feighery, E. L., Tencati, E. M., Butler, J. L. and Weiner, L. (1995). Community mobilization to reduce point-of-purchase advertising of tobacco products. *Health Education Quarterly*, 22(4):427-442.

Rohrbach, L. A., D'Onofrio, C. N., Backer, T. E. and Montgomery, S. B. (1996). Diffusion of school-based substance abuse prevention programs. *American Behavioral Scientist*, 39(7):919-934.

Sussman, S. and Johnson, C. A. (1996). Drug abuse prevention: Programming and research recommendations. *American Behavioral Scientist*, 39(7), special issue.

U.S. Department of Health and Human Services (1994). *Preventing tobacco use among young people: A report of the surgeon general*. U.S. Department of Health and Human Services, Public Health Service, Centers for Disease Control and Prevention, National

Center for Chronic Disease Prevention and Health Promotion, Office of Smoking and Health: Atlanta, GA.

Vartiainen, E., Pallonen, U., McAllister, A. L. and Puska, P. (1990). Eight-year follow-up results of an adolescent smoking prevention program: The North Karelia Youth Project. *American Journal of Public Health*, 80:78-79.

CHAPTER 11

Alcohol and Tobacco Legislative Policies in Multicultural Communities

Ruth Roemer

Recent evidence released by the U.S. Surgeon General reveals an alarming rise in tobacco use among minority teen-agers in the United States (USDHHS, 1998). Examining smoking rates among four groups, African Americans, American Indians and Alaska Natives, Asian/Pacific Islanders, and Hispanics, the report finds that cigarette use increased among all four groups but was significantly higher for African Americans and Hispanics. Especially distressing is the rise in smoking rates among African-American youth, since declines in this group in the 1970s and 1980s had been considered a public health success. But from 1991 to 1997 smoking rates among African-American teenagers have increased 80 percent, and African-American men die from lung cancer at a rate 50 percent higher than Whites. Each year approximately 45,000 African Americans die from totally preventable smoking- related diseases.

New evidence contained in tobacco industry documents released at Congressional hearings before the House Judiciary Committee in February 1998 provides a partial explanation for this threat to multicultural communities. These documents show how the major tobacco companies ran advertising campaigns in magazines, on billboards and buses, and in other media to attract African Americans, especially, to mentholated brands like Salem and Kool (Meier, 1998). For example, a 1973 document of Brown and Williamson showed that 17 percent of the company's promotional budget for Kools was spent on marketing to African Americans, who constituted only 10 percent of the population. Urging more spending on advertising on buses and subways, the document states, "With

231

this additional transit effort, Kool will cover the top 25 markets in terms of absolute Negroes."

Ethnic minority communities also suffer an enormous burden of alcohol-related morbidity and mortality (Jones-Webb, et al., 1995). Drinking by youth correlates with increases in other high-risk behavior (ONDCP, 1998). Drinking greatly increases the risk of being involved in a car crash. More than 2,300 youths aged fifteen to twenty died in alcohol related crashes in 1996 (Wright, 1997). Alcohol use is a significant risk factor not only for motor vehicle crashes but also for boating and recreational activities, injuries, assaults, suicides and homicides, as well as for diseases such as cancer and liver cirrhosis (*Seventh Special Report*, 1990). Leaders in the field of prevention research agree that "alcohol related problems are a major threat to public health and safety, a threat to which policy makers and the prevention community are impelled to respond" (Holder, et al., 1995).

This chapter concerns the response of legislation to combat the preventable morbidity and mortality caused by alcohol and tobacco use. Such legislation faces strong and well-financed opposition from the alcohol and tobacco industries, which are deeply committed to both increasing sales in existing markets and extending their markets to new users of their products. In pursuit of this objective, the alcohol industry does not acknowledge that alcohol itself is a problem but rather that alcoholics are the cause of alcohol related problems (Ashley and Rankin, 1988). The tobacco industry, despite the enormous wealth of evidence to the contrary, continues to deny that smoking causes disease (Hilts, 1994). As Ashley and Rankin point out in their seminal article on prevention of alcohol problems, ". . . promotional activities are purported only to serve objectives related to beverage or brand preference, not to have an effect on consumption, a view similar to that held by the tobacco industry of its products" (Ashley and Rankin, 1988).

Both industries are engaged in activities to expand consumption and to make drinking and smoking acceptable social behavior—a reality that legislative efforts must confront.

While the circumstances and risks associated with use of alcohol and tobacco differ, and therefore call for differing laws and regulations, there are several similarities in the legislative responses to control alcohol abuse and tobacco use. First, in both cases the types of legislative policies that are available fall into two main categories: (1) to control the supply and (2) to control the demand. Second, in both cases, it is important to design policies that are effective in deterring young people from drinking and smoking. Third, success in both fields will depend on changing the social environment concerning use of alcohol and tobacco. Fourth is the necessity not only of enacting but enforcing legislation to control use of both alcohol and tobacco. And, fifth, is the need to support policies—education, employment, health, and recreation—that promote healthful lifestyles.

We begin with a discussion of the role of legislation in health promotion and disease prevention. Then we turn to a review of the types of legislation available for sound alcohol policy and evaluation of their effectiveness. Next is an analysis of tobacco control legislation of various types and worldwide experience in this field. Finally, taking account of the gravity of alcohol-related problems and the rising rates of tobacco use among ethnic minorities, we suggest some legislative priorities for multicultural communities.

ROLE OF LEGISLATION IN HEALTH PROMOTION AND DISEASE PREVENTION

Why legislation, you may ask, to discourage alcohol abuse and combat alcohol problems? Why legislation to prevent smoking by young people and to encourage smokers to stop? Why legislation, rather than education, to bring about behavior change?

Certainly education and public information are essential to behavior change. But for effective prevention policies legislation is an absolute necessity. As the Institute of Medicine stated in its landmark report, *Alcohol and Public Policy*, in 1981, "Drinking practices can be affected principally by law and by education" (Moore and Gerstein, 1981).

The report concludes that legal action to reduce drunk driving has been effective when the law has been enforced and the public knows it will be enforced. Although education, information, and training to reduce alcohol problems have had a checkered history, in recent years promising initiatives in health education combine mass communication principles with behavior modification techniques.

The message is even stronger in the case of tobacco control. An expert committee of the World Health Organization early recognized the necessity for legislation if the tobacco epidemic is to be controlled:

> It may be tempting to try introducing smoking control programmes without a legislative component, in the hope that relatively inoffensive activity of this nature will placate those concerned with public health, while generating no real opposition from cigarette manufacturers. This approach, however, is not likely to succeed. A genuine broadly defined education programme aimed at reducing smoking must be complemented by legislation and restrictive measures . . . (WHO, 1983).

Opposition to legislation by the alcohol and tobacco industries is based on the issues of liberty and choice. The alcohol industry contends that government should not seek to shape drinking practices, that is not the role of government in a free society. The tobacco industry says that smoking is a matter of choice for adults. In answer to these contentions, we should note that the role of government is to protect the health, welfare, and safety of its people. Government has the responsibility to protect the health of the people, particularly of children, to preserve the quality of the environment, to regulate trade and commerce, and to enhance the general welfare by social controls that, for example, prevent drunk driving and provide smoke-free public places (Moore and Gerstein, 1981, pp. 55-58; Roemer, 1993).

The specific purposes of legislation on alcohol and tobacco control are as follows:

1. To prohibit conduct injurious to health.
2. To authorize and finance programs and services to protect and promote health, including treatment programs for alcoholism, cessation programs for tobacco addiction, and education programs on alcohol and tobacco.
3. To control the manufacture, promotion, and sale of alcohol and tobacco products.
4. To create an atmosphere in which moderate use of alcohol (defined as no more than two drinks a day) (Toomey, et al., 1993) and nonsmoking are the accepted social norms.
5. To promote public attitudes that immoderate drinking and tobacco use are dangerous, unhealthful, and socially unacceptable.
6. To dissuade young people from alcohol abuse and from taking up smoking and permit young people to grow up free from the enticements to drink excessively and to smoke.
7. To protect drivers and pedestrians from drunk drivers.
8. To protect the health of nonsmokers and their right to breathe clean air and decrease the opportunities for smokers to smoke.
9. To encourage those who drink not to drive, pregnant women to abstain from alcohol use, smokers to stop smoking, young people not to start drinking and smoking, workers exposed to industrial hazards not to smoke, workers in occupations where responsibility is taken for the lives of others (airline pilots, transport workers) or in occupations that serve as models for others (health services personnel, teachers) not to drink or smoke.

Legislative policies on both alcohol and tobacco may be divided into two types: (1) supply side measures to control the manufacture, promotion, and sale of the products and (2) demand side measures to effect behavioral changes among drinkers and smokers. These laws affect everyone, of course, but may have special significance for racial/ethnic minority groups.

LEGISLATIVE COMPONENTS OF ALCOHOL POLICY

The contemporary approach to alcohol-related problems is a public health approach—a prevention approach focused on the population as a whole, rather than an individualized, personalized approach focused on the heavy drinker (Moore and Gerstein, 1981, pp. 52-55; Toomey, et al., 1993, p. 279). The reasons given for a population-directed approach are as follows: (1) we do not have the resources to cure all at risk; (2) those at high risk are not always identifiable, and membership in high risk groups is continually changing; and what may be surprising to the reader as it was to the author, (3) the majority of problems related to alcohol use are attributable to moderate rather than heavy alcohol consumers (Moore and Gerstein, 1981, pp. 52-55; Toomey, et al., 1993, p. 279).

Supply Side Measures on Alcohol Control

The following types of legislation are designed to control the manufacture, promotion, and sale of alcohol—the supply side.

- structure of the distribution system (state monopolies, privatized licensing systems)
- restrictions on legal availability (times and places that alcohol is available and number, kinds, and location of outlets selling alcohol)
- controls on product contents and packaging (warning labels)
- marketing control policies (advertising, warnings, social availability)

Structure of the Distribution System

Distribution systems for alcoholic beverages range from state monopolies to privatized license systems. State alcoholic beverage control agencies vary in the degree of control over off-premise retail sales of spirits, price regulations, and the number and severity of penalties for illegal alcohol sales (Toomey, et al., 1993, pp. 282-283).

The effect of privatization has been studied mainly by examining the result of introducing wine sales in grocery stores (Holder and Wagenaar, 1990; Wagenaar and Holder, 1991, 1995). This issue, however, is difficult to isolate because privatization is generally associated with other changes in alcohol availability, such as increased number of sales outlets, longer sale hours, use of credit cards, and increased price promotions and advertising. Although recent studies have produced mixed results on whether privatization of wine and distilled spirits distribution increases consumption, authorities conclude that, "[S]tudies using robust research designs indicate that privatization of alcohol distribution systems increases per capita alcohol consumption" (Toomey, et al., 1993, p. 283).

In view of the evidence that privatization increases wine sales particularly, and the fact that privatization of distribution systems cannot be reversed, it is suggested that states with monopoly distribution systems may wish to refrain from privatization until its effects are fully understood (Toomey, et al., 1993, p. 283).

Restrictions on Availability

A major type of alcohol legislation concerns restrictions on the availability of alcohol and alcohol consumption. Since state and local jurisdictions have authority to regulate retail sales of alcohol through licensing or other regulations (Gorovitz, et al., 1998; Moore and Gerstein, 1981, p. 74), controls have been placed on numbers and location of outlets, types of outlet, and times of sale. Evidence concerning the effectiveness of such limitations, however, though extensive, is mixed (Ashley and Rankin, 1988, pp. 247-251; Moore and Gerstein, 1981, pp. 73-76; Toomey, et al., 1993, pp. 283-285). In addition, statutes on minimum drinking age have an important impact on legal availability, an issue discussed below in connection with demand for alcohol.

Without reviewing the many studies of these kinds of restrictions, we may note two studies of density of on-premises and off-premises sales outlets—an issue that has gained prominence in recent years in connection with inner city urban riots and their aftermath. A study of seventy-four cities in Los Angeles County found that the rate of violent crime was significantly associated with density of both on-sale and off-sale outlets (Scribner, et al., 1995). A 1 percent increase in the density of alcohol outlets was found to be associated with a .26 percent increase in the rate of violent offenses. By contrast, a study of 223 municipalities in New Jersey found no geographic association between the rate of assaultive violence and the density of alcohol outlets (Gorman, et al., 1988). This finding, however, may be explained by differences in several variables. The New Jersey municipalities have a lower rate of assaultive violence, a lower alcohol outlet density, fewer off-sale outlets, a lower percentage of Latino residents, and much smaller population size. Clearly, further research is needed to ascertain the relationship between alcohol outlet density and violent crime.

Even without definitive research, however, it is apparent that numerous liquor stores in or near a residential community and ready availability of alcoholic beverages in grocery stores, not to mention pervasive advertising of alcohol, send a message to young people that alcohol consumption is an accepted social norm. The influence of liquor stores on nearly every corner in inner city communities—as contrasted with upper income neighborhoods—cannot be ignored.

Other legislation designed to reduce availability restricts the location of sales outlets near public transportation, churches, schools, and residential areas. Also, legislation restricting drinking in public places—in parks, plazas, and school grounds and at places and events where non-drinkers are present—is becoming more common. But evaluation of these strategies requires more research (Toomey, et al., 1993, pp. 281-282). Restrictions on hours of sale seem to have little impact on alcohol-related problems, merely shifting the time when these problems occur (Toomey, et al., 1993, p. 285). Perhaps these kinds of restrictions serve mainly as educational expressions to prevent alcohol-related problems.

In connection with restrictions on outlets are state or local requirements for server training for persons who serve or sell alcohol and state "dram" shop laws that impose liability on alcohol sellers and servers for damages caused by illegally served persons—intoxicated persons and minors. This type of legislation seems promising in increasing knowledge about ways to reduce intoxication and interventions to prevent harm. Statewide mandatory training and increased server liability appear to be effective in reducing alcohol-related motor vehicle crashes, but continuing research is recommended (Toomey, et al., 1993, pp. 285-286; Moore and Gerstein, 1981, pp. 253-254).

Controls on Product Contents and Packaging

The principal legislation in this field is the federal requirement that all alcoholic beverage containers distributed in the United States contain the following health warning:

> GOVERNMENT WARNING: (1) According to the Surgeon General, women should not drink alcoholic beverages during pregnancy because of the risk of birth defects. (2) Consumption of alcoholic beverages impairs your ability to drive a car or operate machinery, and may cause health problems.

For some beverages the labels must also provide information on alcoholic content. Wine is labeled for percent alcohol, and distilled spirits are described by the proof system. The warning label has been criticized as too long, not sufficiently clear, and difficult to read. The content requirement has been questioned as perhaps less effective than communicating alcohol content in terms of "standard drinks." Nevertheless, consumers are entitled to have this information, and they show considerable awareness of the warnings (Toomey, et al., 1993, pp. 286-288).

Marketing Control Policies

The principal marketing controls on alcohol concern advertising, messages in the media, and warning labels (discussed above).

Alcohol is one of the world's largest advertising categories. Expenditures for alcohol advertising rose sixfold from the mid-1960s to the mid-1980s, reaching the sum of $3 billion worldwide (Holder and Edwards, 1995, p. 193). The dominant theme for alcohol advertising, as for tobacco advertising, is to associate the product with a lifestyle of wealth, prestige, success, or social approval. The industry in the United States has agreed to a voluntary ban on advertising distilled spirits on television, but advertising in the print media and on billboards has been a prominent feature of U.S. society. No warning labels are required on alcohol advertising as they are on tobacco advertising. Currently, the density of alcohol-related billboards is much greater in African-American and Hispanic communities than in areas that are predominantly White (Altman, et al., 1991).

In response to public criticism that poor and minority neighborhoods are inundated with tobacco and alcohol billboards, in June 1989 the Outdoor Advertising Association of America adopted a voluntary code for advertising designed to assure that tobacco and alcohol billboards are at least 500 feet from schools, churches, and hospitals and limiting the number of such billboards. But this voluntary code is often ignored (Hackbarth, et al., 1995).

Concerned about the saturation of minority neighborhoods with alcohol and tobacco billboards, the American Lung Association of Metropolitan Chicago, together with other health advocacy and community groups, undertook a study in 1990 of the number and themes of all billboards in Chicago. The study found that there were 27.8 alcohol billboards per 10,000 population in minority wards, compared with 8.5 per 10,000 in White wards. The number of alcohol billboards in White wards ranged from one to fifteen, with a mean of seven. In contrast, in minority wards the range was from 1 to 111, with a mean of 38. On average, minority wards were burdened with more than five times as many alcohol billboards as White wards. The findings were similar for tobacco billboards. Minority wards had an average of three times as many tobacco billboards as White wards (Hackbarth, et al., 1995, pp. 220-223). With this proof that the alcohol and tobacco industries have targeted minority communities in Chicago, the city of Chicago banned outdoor alcohol and tobacco billboards. In a challenge to the ordinance by the advertising industry, a district court set aside the ordinance on the ground of federal preemption (*Federation of Advertising Representatives, Inc. v. City of Chicago*—F. Supp.2d—(1998). An appeal is pending.

Another billboard study in Los Angeles in 1989 compared the density of alcohol advertisements in two districts of the city where 53.3 percent of the residents were African American and two suburban districts with 2.9 percent African-American residents. The density of alcohol advertisements was sixteen times greater in the city than in the suburbs (Ewert and Alleyne, 1992).

But a new wave of local legislation banning alcohol and tobacco billboards within 1,000 feet of schools and parks is sweeping the country. The movement started in Baltimore, Maryland and has now reached California, as discussed below in connection with tobacco advertising.

One way in which use of alcohol is subtly promoted is through entertainment. The film industry uses drinking as a background feature, and few negative effects are shown (Holder and Edwards, 1995, ch. 8). This practice suggests that advertising and various forms of promotion by the alcohol industry may have the normative effect of making alcohol use accepted social behavior—a long-held goal of the alcohol industry, as mentioned earlier.

Demand Side Measures on Alcohol Control

The following types of measures are designed to change behavior and thus affect the demand for alcohol:

- minimum legal drinking age laws
- legislation on drinking and driving
- taxation and price
- public intoxication laws
- information and education
- reducing environmental risk

Minimum Legal Drinking Age Laws

When Prohibition was repealed, all states designated twenty-one as the minimum age for purchasing and consuming alcohol, but when the age of majority was lowered to eighteen, many states lowered their minimum legal drinking age to eighteen. Several studies in the 1970s showed that traffic crashes increased significantly among teenagers in these states. On the basis of this evidence and action by citizen advocacy groups, sixteen states raised their minimum drinking age to twenty-one. The rest followed suit when the Federal Government passed the Uniform Drinking Age Act, which provided for a decrease in Federal highway funds to states that failed to establish twenty-one as the minimum legal drinking age (Toomey, et al., 1996). This experience provided a natural experiment for investigating the effect of minimum age drinking laws.

Many studies of minimum age drinking laws have shown significant reduction in car crashes and other problems among youth when the minimum legal drinking age was raised to twenty-one (Toomey, et al., 1996; Wagenaar, 1995). The National Highway Traffic Safety Administration found that raising the minimum age to twenty-one saved the lives of more than 1,000 young people each year (NHTSA, 1989).

Despite proof in numerous studies that a minimum legal drinking age of twenty-one saves lives, enforcement has been weak, and the rate of enforcement varies greatly among states (Wagenaar and Wolfson, 1994). Teenagers can easily buy beer and other liquor. Enforcement systems penalize underage drinkers more than the establishments that sell alcohol to them. For every 1,000 teenagers arrested for alcohol possession only 130 establishments that sell alcohol to them have actions taken against them (Toomey, et al., 1996, p. 215). Various strategies can strengthen enforcement of these effective laws: administrative suspension of licenses to sell alcohol; increased numbers of enforcement personnel for Alcohol Beverage Control agencies; regular sting operations in which an underage person attempts to purchase alcohol; and community support for prevention of youth drinking (Wagenaar and Wolfson, 1994, pp. 46-50).

Laws on Drinking and Driving

As of 1995, all but two states (Massachusetts and South Carolina) have "per se" laws making it a crime to drive with a blood alcohol concentration level

(BAC) at or above a prescribed level—usually .08 or .10 percent. Most states specify a much lower BAC level for young drivers below the age of twenty-one or eighteen (IIHS, 1995). A "per se" law provides that finding a specified blood alcohol content level is a conclusive presumption of guilt. The criminal penalties specified in the law are mandatory, and license suspension or revocation generally follows conviction. In thirty-nine states and the District of Columbia an administrative license suspension may also be imposed right after arrest if the driver fails or refuses to take a chemical test. While studies of the deterrent effect of Driving Under the Influence (DUI) laws are inconclusive, indications are that strict enforcement, a high perceived risk of arrest, and public information and education campaigns can deter drinking and driving (Reed, 1981).

Taxation and Price

An important strategy to reduce alcohol consumption and problems caused by it is to raise the price by means of increased Federal excise taxes and state taxes. Abundant evidence demonstrates that higher prices and taxes are associated with lower drinking rates, although the effect of price on consumption levels seems to vary by beverage class. Adult consumers are more sensitive to increased wine and spirits prices, and youth to increased beer prices (Ashley and Rankin, 1988, pp. 244-247; Moore and Gerstein, 1981, pp. 68-73; Toomey, et al., 1993, p. 280).

Unfortunately, federal excise taxes on alcoholic beverages remained constant from 1951 to 1985 and were raised only moderately in 1985 for distilled spirits and in 1991 for all classes of alcoholic beverage (Toomey, et al., 1993, p. 281). Thus, prices have not kept pace with the rate of inflation, making alcohol a cheap luxury. Clearly, this result is at variance with the consensus of researchers that price increases are one of the most important measures in an effective prevention policy.

Public Intoxication Laws

The criminal law operates to regulate drinking behavior through statutes on public intoxication, drunk and disorderly conduct, and vagrancy, but these laws have the objective of controlling the peace and quiet of the community rather than drinking. Recognition that the criminal law offered no solution to alcohol abuse led to a movement for decriminalization and substitution of treatment approaches for punitive approaches.

Several court decisions reversed convictions of chronic alcoholics for public intoxication on the ground that alcoholism is a disease and conviction for public intoxication would be cruel and unusual punishment in violation of the Eighth Amendment (*Driver v. Hinant*, 1966; *Easter v. District of Columbia*, 1966; *Robinson v. California*, 1962). But in 1968 the U.S. Supreme Court upheld a conviction for public intoxication despite clear evidence that the defendant was an alcoholic. A justification for the decision that the conviction did not amount to cruel and unusual punishment was that although the defendant may have been under a compulsion to drink he was not under any compulsion to appear in public in an intoxicated condition (*Powell, v. Texas,* 1968).

This case ended efforts through the courts to substitute treatment for punishment of alcoholics. It led the states to enact laws providing for detoxification centers for voluntary use, referral to detoxification units of alcoholics taken into custody, and civil commitment to mental hospitals when necessary. At the Federal level, Congress enacted the Alcoholism Rehabilitation Act of 1968, which expanded community mental health centers, established the Institute on Alcohol Abuse and Alcoholism within the National Institutes of Health, and provided grants to the states for prevention, treatment, and rehabilitation programs. Thus, Federal and State laws are providing more constructive solutions to public drunkenness than public intoxication and vagrancy statutes.

Information and Education

Public information is essential to enact legislation and to implement it. Legislation is essential to authorize programs and funding for public information. Thus, effective alcohol policy depends on the symbiotic relationship between public information and legislation. For example, laws on minimum legal drinking age and drinking and driving require support of the people for passage and enforcement, and this support depends on knowledge by the people of the crucial importance of these laws to the welfare of youth and society in general.

Educational programs in schools, likewise, require legislation to authorize and fund them. The Institute of Medicine points out, as mentioned earlier, that drinking practices may be influenced by both law and by education and that education, information, and training programs are important complements to legal approaches (Moore and Gerstein, 1981, p. 89). In analyzing experience with these three types of program, the IOM Report concluded that (1) the behavior and health risks that are targeted should be clearly defined, (2) emphasis should be placed on new knowledge, skills, and maintenance of these skills, and (3) reliance should be placed on the professional skills of people trained in behavioral and communication sciences rather than on commercial advertisers and voluntary groups (Moore and Gerstein, 1981, p. 96).

Reducing Environmental Risk

Recognition that the best prevention policy will still not reach all alcohol problems has resulted in proposals for reducing environmental risk for persons who drink. The strategies suggested are physical safety measures and social safety measures (Moore and Gerstein, 1981, ch. 6). Physical safety measures include use of non-flammable materials, improving automobile engineering, use of passive restraints in cars (e.g., air bags), and improved consumer products. Social safety measures include use of designated drivers, server training to protect customers (discussed previously), checks by supervisors of workers reporting for potentially dangerous work, and the enormous challenge of reducing hostility and violence in our society.

LEGISLATION TO COMBAT THE TOBACCO EPIDEMIC

The first Surgeon General's report to deal exclusively with tobacco use among racial/ethnic minority groups, released in 1998, contains alarming news, as mentioned at the outset of this chapter. Its principal conclusions are:

1. Cigarette smoking is a major cause of disease and death in each of the four population groups—African Americans, American Indians and Alaska Natives, Asian/Pacific Islanders, and Hispanics, with African Americans bearing the greatest risk burden.
2. Tobacco use varies among the four groups. Among adults, American Indians and Alaskan Natives have the highest prevalence of tobacco use. African-American and Southeast-Asian men also have a high prevalence of smoking, and Asian-American and Hispanic women have the lowest prevalence.
3. Among adolescents, cigarette smoking prevalence increased in the 1990s among African Americans and Hispanics after several years of substantial decline among all four racial/ethnic groups. This increase is particularly striking among African-American youths, who had the greatest decline of the four groups in the 1970s and 1980s.
4. Multiple factors determine patterns of tobacco use—socioeconomic status, cultural characteristics, acculturation, stress, biological elements, targeted advertising, price of tobacco products, and varying capacities of communities to launch effective control initiatives.
5. Rigorous surveillance and prevention research are needed on the changing cultural, psychosocial, and environmental factors that influence tobacco use to improve understanding of racial/ethnic smoking patterns and identify strategic tobacco control opportunities (USDHHS, 1998, p. 6).

The data in this report sound an alarm for African-American and Southeast-Asian men, for American Indian and Alaska-Native women of reproductive age, and for African-American and Hispanic adolescents, all of whom have a high prevalence of tobacco use.

The increase in smoking among African-American youth is particularly disturbing because this group had had the greatest decline in smoking in the 1970s and 1980s (USDHHS, 1998, p. 12). In fact, the trend of lower smoking prevalence among African-American adolescents in the 1970s and 1980s has continued as these individuals age and become young adults—a finding that speaks loudly for enforcement of the Food and Drug Administration's regulations to reduce access to and appeal of tobacco to youth. In addition to the recent increases among African American high school seniors, smoking among eighth grade African-American students increased from 5.3 percent in 1992 to 9.6 percent in 1996 and among ninth grade African-American students from 6.6 percent in 1992 to 12.2 percent in 1996 (USDHHS, 1998, pp. 30-31).

Especially significant is the report's exploration of possible interactions between the use of alcohol or other drugs and changes in cigarette smoking among African-American and White adolescents. Several recent studies have confirmed the finding of the 1994 Surgeon General's report, *Preventing Tobacco Use among Young People*, that youth tobacco use is associated with various health compromising behaviors, including being involved in fights, carrying weapons, engaging in higher-risk sexual behavior, and using alcohol and other drugs (USDHHS, 1998, p. 44).

Also important is the finding that declines in smoking prevalence were greater among African-American, Hispanic, and White men who were high school graduates than among those with less formal education. Educational attainment, however, explains only some of the differences in smoking behaviors (current smoking, heavy smoking, ever smoking, and smoking cessation) between Whites and the four racial/ethnic minority groups. Other biological, social, and cultural factors are thought to account for these differences (USDHHS, 1998, p. 94; Yang, 1998a).

This report is a goldmine of well-documented information on tobacco use among the four racial/ethnic minority groups. It provides policy makers with a wealth of data to design effective strategies to control the tobacco epidemic.

One of the most effective strategies for prevention and control of tobacco use is legislation. As mentioned above, a WHO expert committee in 1983 recognized the absolute necessity for legislation if tobacco use, the largest single cause of preventable mortality and morbidity, is to be reduced (WHO, 1983).

Important as legislation has proved to be in combating the tobacco epidemic, it should be emphasized that legislation is only one component in a comprehensive attack on the tobacco epidemic. Legislation is essential to establish and promulgate public policy, to enlist the resources of all government departments, to strengthen the activities of voluntary organizations and citizens' groups, and to contribute to the development of a non-smoking environment. Also essential are prevention activities, public information, educational campaigns, smoking cessation programs, outreach to high risk populations, a tax and price policy based on health needs, economic strategies to decrease tobacco production, research on biological, behavioral, economic, and social aspects of tobacco use, and monitoring the effects of tobacco control strategies (Roemer, 1993, pp. 7-8).

As in the case of alcohol control, we analyze here tobacco legislative policies under the two main rubrics of supply side measures and demand side measures.

Supply Side Measures for Tobacco Control

The following types of legislation are designed to control the manufacture, promotion, and sale of alcohol—the supply side.

Advertising and Promotion Bans

The importance of advertising to the tobacco industry is reflected in the size and growth of its expenditures for this purpose. Between 1975 and 1983, the amount of money spent to promote cigarettes increased from $490 million to $1.9 billion (Tye, et al., 1987). By 1988, advertising and promotional expenditures in the United States alone had reached $3.27 billion (CDC, 1990). By 1991, tobacco expenditures for advertising had risen to $4.65 billion (Lynch and Bonnie, 1994, p. 105). R.J. Reynolds budgeted $75 million a year to advertise and promote the cartoon character Joe Camel on billboards, T-shirts, posters, and mugs.

Advertising themes associate smoking with pleasure, sports, beautiful scenery, sexual attractiveness, and social and professional success. So pervasive is this positive message that it overpowers any effect from the health warnings required on billboards and in print. As Richard Kluger states in his comprehensive history of the tobacco industry, *Ashes to Ashes,*

> [T]he image merchants of Madison Avenue were more capable of upstaging the warning message from the Surgeon General. The FTC regulators, mostly lawyers, had naturally been inclined, as wordsmiths, to dwell on the textual content of cigarette ads rather than their visual aspects. But even untutored analysis of the industry's print advertising discussed how effectively it had used overpowering graphics—bold imagery, lush landscapes, huge scale, vivid coloration, sharp contrast, simulated movement—to divert the reader's eye from the health warning (Kluger, 1996, pp. 443-444).

Although the industry contends that its advertising is not designed to recruit smokers but rather to encourage smokers to switch brands, the facts on brand-switching and the sheer volume of expenditures on advertising belie this contention. In pointing out that only about 10 percent of smokers switch brands in any one year, Tye and colleagues estimated that total advertising expenditures of $1.9 billion in 1983 would mean an expenditure of $345 per switcher. If each switcher also switched companies, each would account for an increase in revenue of $347, but in fact such brand-switching is to different brands within the same company, thus generating no new revenue. The industry's contention is clearly fallacious (Tye, et al., 1987, pp. 493-494).

Evidence has accumulated that the industry has targeted women, children, and minority groups. The industry has targeted women by using images that depict smoking as glamorous, sophisticated, romantic, sexy, liberating, and slimming, even naming one brand "Virginia Slims"; by advertising cigarettes in women's magazines, which discourages publication of the health hazards of smoking; and by sponsoring female sports events, such as tennis (Chollat-Traquet, 1992, pp. 5-6).

The appeal of cigarette advertisements to children was shown by experience with the Joe Camel ads. Children are exposed to cigarette advertising, and those as young as three years were able to recognize the Joe Camel cartoon character as representing cigarettes. One well-known study found that 30 percent of three year olds and 91 percent of six year olds could identify Joe Camel as a symbol of smoking (DiFranza, et al., 1991; Fischer, et al., 1989; Fischer, et al., 1991; Lynch and Bonnie, 1994, ch. 4). Convincing evidence has demonstrated that tobacco advertising and promotions play a decisive role in causing children to use tobacco. One study of this age group in 1990 found that 32.8 percent of children who smoked reported smoking Camel cigarettes (DiFranza, et al., 1991; DiFranza, 1994). Outdoor advertising has also targeted African-American communities. A billboard survey conducted in Los Angeles in 1989, mentioned earlier, compared density of cigarette advertisements in two districts of the city where 53.3 percent of the residents were African American and two suburban districts with 2.9 percent African-American residents. The density (number of advertisements per mile) of cigarette advertisements was 4.6 times greater in the city than in the suburbs (Ewert and Alleyne, 1992).

The most flagrant examples of targeting racial/ethnic minority communities has occurred in connection with the industry's efforts to introduce brands targeting African Americans. In the 1980s, in Philadelphia, the Coalition against Uptown Cigarettes mobilized broad community support and forced R.J. Reynolds to cancel test marketing of a cigarette aimed at the African-American market. In 1995, a new mentholated cigarette packaged in the Afrocentric colors red, black, and green with a prominent symbol "X" associated with the African-American leader, Malcolm X, was withdrawn from the Boston market after protests by community leaders. In 1997, the "Just Say No to Menthol Joe Community Crusade" was launched across the nation to force R.J. Reynolds to withdraw its new menthol version of Camel. Camel Menthol clearly targets African Americans and young women, who are the most common smokers of menthol cigarettes. Among African American smokers, 76 percent smoke menthol cigarettes compared with 23 percent of White smokers. African-American adolescents most frequently purchase mentholated brands (Newport and Kool) (Advocacy Institute, 1997).

Churches, schools, and civic groups have mobilized to obtain the removal of billboards. In Chicago, an anonymous "Mandrake" painted over tobacco and alcohol billboards in ethnic neighborhoods. In New York City the Reverend Calvin Butts led his parishioners on walking tours to document and whitewash billboards advertising tobacco and alcohol (USDHHS, 1998, pp. 293-297). Clearly, billboards are one of the most effective ways of reaching a targeted group. The billboard industry's own marketing materials stress the unavoidability of billboards thus, "Outdoor is right up there. Day and night. Lurking. Waiting for another ambush" (Kessler, et al., 1996).

In recent years the tobacco industry has decreased its expenditures for advertising and has increased its spending for promotional activities. In 1995, 89 percent of its advertising and promotional expenditures were for promotion, including coupons, give-aways of free promotional gear and cigarettes, and, most importantly, sponsorship of sports and cultural events (USDHHS, 1998, p. 293). As the Surgeon General's report, *Tobacco Use among U.S. Racial/Ethnic Minority Groups*, points out, the tobacco companies have been creative in supporting cultural and sports events. They have reached out to racial/ethnic communities with Mexican rodeos, American Indian powwows, Tet festivals, Chinese New Year festivities, Cinco de Mayo festivities, etc. (USDHHS, 1998, p. 218). The Report notes the significance of the industry's support for sports events for some young people, particularly African Americans, who perceive athletic ability as a means of personal achievement (USDHHS, 1998, p. 219).

In twenty-seven countries, national legislation imposes a total ban on advertising and promotion of tobacco, and many additional countries impose strong, partial bans (Roemer, 1993, pp. 32, 38). In the United States, federal legislation bans tobacco advertising only on television and radio (The Federal Cigarette Labeling and Advertising Act, 1965; The Little Cigar Act, 1973), with the industry free to advertise on billboards, in the print media, and through promotion of cultural and sports events.

An imaginative strategy has opened a way for local communities to combat the blight of tobacco and alcoholic beverage billboards that incite young people to smoke and to drink. In 1994, the City of Baltimore passed an ordinance completely banning "publicly visible" cigarette and alcoholic beverage advertisements except on "property adjacent to an interstate highway," in heavy industrial zones, and at Baltimore Memorial Stadium (Baltimore, Md., Ordinance, 1994). This action was taken as a measure to assist enforcement of the state's minors' access law banning the sale of cigarettes to minors. The City of Baltimore was sued by a billboard company, Penn Advertising, which sought to enjoin enforcement of the tobacco ordinance on First Amendment and preemption grounds. This challenge was defeated in the federal district court, which ruled that the First Amendment had not been violated and that the federal cigarette labeling acts had not preempted Baltimore's right to regulate and prohibit alcohol and tobacco billboard advertising in order to assist enforcement of its ban on sales of alcohol and tobacco to minors. In 1995, the Fourth Circuit Court of Appeals unanimously affirmed the federal district court's judgment (*Anheuser-Busch, Inc. v. Schmoke*, 1995; *Penn Advertising of Baltimore, Inc. v. Mayor of Baltimore*, 1995, cert.den.117 Sup. Ct. Rptr. 1569, 1997), and the United States Supreme Court has refused to review the decisions of the Fourth Circuit.

In a brilliant analysis of these events and cases, Professor Donald Garner opens his article with the following delightful statement giving due credit for the launching of this successful initiative:

When, in 1990, the improbably named Rev. Calvin Butts led his Abyssinian congregation in a widely reported campaign to whitewash tobacco and alcohol billboards that litter the streets of Harlem, he inspired a national movement. As activists in other cities emulated his tactics, state and local politicians were prompted to take a fresh look at the long-standing problem of intrusive tobacco advertising (Garner, 1996).

After reviewing the First Amendment and preemption issues involved in these two cases, Professor Garner concludes, "A billboard ban thus offers local communities a legal avenue to help curb the rising tide of juvenile smoking without raising taxes, creating bureaucracy, or angering smokers."

Following these landmark cases upholding the Baltimore ordinances, thirty-nine cities have enacted or have pending ordinances restricting tobacco billboards (Americans for Nonsmokers' Rights, 1998). For example, such ordinances have been enacted in Long Beach, Oakland, Compton, Covina, and Los Angeles County in California; Albany, New York City, and Yonkers in New York; and Seattle-King County and Tacoma-Pierce County in Washington. The standard restriction has become a ban within 1,000 feet of schools and parks.

These local ordinances have been reinforced by regulations of the Food and Drug Administration (being challenged in the courts as of 1998) that ban billboards advertising tobacco products within 1,000 feet of schools and playgrounds, limit in-store advertising, restrict billboards to black-and-white text, limit advertising to black-and-white text in publications with significant readership under age eighteen, prohibit brand logos on promotional items, and prohibit sponsorship of sporting or entertainment events using brand or product identification (Code of Federal Regulations, 1996). The Federal Regulations are particularly important because they apply nation-wide in all communities and among all racial/ethnic groups. Moreover, they are broader than local billboard ordinances because they restrict promotional strategies aimed at children as well as billboard advertising.

Health Warnings

We have mentioned earlier the power of tobacco advertising images to overwhelm the health warnings printed in small type on billboards and advertisements in the print media. In addition, cigarette ads aimed at ethnic communities have been printed in Vietnamese, Chinese, or Spanish except for the Surgeon General's warning, which was printed in English.

In 1996, Anh Le, a Vietnamese American health worker with the Vietnamese Community Health Promotion Project at the University of California, San Francisco, launched a grass roots effort to change what he termed a deliberate and continuing effort to mislead and deceive the public and to recruit new smokers (Fernandes, 1998). As a result of a barrage of letters protesting this practice of the tobacco industry, sent by Asian American youngsters to the Federal Trade Commission, the FTC issued an amendment to its policy on advertising disclosures requiring the Surgeon General's warning on tobacco advertisements to be in the language of the ad's target audience. The FTC announced that it was "clarifying its original intent... that all American consumers, regardless of the language they speak, have access to important information regarding the products they purchase" (Fernandes, 1998).

Warning labels are an important way to educate people about the health hazards of tobacco use. To be effective they must be strong and changing so as not to be ignored as weak and hackneyed. The United States has four rotating warnings on cigarette packages in effect since 1984. There is no warning that tobacco is addictive. All smokers would benefit from new and strengthened health warnings.

Control of Harmful Substances in Tobacco

After extensive investigation of tobacco products and nicotine's addictiveness, the Food and Drug Administration determined in 1995 that nicotine in cigarettes and smokeless tobacco products is a drug and that these products are drug delivery devices subject to regulation as "combination products" under the Federal Food, Drug, and Cosmetic Act (USFDA, 1996).

Upholding jurisdiction over cigarettes and smokeless tobacco will authorize the Food and Drug Administration to regulate the contents of tobacco products and harmful substances in them. At present there is no regulation of additives to tobacco but only a requirement in the Comprehensive Education Act of 1984, P.L. 98-474, that manufacturers provide the Secretary of the Department of Health and Human Services with a list of all ingredients. The Secretary's authority is limited to conducting research on additives and reporting to Congress findings on their potential health effects (USDHHS, 1989).

Public support for regulation of nicotine and additives in tobacco is reflected in a survey of youth access to tobacco conducted by the Robert Wood Johnson Foundation. In favor of requiring tobacco companies gradually to reduce the amount of nicotine in cigarettes were 77.7 percent of African-American and 84.8 percent of Hispanic respondents. In favor of requiring tobacco companies to list additives on package labels the way food and drug companies are required to list ingredients were 88.9 percent of African American and 90.4 percent of Hispanic respondents (USDHHS, 1998, p. 298).

Economic Strategies

The principal economic strategies for combating the tobacco epidemic are beyond the scope of this chapter. They involve abolition of tobacco subsidies, tobacco trade policies, and decrease in tobacco production through crop substitution, off-farm alternative employment for tobacco farmers, and payment of tobacco farmers displaced by reduction in demand. Most important is tobacco tax policy discussed below in connection with "Demand side measures."

Demand Side Measures for Tobacco Control

The following types of legislation are designed to change behavior and thus reduce the demand for tobacco products:

* tax and price policies
* smoke-free public places, public transport, and workplaces
* preventing young people from smoking
* health education

Tax and Price Policies

A wealth of evidence demonstrates that increasing taxes and prices of cigarettes decreases consumption, especially among young people (Roemer, 1993, pp. 85-96; Toder, 1985; USDHHS, 1998, pp. 292-293). Analysis of tobacco consumption habits of ninth graders in the United States and Canada compiled in 1990 and 1992 as part of the Community Intervention Trial for Smoking Cessation (COMMIT) found smoking by youth in the communities studied quite responsive to differences in retail cigarette prices. After controlling for differences in age, ethnic and racial group, gender, and parental smoking, the investigators found that the likelihood of a ninth grader's smoking cigarettes is reduced in markets where prices are high (Lewit, et al., 1994). The importance of tax policy for decreasing smoking among young people is shown in a careful analysis by Warner, who concludes:

> An 8-cent decrease in the federal excise tax would increase the ranks of teenage smokers by a tenth, assuming the decrease was fully passed on to consumers. A 16-cent tax increase would diminish the population of teenage smokers by fully 17%. The former would lead approximately 460,000 teenagers in the direction of cigarette habits; the latter would lead 820,000 teenagers away from dependency on cigarettes (Warner, 1986).

A recent study by the Centers for Disease Control and Prevention (CDC) found that, compared to White smokers, Hispanics are fourteen times more likely and African Americans twice as likely to reduce or quit smoking when cigarette prices rise. Rebutting the argument that these smokers have less money and therefore are more responsive to price rises, the study controlled for income and found that people of the same income level in these groups are more likely to quit. Moreover, younger Hispanic and African American smokers ages eighteen to twenty-four are four times more responsive to cigarette price increases than those age forty or older (Yang, 1998b).

Opponents of increased tobacco taxes contend that such taxes are regressive because they impinge more heavily on the poor than on the rich (USDHHS, 1998, p. 292). Warner has pointed out a number of factors, however, that make tobacco taxes not clearly regressive and certainly not highly regressive (Warner, 1984). Moreover, not all components of a tax policy need be progressive in order to have an overall progressive tax policy; a regressive component can be compensated for by other measures in the tax policy. Also, a tax that reduces tobacco consumption, even if it is somewhat regressive, benefits the health of individuals who are thereby induced to quit smoking. Finally, some proportion of increased taxes should be dedicated to public information and education on tobacco.

To be an effective deterrent of tobacco use, taxes and prices must be raised substantially and repeatedly to keep pace with inflation, as shown by experience in Finland (ACHE, 1985; Roemer, 1993, p. 91). Otherwise, cigarettes become a cheap luxury. An increase in the Federal cigarette tax is long overdue. Even in California, where a $0.25 per package increase in the state excise tax in 1988 resulted in an 8 to 10 percent short-term reduction and 10 to 13 percent long-term reduction in per capita cigarette consumption (Novotny and Siegel, 1996), further tax and price increases are necessary to halt the rise in teen smoking.

Smoke-Free Public Places, Public Transport, and Workplaces

The finding by the Environmental Protection Agency that environmental tobacco smoke is a human lung carcinogen that is responsible for 3,000 lung cancer deaths annually in the United States, as well as many other respiratory diseases, makes control of smoking in public places and workplaces a high priority (USEPA, 1993). Nonsmokers living with smokers suffer a 30 percent increase in risk of death from ischemic heart disease or myocardial infarction. Passive smoking accounts for an estimated 53,000 deaths annually and is the third leading cause of death in the United States after active smoking and alcohol (Glantz and Parmley, 1991).

The recent Surgeon General's report summarizes the limited data that exist on the exposure to tobacco smoke of the many individuals from racial/ethnic groups, who work in service industries and blue collar jobs where cigarette smoking is usually allowed. Thirty-two percent of nonsmoking Hispanics are exposed to ETS at indoor workplaces, compared with 19.1 percent of African Americans and 19 percent of Whites. Exposure to tobacco smoke at home is also a problem, although a majority of Asian Americans, Pacific Islanders, and Hispanics in a 1992-93 survey did not allow cigarette smoking in their homes (USDHHS, 1998, p. 287).

Legislation to control smoking in public places and public transport has fortunately become commonplace. State clean indoor air acts have restricted smoking in educational institutions, government buildings, private worksites, and restaurants. Local ordinances have banned smoking in restaurants, bars, and even some outdoor public places, such as parks and beaches. Most important have been local ordinances requiring private worksites to adopt written smoking policies. In the event of conflict between the concerns of smokers and nonsmokers, those of nonsmokers must take precedence (Roemer, 1993, ch. 10; USDHHS, 1998, p. 288). Public places are also workplaces, so that banning smoking in public places protects both visitors and the people who work there. Since people spend much more time at work than in a post office or on a bus, legislation to provide for smoke-free work environments is exceedingly important.

Preventing Young People from Smoking

The increase in smoking prevalence in the 1990s among African-American and Hispanic adolescents, after years of smoking decline, is a matter of great concern. Particularly disturbing, as mentioned earlier, is the increase among African-American youths who had had the greatest decline of the four racial/ ethnic groups (African Americans, American Indians and Alaska Natives, Asian Americans and Pacific Islanders, Hispanics) in the 1970s and 1980s. The prevalence of smokeless tobacco use, however, has remained fairly constant among African Americans, and African-American adolescent males are less likely than White adolescent males to use smokeless tobacco (USDHHS, 1998, pp. 28, 36, 44).

Investigating possible behavioral, sociodemographic, and attitudinal explanations for the lower prevalence among African-American youths in the 1970s and 1980s and for the recent rise, the Surgeon General's report analyzes evidence related to use of other drugs, age of smoking initiation, background and lifestyle factors, and other risk behaviors all very important insights for policy makers (USDHHS, 1998, pp. 36–44).

Among American Indian and Alaska Native youths, smoking and use of smokeless tobacco are high. The prevalence of previous-month smoking during 1990-94 was 39.4 percent among American Indian and Alaska Native females and 41.1 percent among males. Moreover, the prevalence of daily smoking increased for both females and males as they moved from junior high school to high school, but the increase was greater for American Indian and Alaska Native females than for males. The prevalence of regular use of smokeless tobacco in 1990 in this group was 55.9 percent among ninth and tenth graders (USDHHS, 1998, pp. 49-50). Asian American and Pacific Islander youths have a lower smoking prevalence than youths in the other racial/ethnic groups, except African Americans (USDHHS, 1998, p. 59).

Data on tobacco use among Hispanic youth are limited, but studies indicate that rates of smoking for Hispanic youths have been lower than for Whites and higher than for African Americans since the early 1980s and that rates of smoking have increased in the 1990s (USDHHS, 1998, pp. 72-74).

Table 7 of the Surgeon General's report, *Tobacco Use Among U.S. Racial/Ethnic Minority Groups,* reproduced here, shows the trend in smoking among male and female high school seniors for all four racial/ethnic groups.

Table 7. Trends in the Percentage of High School Seniors Who Were
Previous-Month Smokers, by Race/Ethnicity and Gender,
Monitoring the Future Surveys, United States,
1976-1979, 1980-1984, 1985-1989, 1990-1994

	1976-1979	1980-1984	1985-1989	1990-1994
Males				
African American	33.1	19.4	15.6	11.6
American Indian and Alaska Native	50.3	39.6	36.8	41.1
Asian American and Pacific Islander	20.7	21.5	16.8	20.6
Hispanic	30.3	23.8	23.3	28.5
White	35.0	27.5	29.8	33.4
Females				
African American	33.6	22.8	13.3	8.6
American Indian and Alaska Native	55.3	50.0	43.6	39.4
Asian American and Pacific Islander	24.4	16.0	14.3	13.8
Hispanic	31.4	25.1	20.6	19.2
White	39.1	34.2	34.0	33.1

Note: The Institute for Social Research usually reports the N (weighted), which is approximately equal to the sample size. Cases are weighted to account for differential probability of selection and then normalized to average 1.0. For males, the ranges of the N (weighted) for each of the cells in this table are 2,916-4,393 for African Americans, 342-587 for American Indians and Alaska Natives, 242-1,166 for Asian Americans and Pacific Islanders, 893-2,808 for Hispanics, and 24,931-31,954 for Whites. For females, the ranges of the N (weighted) for each of the cells in this table are 3,982-5,716 for African Americans, 299-586 for American Indians and Alaska Natives, 223-1,143 for Asian Americans and Pacific Islanders, 940-2,723 for Hispanics, and 25,627-31,933 for whites.
Sources: Bachman, et al., (1991a). Institute for Social Research, University of Michigan, unpublished data.

Clearly, the high prevalence of tobacco use among adolescents in all four groups makes urgent the implementation of the 1996 Food and Drug Administration's Regulations Restricting the Sale and Distribution of Cigarettes and Smokeless Tobacco to Protect Children and Adolescents mentioned earlier (Code of Federal Regulations, 1996; Kessler, et al., 1996).

The regulations restricting access to children and adolescents are as follows:

1. The sale of cigarettes and smokeless tobacco products to children and adolescents younger than age eighteen is a federal offense, and retailers must check a photo identification of anyone twenty-six or younger.

2. The minimum package size is twenty cigarettes, and retailers are prohibited from selling or distributing individual cigarettes or "kiddie packs."
3. Cigarette vending machines are banned except in very limited locations where the retailer or operator ensures that no person younger than eighteen is present or permitted to enter.
4. Self-service displays of tobacco products are banned except where the retailer ensures that no person under eighteen is present at any time.
5. Free samples of cigarettes and smokeless tobacco are prohibited.

The regulations also contain provisions designed to reduce the appeal of advertising to children and adolescents, while preserving the components of advertising and labeling that can provide product information to adult smokers. These provisions are as follows:

6. Advertising in all media are limited to black-and-white, text-only format.
7. Outdoor advertising is prohibited within 1,000 feet of schools and playgrounds.
8. Advertisements in publications read primarily by adults and advertisements placed in adult-only locations are exempt from restrictions.
9. Distribution of promotional materials, such as T-shirts, caps, and sporting goods, with tobacco brand names or logos is prohibited.
10. Brand names and logos and other identifiers of tobacco products may not be used in sponsorship of sports and cultural events. The name of the tobacco company may, however, be used in sponsorship.

In April 1997, a Federal District Court in North Carolina upheld the authority of the Food and Drug Administration to regulate tobacco products but not its authority to regulate tobacco advertising and promotion. On August 14, 1998 a panel of three justices of the Fourth Circuit Court of Appeal issued a 2-1 ruling that Congress, not the FDA, has the authority to regulate tobacco products. An appeal to the full Fourth Circuit has been filed.

Implementation of the FDA regulations will launch a strengthened movement to prevent teen smoking and use of smokeless tobacco. The ban on tobacco advertising within 1,000 feet of schools and playgrounds in the Federal regulations and also in local ordinances in many communities will promote a smoke-free environment where young people study and play.

In addition to this important development, legislation to authorize, finance, and improve school-based prevention programs is essential. The Institute of Medicine report, *Growing UP Tobacco Free,* concludes that, "School-based prevention programs that identify the social influences prompting youths to smoke and that teach skills to resist such influences have demonstrated consistent and significant reductions or delays in adolescents smoking" (Lynch and Bonnie, 1994, p. 154).

A sobering warning on premature deaths from smoking must be added. According to Peto and Lopez, experts on the scale of the tobacco epidemic, of those who start smoking as adolescents and keep on smoking steadily, one-half will die of smoking-related diseases one-quarter after age seventy and one-quarter in middle age (35 to 69) losing an average of twenty to twenty-five years of nonsmoker life expectancy (Peto, et al., 1994). Young people may know that smoking is dangerous, but they may not know *how* dangerous it is.

Health Education

Two principal types of health education on tobacco are authorized by legislation: (1) requirements and funding for school-based programs and (2) public information on the risks of tobacco use and the importance of cessation.

The fact that smoking prevention varies by educational attainment (USDHHS, 1998, pp. 83-84) adds, of course, to the recognized importance of promoting increased education for racial/ethnic minority groups. More specifically, school-based educational programs should be culturally sensitive and take into account the findings of extensive research on sociodemographic factors involved in tobacco use.

Similarly, public information programs, such as anti-tobacco advertisements, should speak to the various racial/ethnic groups who need to be reached. The decision of the Federal Trade Commission to require health warnings in the language of the advertisement, discussed earlier, corrects a flagrant violation of this principle. Revenues from increased taxes on tobacco should be dedicated at least in part to education and public information on tobacco.

LEGISLATIVE PRIORITIES ON ALCOHOL AND TOBACCO IN MULTICULTURAL COMMUNITIES

The evidence is strong that alcohol controls affect the rates of alcohol-related problems and often affect the consumption patterns of high-risk drinkers (Room, 1984, p. 310). Similarly, the evidence is compelling in the field of tobacco control that specific interventions have positive effects and that legislative restrictions generally reduce consumption and contribute to smoke-free environments (Roemer, 1993, pp. 159-160). In view of the grave impacts of alcohol and tobacco on multicultural communities, legislative strategies are essential components of comprehensive policies to control alcohol and tobacco use.

Although the issues and solutions to alcohol-related problems and the tobacco epidemic differ, certain broad legislative strategies are common to both alcohol and tobacco control. These are:

1. Control of advertising and promotion, which conveys the message, especially to young people, that drinking and smoking are socially acceptable

and associated with pleasure, beauty in nature, sexual attractiveness, and friendship.

2. Increased taxes and prices, which decrease consumption, especially among young people, and may yield revenues for public information and education.

3. Measures to prevent young people from drinking and smoking, such as enforcement of minimum age drinking laws and enforcement of Federal and state laws banning the sale of tobacco to minors.

4. Laws and regulations to create a social environment that prevents alcohol-related problems and promotes a smoke-free society, such as enforcement of drinking and driving laws and laws on smoke-free public places and workplaces.

It is not enough, of course, simply to enact such legislation. The laws must be fully and vigorously implemented. Achieving this result requires strong community support and exercise of political will by governments at the Federal, state, and local levels. Multicultural communities can themselves provide the popular support necessary to encourage government to exercise political will on the side of health and well-being for their people. The partnership of multicultural communities and governments can use the powerful tool of legislation to control the scourge of alcohol-related problems and to combat the tobacco epidemic.

REFERENCES

Advisory Committee on Health Education (1985). *An Evaluation of the Effects of an Increase in the Price of Tobacco and a Proposal for the Tobacco Price Policy in Finland in 1985-87.* Board of Health: Finland, Helsinki.

Advocacy Institute, Smoking Control Advocacy Resource Center (1997). *Communities Launch Protest Against Camel Menthol:* New York, February 28.

Altman, D. G., Schooler, C. and Basil, M. D. (1991). Alcohol and cigarette advertising on billboards. *Health Education Research,* 6:476-490.

Americans for Nonsmokers' Rights (June 18, 1998). *Fact Sheet.*

Anheuser-Busch, Inc. v. Schmoke, 63 F 3d1305 (4th Cir. 1995), cert.den.117 Sup. Ct.Rptr.1569, 137 L.Ed. 2d 715 (1997).

Ashley, M. J. and Rankin, J. (1988). A public health approach to the prevention of alcohol-related health problems. *Annual Review of Public Health,* 9:233-271.

Baltimore, Md., Ordinance No. 307, 1994 restricting the placement of outdoor advertisements for cigarettes and Ordinance No. 288, 1994 restricting the placement of outdoor advertisements for alcoholic beverages.

Centers for Disease Control (1990). *Morbidity and Mortality Weekly Report (MMWR),* 39(16):261.

Chollat-Traquet, C. (1992). *Women and Tobacco* (pp. 5-6). World Health Organization: Geneva.

Code of Federal Regulations (1996). Regulations restricting the sale and distribution of cigarettes and smokeless tobacco to protect children and adolescents. 21 CFR Parts 801, 803, 804, 807, 820, 897. 61 Federal Register 44396.

DiFranza, J. R. (1994) The effects of tobacco advertising on children. In K. Slama (Ed.), *Tobacco and Health* (pp. 87-90). Proceedings of the 9th World Conference on Tobacco and Health, Plenum Press: New York.

DiFranza, J. R., Richards, J. W., Paulman, P. M., et al. (1991). RJR Nabisco's cartoon camel promotes Camel cigarettes to children. *Journal of the American Medical Association*, 266:3149-3153.

Driver v. Hinant, 356 F. 2d 761 (4th Cir. 1966).

Easter v. District of Columbia, 361 F. 2d 50 (D.C. Cir. 1966).

Ewert, D. and Alleyne, D. (1992). Risk of exposure to outdoor advertising of cigarettes and alcohol. *American Journal of Public Health*, 82(6):895-896.

The Federal Cigarette Labeling and Advertising Act, 1965, as amended by the Public Health Cigarette Smoking Act, 1969 and the Comprehensive Education Act, 1984, Public Law 89-22.

Fernandes, E. (1998) Multilingual tobacco warning. *San Francisco Examiner*, July 6: A1.

Fischer, P. J., Richards, J. W., Berman, E. J. and Krugman, D. M. (1989) Recall and eye tracking study of adolescents viewing tobacco advertisements. *Journal of the American Medical Association*, 261:84-89.

Fischer, P. J., Schwartz, P. M., Richards, J. W., Jr., Goldstein, A. V. and Rohan, T. H. (1991). Brand logo recognition by children aged 3 to 6 years: Mickey Mouse and Old Joe the Camel. *Journal of the American Medical Association*, 266:3145-3148.

Garner, D. W. (1996). Banning tobacco billboards: The case for municipal action. *Journal of the American Medical Association*, 275(16):1263-1269.

Glantz, S. A. and Parmley, W. W. (1991). Passive smoking and heart disease: Epidemiology, physiology, and biochemistry. *Circulation*, 83(1):1-12.

Gorman, D. M., Speer, P. W., Labouvie, E. W. and Subaiya, A. P. (1988). Risk of assaultive violence and alcohol availability in New Jersey. *American Journal of Public Health*, 88(1):97-100.

Gorovitz, E., Mosher, J. and Pertschuk, M. (1998). Preemption or prevention?: Lessons from efforts to control firearms, alcohol, and tobacco. *Journal of Public Health Policy*, 19(1):36-49.

Hackbarth, D. P., Silvestri, B. and Cosper, W. (1995). Tobacco and alcohol billboards in 50 Chicago neighborhoods: Market segmentation to sell dangerous products to the poor. *Journal of Public Health Policy*, 16(2):213-229, citing *Billboard Basics: A Primer for Outdoor Advertising*. Outdoor Advertising Association of America (1992).

Hilts, P. J. (1994). Cigarette makers dispute reports of addictiveness. *New York Times*, April 15: 1, 10.

Holder, H., Boyd, G., Howard, J., Flay, B., Voas, R., and Grossman, M. (1995). Alcohol-problem prevention research policy: The need for a phases research model. *Journal of Public Health Policy*, 16(3):324-346.

Holder, H. D. and Wagenaar, A. C. (1990). Effects of the elimination of a state monopoly on distilled spirits retail sales: A time-series analysis of Iowa. *British Journal of Addiction*, 85:1615-1625.

Holder, H. D. and Edwards, G., Eds. (1995). *Alcohol and Public Policy: Evidence and Issues* (p. 193). Oxford University Press: New York.

Insurance Institute for Highway Safety (1995), *FACTS 1995, DUI/DWI Laws.*

Jones-Webb, R., Wagenaar, A. and Finnegan, J. (1995). Designing a survey of public opinions regarding alcohol control policies among Black and White adults. *Journal of Studies on Alcohol,* September 1995:566-572.

Kessler, D., Witt, A. M., Barn, P. S., Zeller, M. R., Natanblut, S. L., Wilkenfeld, J. P., Lorraine, C. G., Thompson, L. J. and Schultz, W. B. (1996). The Food and Drug Administration's regulation of tobacco products. *New England Journal of Medicine,* 335(13):988-994.

Kluger, R. (1996). *Ashes to Ashes, America's Hundred-Year Cigarette War, the Public Health, and the Unabashed Triumph of Philip Morris* (pp. 443-444). Alfred A. Knopf: New York.

Lewit, E. M., Kerrebrock, N. and Cummings, M. (1994). The impact of taxes and regulation on the use of tobacco products by teenagers. In K. Slama (Ed.), *Tobacco and Health* (pp. 217-220). Proceedings of the 9ᵗʰ World Conference on Tobacco and Health, Plenum Press: New York.

The Little Cigar Act of 1973 extended the broadcast ban to little cigars and smokeless tobacco products, Public Law 93-109.

Lynch, B. S. and Bonnie, R. J., Eds. (1994). *Growing Up Tobacco Free, Preventing Nicotine Addiction in Children and Youth.* Committee on Preventing Nicotine Addiction in Children and Youths, Institute of Medicine. National Academy Press: Washington, D.C.

Meier, Barry (1998). Data on Tobacco Show a Strategy Aimed at Blacks. *New York Times,* February 6:1, 14.

Moore, M. H. and Gerstein, D. R., Eds. (1981). *Alcohol and Public Policy: Beyond the Shadow of Prohibition.* National Academy Press: Washington, D.C.

National Highway Traffic Safety Administration (1989). *The Impact of Minimum Drinking Age Laws on Fatal Crash Involvements: An Update of the NHTSA Analyses.* NHTSA Technical Report No. DOT HS 807 349: Washington, D.C.

Novotny, T. E. and Siegel, M. B. (1996). California's tobacco control saga. *Health Affairs,* 15(1):58-72.

Office of National Drug Control Policy (1998). *The National Drug Control Strategy, 1998: A Ten Year Plan* (p. 15). Department of Health and Human Services: Washington, D.C.

Penn Advertising of Baltimore, Inc. v. Mayor of Baltimore, 63 F 3d 1318 (4ᵗʰ Cir. 1995), aff'g 862 F. Supp. 1402 (D Md 1994), cert. den. 117 Sup. Ct. Rptr. 1569, 137 L. Ed. 2d 715 (1997).

Peto, R., Lopez, A., Boreham, J., Thun, M. and Heath, C., Jr. (1994). *Mortality from Smoking in Developed Countries 1950-2000: Indirect Estimates from National Vital Statistics.* Oxford University Press: New York.

Powell, v. Texas, 392 U.S. 514 (1968).

Reed, D. S. (1981). Reducing the costs of drinking and driving. In M. H. Moore and D. R. Gerstein (Eds.), *Alcohol and Public Policy: Beyond the Shadow of Prohibition* (pp. 336-387). National Academy Press: Washington, D.C.

Robinson v. California, 370 U.S. 660 (1962).

Roemer, R. (1993) *Legislative Action to Combat the World Tobacco Epidemic*. Second Edition, World Health Organization: Geneva.

Room, R. (1984). Alcohol control and public health. *Annual Review of Public Health*, 5:293-317.

Scribner, R. A., MacKinnon, D. P. and Dwyer, J. H. (1995). The risk of assaultive violence and alcohol availability in Los Angeles County. *American Journal of Public Health*, 85:335-340.

Seventh Special Report to the U.S. Congress on Alcohol and Health from the Secretary of Health and Human Services (1990). U.S. Department of Health and Human Services, Public Health Service, Alcohol, Drug Abuse, and Mental Health Administration, National Institute on Alcohol Abuse and Alcoholism: Rockville, MD.

Toder, E. J. (1985). Issues in the taxation of cigarettes. In *The Cigarette Excise Tax* (pp. 65-87). Institute for the Study of Smoking Behavior and Policy, Harvard University: Cambridge, MA.

Toomey, T. L., Jones-Webb, R. J. and Wagenaar, A. C. (1993). Policy—Alcohol. *Annual Review of Addictions Research and Treatment*, 3:279-292.

Toomey, T. L., Rosenfeld, C. and Wagenaar, A. C. (1996). The minimum legal drinking age: History, effectiveness, and ongoing debate. *Alcohol, Health and Research World*, 20(4):213-218.

Tye, J. B., Warner, K. E. and Glantz, S. A. (1987). Tobacco advertising and consumption: Evidence of a causal relationship. *Journal of Public Health Policy*, 8(4): 492-508.

U.S. Department of Health and Human Services (1989). *Reducing the Health Consequences of Smoking: 25 Years of Progress. A Report of the Surgeon General* (p. 613). Public Health Service, Centers for Disease Control, Center for Chronic Disease Prevention and Health Promotion, Office on Smoking and Health, DHHS Pub. No. (CDC) 89-8411: Washington, D.C.

U.S. Department of Health and Human Services (1998). *Tobacco Use Among U.S. Racial/Ethnic Minority Groups—African Americans, American Indians and Alaska Natives, Asian Americans and Pacific Islanders, and Hispanics: A Report of the Surgeon General*. U.S. Department of Health and Human Services, Centers for Disease Control and Prevention, National Center for Chronic Disease Prevention and Health Promotion, Office on Smoking and Health: Atlanta, GA.

U.S. Environmental Protection Agency (1993). *Respiratory Health Effects of Passive Smoking: Lung Cancer and Other Disorders: The Report of the U.S. Environmental Protection Agency* (pp. 6, 13). U.S. Department of Health and Human Services, NIH Publication No. 93-3605: Washington, D.C.

U.S. Food and Drug Administration (1996). *Nicotine in Cigarettes and Smokeless Tobacco is a Drug and these Products are Delivery Devices under the Federal Food, Drug, and Cosmetic Act: Jurisdictional Determination* (the 1996 Jurisdictional Determination). Department of Health and Human Services: Washington, D.C.

Wagenaar, A. (1995). Minimum drinking age laws. *Encyclopedia of Drugs and Alcohol*, 2:688-693.

Wagenaar, A. C. and Holder, H. (1991). A change from public to private sale of wine: Results from natural experiments in Iowa and West Virginia. *Journal of Studies on Alcohol*, 52(2):162-172.

Wagenaar, A. C. and Holder, H. D. (1995). Changes in alcohol consumption resulting from the elimination of retail wine monopolies: Results from five U.S. states. *Journal of Studies on Alcohol*, September: 566-572.

Wagenaar, A. C. and Wolfson, M. (1994). Enforcement of the legal minimum drinking age in the United States. *Journal of Public Health Policy*, 15(1):37-53.

Warner, K. (1986). Smoking and health implications of a change in the federal cigarette excise tax. *Journal of the American Medical Association*, 255(8):1028-1032.

Warner, K. E. (1984). Cigarette taxation: Doing good by doing well. *Journal of Public Health Policy*, 5(3):312-318.

World Health Organization, Series 695 (1983). *Smoking Control Strategies in Developing Countries* (p. 43). Report of a WHO Expert Committee. World Health Organization: Geneva.

Wright, J. (1997) *Youth Fatal Crash and Alcohol Facts* (p. 1). National Highway Traffic Safety Administration: Washington, D.C.

Yang, S. (1998a). Nicotine studies find racial factor. *Los Angeles Times*, 7 July:1, 12.

Yang, S. (1998b). Black, Latino smokers quit over price hikes, study says. *Los Angeles Times*, 31 July:A38.

CHAPTER 12

Substance Abuse Prevention in a Multicultural Community: A Community Perspective

Earl Massey, Raquel Ortiz,
and Shana Alex*

The following is a case study of Surviving In Recovery (SIR), a substance abuse prevention and treatment community-based organization that operates in South Central Los Angeles. As such, this chapter will focus less on the theoretical basis of SIR's work and more on the reality of dealing with substance abuse (SA) within one of the most multicultural communities in the United States. Founded in 1992, SIR develops methods of prevention and intervention in response to SA and HIV/AIDS. In order to effectively prevent the spread of SA, SIR focuses mainly on the youth of the community, through both school-based interventions and peer counseling sessions. A focus on families has branched these main programs out into parent education and training sessions, as well. The main goals of the organization are:

1. implementing programs through culturally specific, peer-based approaches;
2. educating community individuals to become aware of the negative environmental influences within their neighborhoods (i.e., over-concentration of liquor stores and cigarette billboards);

*The authors would like to thank Karen Bass, Executive Director of the Community Coalition, and Jennifer Baxter, of Mentor Ohio, for their support and assistance in writing this chapter.

3. empowering people in SA recovery and those infected with HIV/AIDS through personal education and giving them the opportunity to personally educate the community;
4. designing effective, culturally specific intervention and prevention programs within the schools;
5. establishing a system of effective treatment that involves a person's circle of support, particularly family members, friends, and significant others; and
6. developing an effective model to intervene and educate youth and their parents.

In this chapter, the existing programs of SIR will be discussed, along with their benefits to the community and their limitations; this program, while unique in Los Angeles, acts as a case study for further understanding of the concerns of SA prevention community-based groups around the country. The implications for future research and academic/community collaboration will also be discussed.

CURRENT PROGRAMS OF SIR

SIR uses Motivational Intervention Techniques (MIT) as the foundation of their operations that include both intervention programs aimed at recovering addicts and prevention programs geared toward impressionable youth. This flexible method utilizes a therapy-like approach that focuses on the individual's needs. MIT entails friendly, client-oriented, tailored programs that change with the dynamic between the peer counselor and the target individual. Applying these techniques in all the different projects that SIR performs gives a sense of continuity to the disparate programs; all are joined by the MIT philosophy.

For example, the school-based interventions that comprise SIR's foremost undertaking use MIT, in that the program offers open and honest dialogue about SA with groups of students. For the past three years, SIR has worked with three Los Angeles Unified School District (LAUSD) schools, including some in the South Central Los Angeles area, to provide education and limited interventions among students and parents, in conjunction with LAUSD's own Project Impact. Peer speakers, who are themselves recovering addicts who are stable in their recovery, make presentations about SA prevention and youth issues, tailored to the young persons' existing attitudes. SIR provides the training for these speakers, which entails three main components: (1) public speaking training, (2) education about the facts of SA, and (3) practice in using MIT, particularly in dealing with students who are resistant to the initial subject matter. MIT constitutes a culturally congruent approach, particularly for audiences of young Latinos and African

Americans. In addition, information on cultural values and norms is incorporated throughout the speaker's training, allowing them to tailor their presentations further; information such as how a certain groups' socioeconomic environment contributes to the use of gateway drugs (i.e., cigarettes, alcohol, and most recently marijuana) makes the presentation more relevant as a whole. Also, the speakers discuss political policies and the specific ethnic groups that suffer most from the impact of substance abuse and the reality of often unequal treatment under the law. It has been SIR's experience that when the information about drugs is given in a neutral manner by persons who have experienced addiction themselves, it validates that information and often permits the audience to discuss their own experiences. The Speaker's Program provides this training twice per year, not only to potential presenters, but also to every staff member and volunteer within the SIR organization.

Using peers to educate students not only makes the message more meaningful, but also helps to gain the trust of students who may need more intervention than prevention. Peer speakers then become referral services that can steer the young person afflicted with SA to an agency, such as SIR, for help. The adolescent referral program is one of the most utilized components of SIR; outgrowing its current resources, adolescent referrals will soon be handled by an outpatient treatment program sponsored by SIR within South Central Los Angeles. This project will also involve addressing the problem of co-dependency, using a therapist who specializes in family dynamics.

Enlisting parental assistance and other family support for recovering addicts remains vital to the program. In response to the large number of phone calls from concerned parents, SIR has already developed a parental support component of the program co-sponsored by Project Impact. The parental component consisted mainly of: (1) dispensing information about the behavioral patterns and physical problems associated with different types of drug use, and (2) providing a secure environment for the parent to discuss their feelings regarding their child's drug problem. Many parents seemed to gain hope and resilience from both aspects of the program, along with listening to the similar problems that other parents also face.

All of the above services are provided without charge to the community; SIR remains almost completely dependent upon grants and federal funds for financial support. This arrangement allows SIR to treat low-income people in the area without concern about bullying their clients for payment. In order to become more financially self-sufficient, however, SIR has been using some of the funds garnered from marketing both its SA education curriculum and its HIV/AIDS curriculum to schools to invest in the organization's future stability. To date, however, this marketing has not developed to the point of generating significant income that has real impact on SIR's economic situation.

LIMITATIONS OF SIR

Like many other community-based organizations, SIR faces three main problems from which all its other difficulties sprout: (1) lack of adequate funding, (2) lack of the amount of resources needed to fulfill the potential of its programs, and (3) lack of evaluative skills in order to measure SIR's actual impact.

Lack of Adequate Funding

Reliant upon federal money like many other organizations around the country, SIR is particularly sensitive to changes in the political climate. From an example personally experienced by the authors: following the civil unrest in Los Angeles in 1992, SIR's parent organization, the Community Coalition (CC), fought to keep many of the liquor stores that had been destroyed from being rebuilt. The reason: the over-concentration of liquor stores in South Central Los Angeles helped to create the next generation of alcohol-dependent minority groups through the saturation of the environment with pro-alcohol messages, a process which the CC strove to subvert. After the CC won its battle in court, the liquor industry lobbied the new Congress of 1995, successfully eliminating the funding appropriation for not only the CC, but also all community-based organizations of a similar nature around the country. CC had enough clout to fight back, eventually managing to actually increase its Congressional appropriation from the original budget while simultaneously reinstating funding for the other community groups, but the leadership of SIR learned that federal money cannot always be relied upon as a given.

In order to find other sources of funding, however, SIR needs not only someone who has the time to search out the grants, but also has the skills to write successful proposals. Time itself is at a premium; since the staff is either underpaid or volunteer and there is a high turnover rate, the Executive Director often must perform the duties of several staff members while continuing his own job of keeping SIR solvent and running smoothly. Even compensating for the lack of time, however, the Executive Director has not had the opportunity to hone his grant-writing skills in order to apply for outside funding. Currently, SIR is attempting to locate a funding source that will last for two years, until the organization has accumulated enough funds from marketing its curricula and can become virtually self-supporting. SIR is also looking for existing economic models that would engender self-sufficiency.

Lack of Necessary Resources

SIR goals, unfortunately, are almost impossible to achieve without extended community resources. For example, during the course of the parental education program, several needs arose that could not be met. Not only was the program too short to be truly effective, it also lacked any methods with which to cope with the *parental* drug abuses that adversely affect their children. These problems, by necessity of the lack of funding and staff, had to remain unaddressed.

Within the adolescent program, SIR constantly faces the problems of lack of bed space for residential treatment and limited availability of treatment programs, many of which had huge wait-lists. While SIR handles the intervention part of the process, the actual detoxification and treatment must be carried out by another agency, which can lead to problems when SIR cannot place a needy individual in a program. Also, many detoxification programs require payment, which may be beyond the means of most of SIR's clients. This discrepancy has directly led to SIR's plans to open its own treatment facility capable of treating all the community, regardless of economic status. This early intervention and treatment, in turn, will simultaneously create a savings to taxpayers, provide relief for families, and help the persons recovering from addiction.

The program will not only utilize the state-of-the-art methods, such as MIT, but will also be ideologically based on solid research data gathered by the state of California. A research project commissioned by the state (CALDATA, 1994) stated that for every dollar spent on treatment, seven dollars were saved through reduced prison costs, later treatment costs, and healthcare costs; SIR's goal is to put this research data into practice through its treatment program. Based on the organization's experience, the treatment center will focus on adolescents, in order to maximize the effectiveness of the intervention. This program, however, needs the necessary support in order to thrive and properly serve the community in the intended manner. In other words, SIR must find the original dollars needed to save seven in the future.

Lack of Evaluation

Currently, SIR has only one form of comprehensive evaluation in place; at the end of a speaker's program or an adolescent intervention, SIR hands out questionnaires to the participants and asks for candid responses, in order to better serve the community. These questionnaires are carefully read and heeded. When the participants often stated that they required more visual aids during a presentation, SIR diverted some of its resources into equipment that could fulfill this request. However, these forms cannot tell SIR about the impact that their techniques have in the long-term, nor can they gauge the impact that the carefully crafted, culturally congruent messages have on student behaviors.

This problem affects the day-to-day existence of SIR in subtle but unmistakable ways. Without the time or skills to perform evaluations, the Executive Director can become unsure as to which program is most effective, and therefore should be supported, and which may be nothing more than a waste of money. As a further frustration, most funders insist upon hard data that a program actually works to accomplish its goals before deciding to put money into the organization running that program. In other words, without evaluations, SIR has difficulty getting funds, and without funds, SIR has difficulty hiring people to perform evaluations. This cycle can only be halted through a strong partnership with the academic community, providing both SIR and the field of public health promotion with evaluative data.

IMPLICATIONS FOR ACADEMIC/COMMUNITY COLLABORATION

Before discussing what future collaborations may take place between community-based groups like SIR and academia, it is first necessary to relate the current linkages that have worked well for this particular group. In three particular instances, UCLA and SIR have joined together to improve the quality of substance abuse prevention and intervention in South Central Los Angeles. First, the initial partnership with UCLA in 1996 led directly to the initial federal grant that currently sustains SIR. The current project consists of a behavioral change model that derived from a collaborative effort between Dr. Doug Longshore (UCLA) and Earl Massey, Executive Director (SIR).

Second, a joint project with the UCLA Drug Research Department's Dr. Doug Longshore, Loyola Marymount's Dr. Cheryl Grills, and Pepperdine University's Dr. Darryl Rowe gave SIR the necessary initial training in the Motivational Intervention Techniques that became the foundation of SIR's work. As the data from the research project, named Engage and Respond (ER), was analyzed, SIR immediately began using the results in its daily operations. Joining the insights of recovering addicts, academic researchers, community organization professionals, and other community groups such as the Southern Christian Leadership Conference led to the successful development and inception of a service providing agency with unique approaches to substance abuse and HIV/AIDS intervention and prevention.

Third, this chapter, and the opportunity it presents to provide academia with the viewpoint of the community, would not have happened without the collaboration between SIR and the UCLA Office of Public Health Practice. This chapter and other efforts, like those enumerated above, were born out of genuine mutual concern for the community and a recognition of the strengths of both research and practice.

With these positive occurrences in mind, the authors have three major recommendations for enhancing future relationships between researchers and community groups: (1) academia should recognize the need for the practical data that comes from evaluation, (2) the lines of communication must remain open, and (3) both sides should avoid distrust through a constant practice of tolerance, patience, and focus on serving the community.

Recognize the Need for Evaluation

A database search of the literature reveals huge holes in the available data concerning substance abuse, particularly among ethnic groups. SIR and other similar Community Based Organizations (CBOs) can provide a place to gather that kind of real-world information, especially concerning the effectiveness of different types of programs. Also, this kind of research would add a new dimension of understanding to public health literature as models are applied in multi-cultural communities. This statistical knowledge, essential to combating substance abuse, remains unknown to both researchers and practitioners. Despite this lack of hard data, SA prevention programs have become aware, after years of working in the field, of the kinds of programs that seem to work best. However, without the data that can only come from a formal evaluation process, no factual evidence supports their claims.

Keep the Lines of Communication Open

When breakdowns occur between academia and the community, it poisons the work of both sides; research is performed in a vacuum that has little to do with the reality of the outside world, and community groups use outdated techniques that have been shown to be ineffective. Simply facilitating a flow of communication could alleviate this situation. For example, the State-of-the-Art-Review (STAR) Conference that created this book allowed community members, such as the Executive Director of SIR, to learn about the research that is occurring and which might be able to help him improve his organization's methods. Fulfilling his side of the communication flow, he recognized the need to learn from academics and made the conscious effort to become part of an academic conference. The UCLA Office of Public Health Practice, whose mission is to facilitate academic/community relations, kept their side of the communication open by informing community members of the event. This type of collaboration should occur more often.

Language barriers also exist, in that community organizers may not always understand the technical jargon associated with the academic discipline of public health. Researchers should keep their audiences in mind when presenting models or findings to CBOs.

Avoiding Distrust

In the past, distrust that flows from both sides has sometimes stood in the way of healthy relationships between researchers and the community. On the community side, many people feel that their life experiences within the neighborhood have taught them more than an outside researcher could ever possibly tell them. Community people often feel their intellectual and theoretical abilities as well as academic achievements and experience are ignored. This could downplay what knowledge the researchers may bring to the community. This blinds people to the fact of researchers' knowledge of the larger trends and latest models for effective implementation, in essence cutting the community-based groups off from newer information. On the part of the researchers, many seem to think of their community partners as inferiors, discounting the wealth of personal and detailed information that a person gains from daily living in a neighborhood. This huge gap of resentment and arrogance must be bridged in order for constructive and positive work to begin. If each party is not willing to maintain a degree of flexibility in order to achieve their agendas, the process of research will become drawn out and eventually fail, sunk by its own weight.

To illustrate this problem, SIR's partnership with the UCLA Drug Research Department did not begin easily. Initially, the community had quite a bit of mistrust concerning the data that was collected. With suspicions founded on historical examples of mistreatment of African Americans such as the Tuskegee Syphilis Study, those working on the project kept questions regarding the utilization of the information foremost in their minds. Factors that led to the building of trust were:

- The project was born directly out of the community's need. Its focus was to promote drug recovery by motivating actively addicted persons to seek help before death or a prison sentence occurred.
- The study used African-American researchers to perform the training and monitor the project.
- The study employed, with compensation, recovering addicts from the community to carry out the project. By working for the project, the addicts gained some research and data collection skills that could translate into future work. The community particularly felt that this created a "win-win" situation for all involved.
- The research project was aided by CBOs who often act as gatekeepers of information in poor communities, and therefore are already trusted by their constituents.

These factors combined to create a fruitful partnership that permanently assisted the community through training while giving the researchers the hard data they needed.

This partnership has greatly benefited the area by aiding a service-providing agency in its growth and development, thereby leaving a positive entity within the community. Most research projects leave the community after extracting the data without changing the surrounding conditions that were studied. In the case of UCLA/SIR, there has been a genuine, long-term relationship that can be expanded for future partnership projects. SIR's reputation and working history with UCLA have both been built over time through joint academic and community efforts, operating with patience, perseverance and tolerance. This kind of fruitful partnership can only enrich the field of substance abuse prevention, allowing both researchers and practitioners to better combat this pervasive problem.

REFERENCE

California Drug and Alcohol Treatment Assessment (1994). *Evaluating Recovery Services: General Report Submitted to the State of California.* California Department of Alcohol and Drug Programs, Resource Center: Sacramento, CA.

CHAPTER 13

Summary and Implications

Snehendu B. Kar, Kirstin L. Chickering,
and Felicia Sze

This chapter presents a review of the key issues, consensus, and gaps related to substance abuse prevention from a multicultural perspective. Based upon our review of issues, we propose a model for substance abuse research and prevention (Figure 1). The issues reviewed were identified through extensive dialogue among the workshop participants, which included the authors of the State-of-the-Art-Reviews (previous chapters), other academics, and community-based practitioners involved with substance abuse prevention. Rather than summarize all chapters and discussions, we focus here on identifying and discussing the important themes and their implications for substance abuse prevention research and action. These issues are grouped into three categories: (1) multiculturalism and risks prevention, (2) key issues affecting substance abuse prevention, and (3) recommendations—including the importance of a community-based participatory prevention strategy using the new public health paradigm.

Before we elaborate on these common themes, it is essential to briefly articulate why we should concern ourselves with the issues of a multicultural community. There are sound ethical and pragmatic reasons to develop prevention strategies from multicultural perspectives. This multicultural trend and its imperative for substance abuse prevention is repeatedly emphasized in this volume and has been reviewed in detail in the first Chapter. There are two types of justifications for a multicultural approach in our social policy and action including substance abuse prevention: deantological and utilitarian (Kar and Alex[1]). The deantological (or moral) imperative holds that the basic values of our society are

---

[1] Author's names without the year of publication indicates authors of chapters in this volume.

271

instilled in the Bill of Rights which guarantees certain inalienable rights to all Americans. One of these inalienable rights is equal protection for all against threats to their lives. Therefore, it logically follows that: all Americans, regardless of their ethnicity, should have equal access to opportunities and services necessary to protect their health, and substance abuse prevention programs do not have the option to underserve certain ethnic groups because of their race and origin. The utilitarian imperative holds that our collective self-interest dictates that substance abuse programs must focus on all ethnic groups. Notwithstanding the wish and demands of the assimilationists, the demographic reality is that we are becoming a truly multicultural nation. From the utilitarian perspective, we need a multicultural approach for substance abuse for two pragmatic reasons. First, if a program fails in one ethnic group in a multicultural community, the entire community suffers the negative consequences. Second, effective prevention strategies require the active participation of the community at risk; all ethnic groups that are affected must be involved in prevention efforts. Indeed, several ethnic minorities seem to be at greater risk of substance abuse, and in order to protect our self-interest (not as a special favor) we must apportion our program development efforts in accordance with actual risks and needs. We cannot effectively respond to these imperatives unless we understand the factors and forces that affect substance abuse and prevention in various ethnic groups.

MULTICULTURALISM AND RISK PREVENTION

As America prepares to enter the twenty-first century, our society is becoming more culturally diverse and complex than ever before. Substance abuse affects all segments of our society, crossing gender, ethnic, religious, socioeconomic, and geographic lines. In order to address the problem of substance abuse in our increasingly multicultural society, America needs to look beyond its current research paradigms and develop innovative approaches appropriate for culturally diverse and complex communities. In this book, we have begun to explore how substance abuse prevention may be affected by the specific issues and factors in multicultural communities when people of different cultures reside as neighbors. While several chapters in this volume concentrate on different ethnic groups and others focus on generic issues affecting substance abuse prevention, there are many themes pervasive throughout the volume. The issues and concerns on which there was a consensus among the authors and workshop participants include: the problem of definition and measurement of ethnic identity and multiculturalism; the diversity between and within the frequently used ethnic categories; a lack of research on substance abuse prevalence and determinants in many important ethnic groups; the scarcity of research on substance abuse prevention in important ethnic groups; the question of effectiveness and generalizability of standard programs developed for one/dominant ethnic group to other ethnic groups; and the importance of developing culturally appropriate and community based participatory prevention intervention using the new public health paradigm.

Meaning and Measurement of Multiculturalism

A major theme throughout the state-of-the-art-review chapters and workshop discussions is the lack of understanding of the complex dynamics within a multicultural community that effect substance abuse risk and prevention. Several authors raise the question of how to define and measure the construct of multiculturalism. Kar and Alex (Chapter 1) identify three approaches to defining multiculturalism and the problems related to each. The three approaches are: demographic, personal identity, and social relational.

(i) *Demographic* definition uses U.S. Census and other data on people of various ethnic/national origin. This method generally places individuals in one of five ethnic categories: African American, American Indian, Asian American, Latino/Hispanic, and White. Historically, most communities had some minorities, but the American population, at least since the first census was taken in 1790, had a predominantly White majority. Since then, the ethnic composition of our population has changed dramatically. The proportion of ethnic minorities has been increasing so rapidly during the last half of the twentieth century that, today, no single ethnic group holds a majority in many major metropolitan areas. Some researchers use the criterion that when the number of minorities collectively exceed the number non-Hispanic Whites, the community is truly multicultural (American Demographics, 1991). Using this criterion, over 189 counties including the fifteen largest metropolitan areas were multicultural as of 1990 (American Demographics, 1991). Furthermore, the U.S. Census Bureau projects that by the middle of the twenty-first century, non-Hispanic Whites will become one of the minorities, and no single ethnic group will be the majority. But what about those communities where the minorities constitute less than 50 percent of the population—are they qualitatively significantly different than communities with 51 percent minorities? Or are communities with 51 percent or more non-Hispanic Whites not multicultural? There is no clear definition or threshold to determine when a community is multicultural. It can be argued that, from a demographic perspective, most communities are multicultural; some more than others.

(ii) *Subjective ethnic identity* is used by the U.S. Census and other surveys to classify individuals into different ethnic groups. However, this approach is not free from problems. First, subjects must choose from (or be assigned to) a list of fixed ethnic categories, usually the five ethnic categories mentioned previously. This method of categorization excludes many ethnic groups, and, consequently, many respondents do not identify themselves with any of the choices given to them. These respondents are generally grouped into the "other" category, concealing their true ethnic identity. There are other problems as well. For example, individuals may hold a mono-cultural (ethnocentric), a bicultural/hyphenated (e.g., African American or Asian American), or a multicultural identity. Currently, there are scales that measure mono-cultural and bicultural identities, but no acceptable scale is available to measure a multicultural identity. How do we then categorize those who identify with more than two ethnic groups? With the increasing number of inter-ethnic marriages and the children from these unions, along with the children of recent ethnic immigrants who grow up in multi-ethnic communities, the proportion of Americans who hold multicultural identity is likely to be substantial. But due to the lack of appropriate measurement tools and criteria, we do not know what proportion of our population identifies themselves as multicultural. We also do not know whether those who hold a multicultural identity have higher acculturation stress and greater risk of substance abuse than those who hold mono or bicultural identities. At the present time, there is no consensus on how to address this issue and no published study on how multicultural identity affects substance abuse and other risks.

(iii) From a *social relation perspective*, the nature of inter-ethnic relationship in a multicultural community becomes a central issue. Inter-ethnic cohesion or conflicts (including linguistic differences, value clashes, and actual hostility) can significantly affect quality of life and existential stress; it can also make the difference between the success and failure of a community based prevention program. The central concern here is understanding the factors that contribute toward community cohesiveness and/or conflicts. Literature in community empowerment and organization suggests that a cohesive community is more likely be responsive to and organize itself for social action interventions, particularly when those interventions are responsive to their own perceived needs. Conversely, inter-ethnic tensions and conflicts may exacerbate substance abuse and related risks and at the same time decrease the likelihood of effective prevention programs. Several authors and participants emphasized that we know very little about the community level variables that affect substance abuse risk and prevention efforts in general and in a multicultural community in particular (Bhattacharya; Brown and John; Ellickson, Kar, and Alex; Pentz).

Diversity Between and Within Ethnic Groups

Another major problem with analyzing multicultural communities is that the diversity between and within a given ethnic group makes many ethnic classifications of questionable value. For instance, the Asian Pacific Islanders (API), as defined by the Census Bureau, includes descendants of forty-nine separate populations from twenty-nine Asian nations and twenty island cultures from the Far East, South East Asia, Indian Sub-Continent, and Pacific Island (U.S. Bureau of Census, 1990). The API's speak over thirty distinct languages. Asian Pacific Americans represent a mix of recent immigrants, long-term immigrants, and U.S.

born citizens, some of whose families have resided in the United States for up to five generations. In the African-American communities, diversity is the result of family/migration history as well as geographic distribution. Many African Americans are recent immigrants from Africa, which is a stark contrast with the typical portrayal of African Americans as descendants of the slave tradition. In addition, African Americans themselves diverge considerably; the background and socioeconomic conditions of African Americans living in different areas of New York varies according to geographic location of communities (Brown and John). Increasing diversity can also be found within the Latino community, which has long surpassed the time when it was easily divided into three ethnic subgroups. As a result of different historical backgrounds and migration histories, significant diversity is now apparent among many different Latino subgroups (Delgado).

Intergeneration and Gender Role Conflicts

Intergeneration conflicts, gender role conflicts, and poor parent-child relationships are believed to affect deviant behavior, including substance abuse (Bhattacharya; Kar and Alex; Ellickson). Inter-generation and inter-gender differences within a first generation immigrant family make them very different from other families in the same ethnic group who had migrated generations ago (e.g., a fifth generation and first generation Latino). The children of first generation immigrants, born and raised in the United States, often acquire values and behavior that are significantly different from their parents; these children may have much in common with their peers from other ethnic groups, which sets them apart from their parents and grandparents. Consequently, inter-generation conflict and stress is likely to be most pronounced between the first generation immigrants (foreign born) and their children born and raised in the United States. With successive generations, as immigrants become more Americanized, intergeneration conflicts may be lessened (Bhattacharya, 1998; Felix-Ortiz, et al., 1998; Kar, et al., 1998; Smart and Smart, 1994). One study that compared two groups of Asian Americans found that Indo-Americans,* who are predominantly first generation immigrants (75.4% foreign born), had a significantly higher level of intergeneration and gender role conflicts than Japanese Americans (32.4% foreign born), who are more often descendents of immigrants several generations back (Kar, et al., 1998). In contrast, 7.9 percent of Americans are foreign born (Shinagawa, 1998). Indeed, in our study, intergenerational conflict was the single most important source of distress among the Indo-Americans (Kar, et al., 1995, 1996, 1998). Clearly, we need to know more about how intergeneration and gender role conflicts affect substance abuse across and within various ethnic groups and recent immigrants.

*Americans originating from India.

Relative Risks

A common concern throughout this volume is the lack of data on the prevalence of substance abuse and related issues in many ethnic groups. One specific instance is the inordinately low level of research information among Asian/Pacific Islanders in comparison to other groups. Along with this scarcity of research on different ethnic communities, there is a dearth of published data on substance abuse prevalence, determinants, and prevention activities in these communities. When reliable data is available, we find that there are significant differences between ethnic groups in quality of life, health status, and substance abuse (Kar and Alex). Furthermore, substance abuse data on ethnic groups, when available, are not always in the same format and for same timeframe which makes any comparison difficult. In addition, the findings do not always show clear and consistent patterns. For example, while one researcher reports that African Americans and Asian Americans have, in general, lower rates of substance abuse than Whites, Native Americans, and Latinos (Ellickson), others report that African Americans were "much more likely" to use an illicit substance in comparison to their counterparts (Brown and John). Another example is that the sequence of drug use among the Asian Americans is often different than the usual sequence observed among the adolescents as a whole. Unlike most adolescents who begin with tobacco and alcohol and subsequently use other illicit drugs, some Asian-American adolescents often initiate their drug abuse with illicit drugs and subsequently move on to tobacco and alcohol abuse (Subramanian and Takeuchi). Anecdotal and agency reports allude to a difference in substance abuse prevalence rates across different Asian/Pacific Islander ethnic groups such as Japanese Americans, Chinese Americans, Indo-Americans, Filipino Americans, and Vietnamese Americans. With inadequate research in this field, it is difficult to ascertain exactly what the trends are in specific ethnic communities.

There is also evidence that the negative consequences of substance abuse vary significantly by ethnic groups. For instance, African Americans are not only at a greater risk of certain types of substance abuse, they also suffer from greater negative consequences of substance abuse (Brown and John; Sanders-Phillips). These and other evidence lead to three conclusions. First, we do not have reliable measures of relative risks of substance abuse across all important ethnic groups; when data is available, there is a significant difference in prevalence rates. Second, the pattern and effects of substance abuse, including the sequence of risk acquisition and consequences of substance abuse, may vary significantly by ethnicity; but we do not know enough about these processes across major ethnic groups. Third, we do not have sound cross-cultural studies to identify determinants of substance abuse that are common to all or unique to various ethnic groups. Filling in these research gaps will lead to the development of more effective prevention programs.

Culture and Health Behavior

Cultural/ethnic differences in quality of life, health status, and substance abuse risks have been discussed by the authors of this volume and others including Cantril (1965), Cazeres and Beatty (1994), Cruickshank and Beevers (1989), DHHS (1998a, 1998b), Gordon and Newfield (1996), Harwood (1981), Howard (1995), Kar, et al. (1996, 1998), Langton (1995), Orlandi (1992), Paul (1955), Penn, et al. (1995), and Sowell (1996). It is important to recognize that prevention programs from outside do not bypass or neutralize the socio-cultural factors that determine health-related behavior, including substance abuse. Cultural attributes may enhance some risks and protect against others. For instance, some ethnic groups suffer from higher health related risks on almost all counts (e.g., African Americans) and conversely, in spite of their relative poverty, several Asian- American and Latino sub-groups have relatively lower risks on several indicators (Kar and Alex). Asian Americans are often termed as the "model minority," a stereotype which obscures the real risks they face on many other counts (Nakanishi, et al., 1998; Penn, et al., 1995; Kar, et al., 1995/96, 1998; Subramanian and Takeuchi).

Culture may also contain positive attributes, often termed as "cultural capitals" which contribute to socioeconomic achievements and improved quality of life of an ethnic group. Some ethnic groups consistently demonstrate higher accomplishments across nations and compared to other ethnic groups within a multicultural community (Sowell, 1996). Cultural capitals may also serve as protective mechanisms against health risks, including acculturation stress and substance abuse. One example is the lower infant mortality among Latina women in spite of their relative poverty and lower access to health care services (Kar and Alex). Several authors have suggested that religiosity, moral codes, strong family ties, culturally conditioned gender roles, and ethnic identity and pride are among the cultural capitals that may serve as protective mechanisms against substance abuse (Bhattacharya; Brown and John; Ellickson; Kar and Alex; Pentz; Ringwalt, et al.). Prevention interventions must interact with culturally conditioned beliefs, values, knowledge, attitudes, and practices (BVKAP) affecting health risk; in combination with an organized program, these factors affect preventive health behavior and program outcomes. A significant lesson we have learned from successful prevention campaigns is that effective prevention programs should not be based upon the old "hypodermic model" of communication, which held that messages injected by powerful media or sources into a community will be a sufficient cause for changing people's behavior independent of social and cultural influence (Kar and Alex). This hypodermic model conceptualized the public as passive and captive subjects manipulated by a powerful external intervention. Subsequent behavioral science and communication research underscores the importance of several psychosocial factors in risk behavior. These psychosocial factors, including cultural relativity, selective perception and retention, interpersonal influence, group pressure, expectancy, personal efficacy, and value maximizing, help to explain why the old hypodermic model of social action programs must be rejected. We need to have better understanding of the culturally conditioned influences on risk taking behavior to develop effective substance abuse intervention programs.

Culture and Health Behavior Matrix

One framework for looking at culturally conditioned factors that influence health-related behavior is conceptualized in Table 1. The basic tenet of this model is that an individual's culturally conditioned beliefs, values, knowledge, attitudes, and practices (BVKAP) influence his/her health-related behavior through five dimensions/processes: belief about disease etiology, preferred modality of treatment, locus of decision/responsibility, communication and social relations, and accessibility of information and services. These forces influence not only which sources of prevention information will be taken seriously, but also how substance use decisions are made. The cultural beliefs and norms about smoking, drinking, substance abuse, and their consequences, can either reinforce or negate the effects of prevention communication on these matters from outside sources.

Table 1. Health Behavior Matrix: Modern and Traditional Societies

Cultural Beliefs, Values, Knowledge, Attitudes, and Practices	Modern Societies (e.g., U.S., U.K., Canada)	Traditional Societies (e.g., Japan, India)
Disease Etiology	Modern Scientific—believes in germs, genes, toxins, trauma	Unitary Cosmic and Magico-religious—believes in Chi, Yin/Yang, Karma)—and Modern Scientific
Preferred Treatment Modality	Modern Clinical and Surgical-Specialist Driven	Traditional Medical, Spitirual, and Self-Care Augmented by Modern Medicine
Locus of Responsibility	Individual and Personal	Collective, Familial Decision, Hierarchic and Compliant
Communication/ Social Relations	Mass Media: Printed and Electronis; Formal and Impersonal	Informal Personal Network Augmented by Modern Media
Accessibility of Services	Highly Variable, Low/No Access for Disadvantaged	Traditional Services More Accessible and Affordable

Source: S. Kar, et al. (1998). Acculturation and Quality of Life: A Comparative Study of Japanese-Americans and Indo-Americans. *Amerasia Journal*, 24(1):129-142.

Some cultures may conceptualize disease etiology in terms of a cosmic or unitary force and not in terms of specific causal factor (e.g., germs, genes, toxins, and trauma). Consequently, specific regimens recommended by Western medicine do not necessarily fit in those cultural etiologies, and prevention efforts as we know them may not be relevant in such situations. In addition, in some cultures, religion, spirituality, and healing practices are inextricably linked. Many traditional cultures encourage healing practices under the direction of traditional healers, and in some of these cultures, ritualistic use of illicit substances is not uncommon. Ethnic groups also vary significantly in terms of the sources they prefer to use for health related information and decisions (Delgado; Kar and Alex; Ringwalt, et al.; Sanders-Phillips). The role of informal communication networks, traditional healers, and alternative medicine and their effect on substance abuse across cultures is not well understood. Substance abuse prevention and intervention should therefore strive to understand those cultural factors and utilize them to create effective programs; the five dimensions suggested in Table 1 may be a useful framework to examine how traditional and modern cultures view and deal with health related issues including substance abuse.

It is interesting to note that most traditional cultures do not completely reject modern medicine, but rather selectively integrate elements of both traditional healing and modern medicine. While many ethnic groups who have lived in the United States for generations may not be as closely tied to their original cultures as recent immigrants, some of the cultural norms and health related practices may have been sustained throughout the years. These norms and practices must be recognized in order for a program to be effective. In a multicultural community, we need to understand the communication networks and sources of information that are perceived to be most credible by the members of each ethnic groups and incorporate these elements into prevention efforts. In Table 1, we illustrate how these five domains may affect health related behavior in two very different types of societies: those acculturated in modern industrialized societies and those that are acculturated in traditional cultures.

ISSUES AFFECTING
PREVENTION INTERVENTION

A Dual Approach

To be effective, substance abuse prevention interventions must be well designed, sustained over time, and utilize a dual approach: reduction of the demand for substance abuse and reduction of the supply of tobacco, alcohol, and illicit substances in the environment (Bhattacharya; McCaffrey, 1997; Roemer). Such interventions should adopt a dual approach aimed at reducing: a) demand for substance use, and b) supply of drugs in the environment. Effective interventions tend to be those that are school based with strong parental and community support. Several chapters of this volume deal with this issue in greater depth (Brown and John; Delgado; Ellickson; Johnson; Pentz; Ringwalt). Programs directed at adolescents are generally more effective when specific prevention goals are also reinforced by their parents, social norms, and the community at large. Research also suggests that some determinants are more malleable through interventions than others, and that programs that focus on the malleable determinants are more likely to have an effect. Malleable determinants include relevant perceptions, memory, cognition, group influences, and behavioral skills (Johnson). School-based programs that emphasize these malleable factors and social influence are likely to be more successful than those which focus on cognitive changes alone. However, we are less certain about the relative effectiveness of these programs across various ethnic groups for two reasons. First, available school based studies usually report intervention outcomes by age/grade/gender rather than by ethnicity; and second, interventions are neither designed for nor evaluated by different cultural groups. Several authors have argued convincingly for an approach that includes both school and community based interventions simultaneously.

Community Based Prevention

Compared to the impacts of school based interventions, the evidence is less conclusive about the effectiveness of community level interventions across ethnic groups. Indeed, a major concern among the authors and participants of our workshop is that we know very little about the relative risks, socio-cultural determinants, and efficacy of prevention interventions by major ethnic groups. Given our current state of knowledge, two major research questions need to be addressed: To what extent would a "standard" intervention model that is effective among the mainstream population be effective across major ethnic groups? And, what are the attributes of effective interventions by major ethnic groups? Several chapters identified cultural factors that affect substance abuse risks and interventions, some of which have been addressed in the previous section of this chapter. We mention here several additional factors that are conditioned by culture.

The role of culturally conditioned beliefs about health related risks and the lack of fit between these and specific prevention measures prescribed by the Western medicine is likely to have a major impact on substance abuse prevention efforts (Pentz). Substance abuse is a learned behavior that is acquired through prolonged interpersonal interactions with the adolescents' socio-cultural network. To adolescents, it is a rite of passage from childhood to adulthood as well as an assertion of independence. In this context, substance abuse behavior is affected by two sets of perceived socio-cultural norms: perceived prevalence of substance use and perceived social approval of substance abuse (Johnson). Substance use/abuse norms vary across cultures and it is important that interventions aimed at changing individual behavior are supported by the norms of his/her culture. If adolescents are cautioned to refrain from substance abuse behavior at school but at the same time find their parents and other adults in the community behave in ways that contradict with these proscriptions, it sends a mixed message, which is often interpreted as a sign of permissiveness. It is important for school based interventions to be complemented and supported by community norms. Programs that are able to create a synergy between school and community based interventions will ultimately be more effective. Among adults, due to the cumulative effects of poverty, discrimination, and helplessness, some social groups, notably African-American women, suffer from disproportionately high levels of stress and depression; alcohol and substance abuse becomes a self-destructive way to cope with existential trauma (Sanders-Phillips).

Successful community based programs require the active involvement of local leadership and community based organizations (CBOs). Most programs fail to involve local leaders, especially mothers, who have the greatest stake in prevention efforts. When these individuals are involved, it is usually only to seek their support after the program has been designed by professionals. Several authors have made a persuasive case for greater emphasis on community partnership and empowerment for prevention efforts (Bhattacharya; Delgado; Kar, et al.; Pentz; Ringwalt; Roemer). In addition, ethnic groups vary significantly in their choices of health related information sources. We cannot assume that a medium that is popular among the mainstream population will be effective for various ethnic groups. Indeed there is strong evidence that mainstream media do not reach different ethnic groups equally (Kar and Alex). Consequently, community based interventions must be designed to meet the socio-cultural realities of ethnic groups. In order to adjust to multicultural realities, programs must mobilize local leadership and resources. This position is best summarized by the following quote from the former Surgeon General of the United States: "Special population groups often need targeted preventive intervention efforts, and such efforts require understanding the needs and the disparities experienced by these groups. General solutions cannot always be used to solve special problems" (DHHS, 1991).

Religion, Religiosity, and Prevention

Several authors have raised questions about the role of religion, religiosity, and religious leaders in prevention and intervention; however this is still an uncharted area (Eiseman, 1997; Kar and Alex; Pentz; Ringwalt, et al.). While the importance of involving local churches and religious leaders has been frequently noted, especially in the African-American and Latino communities, we do not clearly understand how different religions and religiosity within each faith affect risk behavior. It is difficult to separate the influence of religion from culture in a specific ethnic group; however, several religious groups explicitly discourage alcohol and tobacco use, and some of these groups have significantly low rates of use. An exploratory study of Sephardic Jewish and Hindu women revealed that both groups, notwithstanding acculturation stress experienced by them, had extremely low consumption of alcohol; the author identifies several common attributes of these two religions that function as protective mechanisms against alcohol use (Eiseman, 1997). These religious proscriptions have nothing to do with good or bad health outcomes per se, but rather with morality, or good and evil. The basic tenet is that alcohol use can lead to immoral and evil conduct and hence is not consistent with religious values and practices (Eiseman, 1997). It would be beneficial to study several religious groups with very low prevalence or abstinence from alcohol and tobacco (e.g., Moslems, Mormons, Buddhists, and Sikhs) to determine if there are common precepts that serve as protective mechanisms and how these precepts can be used in designing preventive interventions for other groups without necessarily challenging their respective religious beliefs.

Components of a successful intervention include an understanding of cultural and religious attributes, collaboration with policymakers, and media use to influence social norms. However, we have barely begun to develop interventions that are targeted at high-risk subgroups while simultaneously influencing societal response and norms in support of such interventions (Brown and John; Ellickson; Johnson; Pentz).

Legislation, Public Education, and Empowerment

Several authors and participants emphasized the importance of a strategy that combines legislation, public education, and community empowerment (Bhattacharya; Brown and John; Delgado; Ellickson; Kar and Alex; Pentz; Ringwalt, et al.; Roemer; Sanders-Phillips). Legislation, in combination with public education and community activism, is one of the most effective modalities of prevention intervention. Recent progress in reducing automobile injuries and cigarette smoking rates for the general public in the United States are among the many success stories of legislative intervention supported by public education and appropriate support services. In her chapter, Roemer carefully analyzes the issues and modalities through which effective legislation can reduce both the demand for substance abuse among those at risk and the supply of harmful substances. It is important to emphasize here that there is a cyclic relationship between effective legislation and public education; public education often precedes and generates support for legislation, and legislation in turn can promote public education by generating resource for public education. For instance, the passage of California's Proposition 99 required robust public education and advocacy campaigns; the proposition in turn generated tax revenue used for anti-tobacco media and educational campaigns. Roemer cites examples of the power of "sting" operations by parents to prevent supply (access) of cigarettes to school children, and Rev. Butt's social activism for removing tobacco and alcohol billboards in Harlem. Organized social action for monitoring compliance with legislation and local ordinances has an important role in the legislation-education paradigm. This requires effective community empowerment and leadership development (Bhattacharya; Brown and John; Delgado; Ellickson; Kar, et al.; Ringwalt, et al.; Roemer; Sanders-Phillips).

Our own content analysis of forty case studies of women initiated and women led successful empowerment movements across the world revealed several common elements (Kar, et al., 1997). These include: women and mothers can be a powerful force in grass roots movements for risk prevention; concerns for protecting their children from imminent harm is a motivation strong enough to unite diverse ethnic groups for combined action; professionals, local leaders, and CBOs play important roles as catalysts and allies in social action movement; and empowerment education, legislative action, and advocacy are important steps for sustaining and institutionalizing a grass roots movement. Our analysis also revealed that regardless of the nature of the problem, and level economic development of the community, these grass roots movements used various combinations of seven methods represented the acronym **EMPOWER**. These seven methods are **E**mpowerment training and leadership development; **M**edia use and advocacy; **P**ublic education and participation; **O**rganizing partnerships, associations, cooperative, and coalitions; **W**ork/job training and micro-enterprise; **E**nabling services and assistance; and **R**ights protection and social action/reform.

Communication between Researchers and Community

Decades ago, British philosopher Sir C.P. Snow argued that, in our modern era, scientists and the public live in two distinctly different worlds and that there is a lack of communication between these two cultures (Snow, 1964). This lack of communication adversely effects both cultures and ultimately our society at large. Scientific culture suffers because the public does not fully appreciate the value of scientific knowledge and society suffers because scientific knowledge is not fully utilized by the public and by those who make public policy decisions. Researchers often share their results exclusively with their peers and are not interested in communicating with the general public. In addition, researchers are preoccupied with generating knowledge; with few exceptions, they are seldom involved in planning or implementing community based interventions. Several authors lament the fact that we not only have gaps in our current knowledge, but often what we do know is not well used in intervention planning. The need for better communication between the researchers and interventionists cannot be over emphasized. In Chapter 12, three practitioners succinctly describe the communication gap between the researchers and the practice community (Massey, Ortiz and Alex). They point out that the practitioners and the community often lag behind the new knowledge generated by researchers on prevention strategies, they often lack technical expertise necessary for systematic needs assessment and evaluation of their own programs, and that they are unable to share their problems and experiences with others. There are stereotypes that adversely affect communication and collaboration. Practitioners perceive the researchers as opportunists who use the community for research but do not care about helping the community solve local problems, and that researchers often treat community members as their inferiors. Consequently, mutual lack of respect and communication becomes an insurmountable problem. They also cite examples of successful collaboration with UCLA units, including our Office of Public Health Practice, that have enabled community-based agencies and academic researchers to collaborate on mutually beneficial projects. Joint on-the-job continuing education programs, outreach activities, and workshops are among the mechanisms that enhance communication and mutual trust between the researchers, practitioners, and the community. Since that writing by Snow, in the industrialized societies, the commercial communication sector has emerged as a more powerful force than ever before in our history. The communications industry has a significant influence on setting national agenda, policy and research priorities, research utilization, and especially on the flow of scientific information to the public.

Media as a Risk Factor

It is ironic indeed that modern communication media has itself emerged as a risk factor. Programs on television glamorize sex, drugs, and violence. In so doing, the media create a virtual reality which may be perceived by uncritical viewers (especially young children) as actual norms of our society and therefore acceptable behavior (Kar and Alex). For instance, the tobacco and alcohol industries have used the modern media to promote products that are hazardous to health; at the same time they have reportedly withheld scientific findings that demonstrate adverse effects of their products. There is clear evidence that a higher proportion of tobacco and alcohol advertisements and billboards are aimed at minority communities (Brown and John; Delgado; Johnson; Kar and Alex; Roemer). An example of this is tobacco industry efforts to withhold the fact that tobacco smoking is carcinogenic and that nicotine is addictive (Roemer). Given this situation, it is now more important than ever before for the researchers to be proactive in sharing scientific knowledge with the public. The lack of communication and collaboration between the researchers and the public is not unique to the substance abuse field. The challenge before us is to find effective ways to enhance communication between the researchers and the public so that systematic knowledge about substance abuse and culturally consistent and effective interventions can be generated and utilized. With the rapid expansion of the communications media, particularly the emergence of Internet, concerned research institutions can make information available online (Web sites) for use by the public and community based organizations (CBO).

A Conceptual Model

Figure 1 presents a prevention model that integrates the major findings and recommendations for substance abuse prevention research and intervention discussed in this volume. This prevention model focuses on two major categories of determinants that affect substance abuse behavior. First, the two proximal (or most immediate) antecedents of substance abuse behavior are *demand* for substance use and *supply* or availability of alcohol, tobacco, and other substances. Researchers and policy analysts have argued that interventions that reduce both demand and supply are likely to be more effective than those that focus on only one of these proximal determinants. Indeed, the "Performance Measures of Effectiveness (PME)" system adopted by the Office of the National Drug Control Policy focuses on three clusters of outcomes for evaluating intervention effectiveness; these are reduction in demand for drugs, supply of drugs, and negative consequences of abuse (McCaffrey, 1997). While these three sets of performance measures are sufficient for a summative evaluation, effective prevention interventions should be based upon a sound understanding of the factors that determine the demand for and supply of drugs.

In Figure 1, we present three categories of determinants that affect demand and supply; these determinants, in turn, affect behavior. These three categories of distal determinants are: personal factors, community factors, and program/intervention factors. The authors and participants of our STAR project have repeatedly emphasized that, while substantial research results are available on personal level determinants of substance abuse, community level determinants are not well understood. Similarly, although we have an understanding about the effectiveness of school based programs, we do not know how effective these programs may be in the community across major ethnic groups. We know very little about the determinants of intervention effectiveness in ethnic minorities and multicultural communities. We present examples of factors under each category of distal determinants and wish to emphasize that these are not complete lists. Indeed, one theme that prevails through all the chapters in this volume is that we need to know more about the specific and malleable variables under these categories so that appropriate interventions can be developed to address these determinants. This is particularly true for ethnic minorities and multicultural communities.

The thick solid arrows in Figure 1 indicate the direct effects that are our primary concern; the dotted lines indicate effects of outcomes (feedback) on behavior and its proximal determinants. It is important to note that, theoretically, there could be many more paths of hypothesized relationships and interactions among these five categories (2 proximal and 3 distal) of determinants and behavior. Our aim here is not to present a list of all such possibilities; rather, the aim of this proposed prevention model is to bring into focus the three important categories of distal determinants, which, along with the two categories of

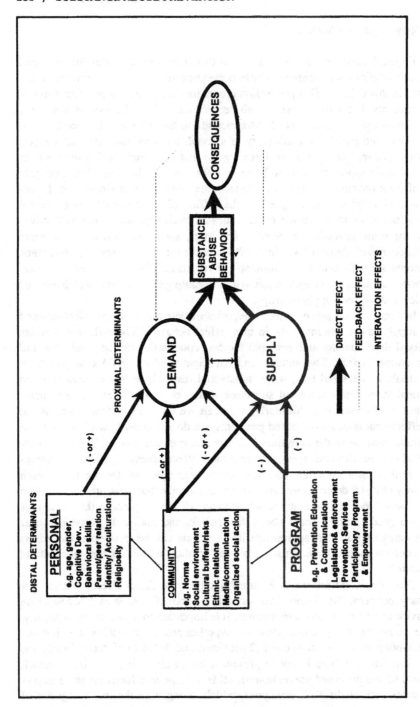

Figure 1. Proximal and distal determinants

proximal determinants, are of critical importance in prevention research and intervention.

RECOMMENDATIONS

Action Research

Over fifty years ago, eminent psychologist Kurt Lewin introduced the "action research" paradigm (Bargal, et al., 1992). "The idea of action research combined two components that he [Lewin] was concerned about, the systematic, preferably experimental, study of social problem, and efforts at its solution" (Bargal, et al., 1992). Lewin was among those who led a movement termed as Research-cum-Action (RCA) model that was extensively used nationally and internationally, especially in agriculture, community development, and health/family planning, with impressive results (Lewin, 1992; Piotrow, et al., 1997; Rogers, 1973). Beginning in the 1950s and 1960s, international donors and foundations (including the Ford and Rockefeller Foundations) sponsored numerous demonstration projects in primary health, family planning, and agriculture and rural reconstruction in Asian, African, and Latin-American countries. More recently, there has been a resurge of interest in participatory action research (PAR), community empowerment, and empowerment evaluation as integral processes in population based public health practice. Through these approaches, researchers and community residents can effectively collaborate as partners in health and human services programs (Fetterman, et al., 1996; Hall, 1979, 1981; Isreal, et al., 1994; Minkler, 1992; Park, et al., 1993; Pilusik, 1996; SPRA, 1982; Tandon, 1981; Yeich and Levine, 1992; Zimmerman, 1995). Participatory action research has also gained acceptance among several researchers in the field of alcohol related problems (Langton, 1995). The four objectives of alcohol related participatory research, which emerged from collective efforts sponsored by the Center for Substance Abuse Prevention (CSAP), are equally applicable to other types of substance abuse research, particularly in multi-ethnic communities (Howard, 1995/in Langton, 1995). These objectives are to: (1) understand how to develop science based intervention in ethnic communities, (2) learn more about the effective process of transfer of technology on promising prevention strategies between ethnic communities, (3) better understand ethnic communities as unique resources for social change, and (4) further develop participatory research methodology in ethnic communities (Howard, 1995).

Most researchers in academic settings are not accustomed to participatory research because their research is generally driven by scientific interests rather than by community priorities. In addition, their research actions are often dictated by those sponsoring the research. Furthermore, because they are primarily motivated to share research information with their peers, researchers tend to disseminate research results via peer-reviewed journal publications, books, and conferences. The community usually serves as the source of data and subject of research; the community may not have any say about the research topic, methods, and may not even have access to the results. Given this situation, many academic researchers are likely to resist a participatory action research model that requires shared control of research with the community. In recognition of this problem, the Institute of Medicine (IOM) asserted that research aimed at solving community problems requires a fundamentally different paradigm and has championed the cause of participatory action research, as was discussed in detail elsewhere (Kar and Alex) (see Chapter 1, Figure 1).

Community Participation and Empowerment for Risk Prevention

The importance of community participation in social change has been well documented in the literature. Over 150 years ago, Alexis deTocqueville observed that, in spite of our rugged individualism, Americans' unique sense of personal efficacy combined with self-interest make us more likely to participate in civic associations and social action to solve our community problems than most other countries (Bellah, et al., 1985; Perkins, et al., 1996). More recently, researchers have attempted to identify additional factors that affect citizens' participation in solving local problems. Research shows that participants' economic investments (e.g., homeownership) and self-interest in protecting such investments act as the driving force for grass roots organizations (Prestby, et al., 1990). Other studies have identified additional factors, which contribute to participation in social action by citizens, including: (1) individual psychological factors (skills, attitudes, and self-identity), and (2) inter-group relationships (including communication and group dynamics, group identity, coalition building, and empowerment) (McKnight, 1994; Zander, 1990; Zimmerman, 1990). Finally, research has shown that levels of community participation by citizens may vary by demographic and geographic variations (Perkins, et al., 1996). These results suggest two significant research questions related to health promotion, including substance abuse risk reduction: Is the desire to protect our children from health hazards, including the dangers of substance abuse, a sufficient motivation for a diverse community to come together for social action to prevent these risks? And, if so, how do we build and sustain an effective partnership with a multicultural community, especially the parents, for successful substance abuse prevention movements?

We do not have decisive answers to these questions. However, numerous case studies illustrate that ordinary citizens, including women and mothers from even the most disadvantaged social strata, can and do organize successful grass roots movements when they are driven by desperate need to protect their children and themselves from imminent harm, (Bair and Cayleff, 1993; Kar, et al., 1997; Pilisuk, et al., 1996; WFS, 1993). Examples of successful grass roots movements led by women include the International Planned Parenthood Federation (IPPF), the Mothers Against Drunk Driving (MADD); the Tri-valley Citizens Against Radioactive Environment (CARE); parents' "sting" operations against cigarette sales to minors and demand for removal of cigarette and alcohol billboards from school environments all in the United States; the Quiche Indian peasant's movement for human rights and safety led by Nobel laureate Rigoberta Menchu in Guatemala; the powerless mothers' movement demanding information about their sons who "disappeared" under military junta rule in Argentina (Madres de Playa Mayor); the poor women's movement against economic discrimination and sexual harassment known as the Self-Employed Women's Association (SEWA) in India (Kar, et al., 1997).

It is important to remember that fault lines existing within many multicultural communities can lead to rifts between different groups and discourage collective participation. For example, in South Central Los Angeles, historical tensions between Black, Hispanics, and Asians (particularly Korean shop-owners) has been well-recognized, particularly since the civil unrest of 1992 (Skerry, 1995). When economic scarcity creates a competition for resources, opposing groups tend to break down along ethnic lines. In order to enlist the support of an entire multicultural community, these forces must be reckoned with in developing substance abuse prevention programs. The question before us is: What can bring a diverse group together for collective action?

In our own efforts organizing a multicultural and highly distressed community in South Central Los Angeles during the last five years, we have discovered that an extremely diverse community can unite for collective action when two powerful forces converge. One such unifying force is the parents' desire to protect their children from "harms" which they defined as drugs, violence, and unsafe sex. The second unifying force is our community based public health practice project which offered a real opportunity for the parents to participate in a prevention program to protect their children and at the same time receive employable skill development training for themselves. This combination of participation in community change and real skill development helped the residents to feel empowered. We found that motivation to protect their children from harm and a real opportunity to enhance their income potential can override ethnic fault-lines and empower communities to tackle problems, such as substance abuse, with the knowledge that all ethnic groups are working towards a common goal (Kar, et al., 1997).

Synergy between Substance Abuse Prevention and Public Health

Another impediment to the implementation of community-based prevention programs has been the lack of coordination between the fields of substance abuse and public health. For years, these two disciplines have tended to conduct research and develop programs independent of one another. Furthermore, the field of substance abuse has historically been more closely linked with the clinical fields than with public health. This situation is further exacerbated by the fact many schools of public health overlook this area and do not require courses on multiculturalism or substance abuse. Substance abuse research institutions, on the other hand, do not reach out to schools of public health for collaborative research and teaching. As a result, few public health graduates end up working in the field of substance abuse. However, this scenario is slowly changing as substance abuse is increasingly being viewed as a public health problem.

There is much to be gained by integrating the fields of public health and substance abuse, particularly as the focus shifts to community-based prevention programs. Schools of public health can play an important role in effectuating this change. First and foremost, schools of public health can recruit faculty members with expertise in substance abuse to teach courses and supervise student internships. The importance of the M.P.H field placement requirement should not be overlooked—a recent student survey at UCLA indicated that 79 percent of students consider the internship to be an integral component of the M.P.H. training (Chickering, et al., 1998). As more students become exposed to this area of public health, more public health graduates will find jobs in this field. This will help to fill a leadership gap because, at the present time, the majority of people working in community-based substance abuse prevention do not have formal training in public health. Schools of public health can also offer direct assistance to community-based organizations (CBOs) by providing training, such as in-service seminars or certificate programs, to agency staff. Trainings may include topics such as basic research methods, grant-writing, program planning, and evaluation. Community-based agencies can also effectuate change and actually assist schools of public health better to train their students. By offering internships/field placements to graduate students, community-based organizations can help to ensure that graduate training programs remain practical and culturally relevant. The areas of critical need for technical support from universities to communities and CBOs has been clearly and forcefully articulated by the practitioners (Massey, Ortiz, and Alex)

Clearly, researchers need to make a concerted effort to not only share their findings, but to translate them into culturally relevant terms for the communities at stake. Schools of public health can also take this one step further and assist local communities to address the problems that have been identified. By forming partnerships, schools of public health, schools of social welfare, and local agencies can share information on a consistent basis and develop more effective programs. Such partnerships may include joint grant writing efforts and program development, task forces, workshops, coalition building, policy development, and the production of manuscripts, guidebooks, or prevention materials.

In sum, the key issues related to substance abuse and prevention in a multicultural community are: (1) difficulty defining and measuring multiculturalism, especially the construct of multicultural identity, (2) lack of knowledge about relative risks or prevalence of substance abuse by major ethnic groups; for instance the *Health, United States 1998* and other national surveys do not provide data for Asian Americans who may be vulnerable to substance abuse due to high acculturation stress, (3) inadequate understanding of the determinants and sequelae of substance abuse that are common to all ethnic groups and unique to each, (4) cultural themes, values, and processes that affect risk behavior, protective mechanisms, and prevention, (5) effectiveness of "standard" prevention models developed with mainstream population for specific ethnic groups, (6) need for effective and comprehensive community based prevention and empowerment models that are based on the lessons learned from two interrelated fields: substance abuse and public health, and (7) need for participatory action research for social action to augment standard research in substance abuse prevention. The new public health model, which has evolved as a result of changes in risk patterns and social trends, serves as an important paradigm for community based substance abuse prevention in partnership with the public (Kar and Alex). A synergy between the two related fields, substance abuse prevention and public health, would be an important force to deal with the challenges ahead.

REFERENCES

American Demographics (1991). *American Diversity, Desk Reference Series, #1*. Ithaca, NY: American Demographics Magazine.

Bair, B. and Cayleff, S., Eds. (1993). *Wings of Gauze, Women of Color and the Experience of Health and Illness*. Wayne State University Press: Detroit, MI.

Bargal, D., Gold, M. and Lewin, K., Eds. (1992). Special Issue: The heritage of Kurt Lewin—Theory, research, and practice. *Journal of Social Issues*, 48:2.

Bellah, R., et al., Eds. (1985). *Habits of the Heart: Individualism and Commitment in American Life* (Chapter 1). University of California Press: Berkeley, CA.

Bhattacharya, G. (1998). Drug use among Asian-Indian adolescents: Identifying protective/risk factors. *Adolescence*, 33(129):169-184.

Cantril, H. (1965). *The Pattern of Human Concerns*. Rutgers University Press: New Brunswick, NJ.

Cazeres, A. and Beatty, L. A., Eds. (1994). *Scientific Methods for Prevention Intervention Research*, NIDA Research Monograph 139, NIH Publication No. 94-3631.

Chickering, K. L., Malik, T., Halbert, R. J. and Kar, S. B. (1998). Re-inventing the field training experience: Building a practical and effective graduate program at the UCLA School of Public Health. *American Journal of Public Health* (in press).

Cruickshank, J. K. and Beevers, D. G. (1989). *Ethnic Factors in Health and Disease*. Butterworth-Heinemann: Oxford.

DHHS: U.S. Department of Health and Human Services (1991). *Healthy People 2000: National Health Promotion and Disease Prevention Objectives*. U.S. Dept. of Health and Human Services, Public Health Service: Washington, D.C.

DHHS: U.S. Department of Health and Human Services (1998a). *Tobacco Use Among U.S. Racial/Ethnic Groups—African Americans, American Indian and Alaska Natives,*

Asian Americans and Pacific Islanders, and Hispanics: A Report of the Surgeon General. Atlanta, Centers for Disease Control and Prevention.

DHHS: U.S. Department of Health and Human Services (1998b). *Health, United States, 1998.* DHHS Pub. No. 98-1232, Center for Disease Control and Prevention, National Center for Health Statistics: Hyattsville, MD.

Eiseman, S. (1997) (unpublished paper). Multicultural factors pertaining to use of beverage alcohol among Sephardic Jewish women and Hindu women from India. STAR Workshop, UCLA.

Félix-Ortiz, M., Fernandez, A. and Newcomb, M. (1998). The role of intergenerational discrepancy of cultural orientation in drug use among Latina adolescents. *Substance Abuse & Misuse,* 33(4):967-994.

Fetterman, D., Kaftarian, S. and Wandersman, A., Eds. (1996). *Empowerment Evaluation, Knowledge and Tools for Self-Assessment and Accountability.* Sage Publications: Thousand Oaks, CA.

Gordon, A. and Newfield, C., Eds. (1996). *Mapping Multiculturalism.* University of Minnesota Press: Minneapolis, MN.

Hall, B. (1979). Knowledge as a commodity and participatory research. *Prospects,* 9:4-20.

Hall, B. (1981). Participatory research, popular knowledge, and power: A personal reflection. *Convergence,* 14:6-17.

Harwood, A., Ed. (1981). *Ethnicity and Medical Care.* Harvard University Press: Cambridge, Massachusetts and London, England.

Howard, J. M. (1995). Alcohol prevention research in ethnic/racial communities: Framing the research agenda. In P. A. Langton (Ed.), *The Challenge of Participatory Research: Preventing Alcohol-Related Problems in Ethnic Communities,* SAMSHA, DHHS Publication No. (SMA) 3042:441.

Isreal, B. A., Checkoway, B., Schulz, A. and Zimmerman, M. (1994). Health Education and community empowerment—Conceptualizing and measuring perceptions of individual, organizational and community control. *Health Education Quarterly,* 21(2):149-170.

Kar, S. B., Campbell, K., Jimenez, A. and Gupta, S. (1995). Invisible Americans: An exploration of Indo-American quality of life. *Amerasia Journal,* 21(3):25-52.

Kar, S. B., Chickering, K. and Pascual, C. (1996). *Public Health Practice in a Multicultural and Underserved Los Angeles Community: A Case Study* (Monograph). Bureau of Health Professionals/Public Health Service: Washington, D.C.

Kar, S. B., Pascual, C. and Chickering, K. (1997). *Empowerment of Women for Health Promotion: A Meta Analysis.* Paper presented at the 47th Annual Meeting of Comparative International Education Society (CIES): Mexico City, Mexico.

Kar, S., Jimenez, A., Campbell, K. and Sze, F. (1998). Acculturation and quality of life: A comparative study of Japanese-Americans and Indo-Americans. *Amerasia Journal,* 24(1):129-142.

Langton, P. A., Ed. (1995). *The Challenge of Participatory Research: Preventing Alcohol-Related Problems in Ethnic Communities.* SAMSHA, DHHS Publication No. (SMA) 3042.

Lewin, K. (1992). In D. Bargal, M. Gold and K. Lewin (Eds.), Special Issue: The heritage of Kurt Lewin—Theory, research, and practice. *Journal of Social Issues,* 48:2.

McCaffrey, B. R. (1997). *Performance Measures of Effectiveness (PME): A System for Assessing the Performance of the National Drug Control Strategy*, Office of National Drug Control Policy, Washington D.C.

McKnight, J. L. (1994). Two tools for well-being: Health systems and communities. *American Journal of Preventive Medicine*, 10(3):23-25.

Minkler, M. (1992). Community organizing among the elderly poor in the United States— A case study. *International Journal of Health Services*, 22(2):303-316.

Nakanishi, D., et al. (1998). *1998-99 National Asian Pacific American Political Almanac*. UCLA Asian American Studies Center: Los Angeles, CA.

Orlandi, M. O., Ed. (1992). *Cultural Competence for Evaluators, A Guide for Alcohol and Other Drug Prevention Practitioners Working with Ethnic/Racial Communities*, DHHS Publication No. (ADM) 92-1884.

Park, P., Brydon-Miller, M., Hall, B. and Jackson, T., Eds. (1993). *Voices of Change: Participatory Research in the United States and Canada*. Ontario Institute for Studies in Education: Canada.

Paul, B. D., Ed. (1955). *Health, Culture, and Community: Case Studies of Public Reactions to Health Programs*. Russell Sage Foundation: New York.

Penn, N. E., Kar, S. B., Kramer, J., Skinner, J. and Zambrana, R. (1995). Ethnic minorities, health care systems, and behavior. *Health Psychology*, 14(7):641-646.

Perkins, D. D., Brown, B. B. and Taylor, R. B. (1996). The ecology of empowerment: Predicting participation in community organizations. *Journal of Social Issues*, 52(1):85-110.

Pilisuk, M., McAllister, J. and Rothman, J. (1996). Coming together for action—The challenge of contemporary grassroots community organizing. *Journal of Social Issues*, 52(1):15-37.

Piotrow, P. T., Kincard, D. L. and Rinehart, W. (1997). *Health Communication: Lessons from Family Planning and Reproductive Health*. Praeger Publishing Group: Westport, CT.

Prestby, J. E., Wandersman, A. F., Floring, P., et al. (1990). Benefits, costs, incentive management and participation in voluntary organizations: A means for understanding and promoting empowerment. *American Journal of Community Psychology*, 18:117-149.

Rogers, E. M. (1973). *Communication Strategies for Family Planning*. Free Press: New York.

Shinagawa, L. H. (1998). The impact of immigration on the demography of Asian Pacific Americans. In D. Nakanishi, et al. (Eds.), *1998-99 National Asian Pacific American Political Almanac*. UCLA Asian American Studies Center: Los Angeles, CA.

Skerry, P. (1995). The Black alienation: African Americans vs. immigrants. *New Republic*, 212(5):19-21.

Smart, J. and Smart, D. (1994). The rehabilitation of Hispanics experiencing acculturative stress: Implications for practice. *Journal of Rehabilitation*, 60(4):8-14.

Snow, C. P. (1964). *The Two Cultures: And a Second Look*. 2nd ed. University Press: Cambridge.

Society for Participatory Research in Asia (1982). Participatory research: An introduction. *Participatory Research Network*, series no. 3: New Delhi, India.

Sowell, T. (1996). *Migrations and Cultures: A World View*. Basic Books: New York.

Tandon, R. (1981). Participatory research in the empowerment of people. *Convergence*, 14:20-29.

U.S. Census Bureau (1990). *1990 Census*. Department of Commerce, U.S. Census Bureau Website.

Women's Feature Service (1993). *The Power to Change*. Zed Books Ltd.: London, England.

Yeich, S. and Levine, R. (1992). Participatory research's contribution to a conceptualization of empowerment. *Journal of Applied Social Psychology*, 22:1894-1908.

Zander, A. (1990). *Effective Social Actions by Community Groups*. Jossey-Bass: San Francisco, CA.

Zimmerman, M. A. (1990). Towards a theory of learned hopefulness: A structural model analysis of participation and empowerment. *Journal of Research in Personality*, 24: 71-86.

Zimmerman, M. A. (1995). Psychological empowerment: Issues and illustrations. *American Journal of Community Psychology*, 23(5):569-579.

Contributors

Shana Alex, B.A., is the Program Assistant at the UCLA Office of Public Health Practice. She received her B.A. in American Politics with a minor in Urban Planning and Public Policy from the University of California, Los Angeles, in 1997. Her current research interests include urban policy, Los Angeles regional policy, and national issues of multiculturalism.

Gauri Bhattacharya, D.S.W., A.C.S.W., received her D.S.W. and M.S.W. from the Adelphi University, Garden City, New York, and a master's degree in Economics from Calcutta University, India. Dr. Bhattacharya's research areas include substance abuse prevention, the economics of substance abuse treatment, and timely health care seeking related to HIV/AIDS. She was a Principal Investigator on research projects funded by the National Institute on Drug Abuse on substance abuse prevention among minority adolescents. She is an expert on developing risk reduction and health promotion strategies among Asian and other immigrant groups. Her professional specialties focus on adolescent development, parent-child communication, and substance abuse prevention in multicultural communities; research methodology; and program evaluation. She is a licensed clinical social worker. Dr. Bhattacharya emphasizes on integrating scientific research with clinical practice and public health policy. Recently, she joined as an assistant professor in the School of Social Work at the University of Illinois at Urbana-Champaign.

Lawrence Brown, M.D., M.P.H., serves as the Senior Vice President for Medical Services, Evaluation and Research at the Addiction Research and Treatment Corporation. He has appointments as Attending Physician at Harlem Hospital, Assistant Clinical Professor of Medicine, Columbia University, College of Physicians and Surgeons, and Clinical Associate Professor of Public Health of the Cornell University Medical College. Dr. Brown's scientific contributions have focused upon treatment for drug addiction and drug abuse-related HIV transmission. He has made presentations at national scientific, public health and medical meetings, and authored over forty peer-reviewed articles, over ten chapters, and in excess of 100 published abstracts.

Dr. Dorothy C. Browne is an Associate Professor, Department of Maternal and Child Health, UNC School of Public Health. She received her BA from Bennett College and her MPH, and Dr.P.H. from Harvard University. Dr. Browne began her career at UNC-CH working on a prospective study of stress, social support, and family violence, with her colleague, Dr. Jonathan Kotch (PI). This study, which is on-going, examined the relevance of an ecological model of child abuse and neglect proposed by her and her colleague. This study has provided evidence that social support mediates the relationship between stress and child maltreatment. Until recently, Dr. Browne was the Co-PI for the North Carolina site of a national multisite longitudinal study, an outgrowth of the Stress and Social Support Project, which examines the effects of child maltreatment at various developmental stages. She is currently the PI for Project RAPP, a NIH-funded intervention and research project, examining violence and other problem behaviors among African American adolescents. A major component of this study is examining the roles of ethnic identity, ethnic socialization and discrimination in violence and other risky youth behaviors. Her publications are in the areas of family violence, youth violence and related areas.

Kirstin L. Chickering, M.P.H., is the Program Manager of the UCLA Office of Public Health Practice. For the past ten years, Ms. Chickering has worked both domestically and internationally in the fields of STD/AIDS prevention and control, family planning, and women's health. Her current activities include program development for multicultural populations and empowerment of women for health promotion. She received her M.P.H. in Behavioral Science and Health Education from UCLA and her B.A. in Political Science and French from Duke University.

Melvin Delgado, Ph.D., is currently Professor of Social Work and Chair of Macro-Practice at the Boston University School of Social Work. A faculty member there since 1979, he has also served the University as the Acting Coordinator of the Racism-Oppression Sequence and the Chairperson of the Community Organization, Management and Planning Sequence. He has been the principal investigator on many studies funded by organizations such as the Center on Substance Abuse Prevention, the Carlisle Foundation, the Massachusetts Department of Education, and the National Institutes of Health. In 1994, he received the award for the Greatest Contribution to Social Work Education from the National Association of Social Work, Massachusetts Chapter, and in 1996, he received the Outstanding Contribution to the Boston University School of Social Work Alumni Award.

Phyllis Ellickson, Ph.D., is a Senior Behavioral Scientist at RAND and Director of the Center for Research on Maternal, Child and Adolescent Health. She received her Ph.D. in Political Science from the Massachusetts Institutes of Technology and formerly served on the faculty of the Political Science

Department at UCLA. A nationally recognized expert on drug prevention, she led a multi-site, multi-year drug prevention trial (Project ALERT) that has been widely acclaimed as an exemplary program and research model. She has also published extensively on the patterns and antecedents of adolescent problem behavior, the methodological issues involved in conducting large-scale field trials, and the factors that promote successful program implementation. Her current research focuses on adolescent and young adult health (behavioral and emotional problems); the links between violence, drug use and other public health problems; access to health services; and patterns of adolescent and young adult smoking. She also serves as a faculty mentor for the RAND/UCLA Clinical Scholars Program in Mental Health Services Research.

Dr. Stanley L. John functions in the capacity of Associate Director for Evaluations and Research for the Department of Medical Services, Evaluation and Research at the Addiction Research and Treatment Corporation (ARTC). Since 1997, Dr. John has been a certified Clinical Research Coordinator with the Associate of Clinical Research Professional (ACRP). Dr. John's major contributions have been in the field of HIV clinical trials (Phases III and IV). He has also done some publishing (chapters and abstracts).

C. Anderson Johnson, Ph.D., is the Sidney Garfield Professor of Preventive Medicine in the School of Medicine and is the Director of the Institute for Health Promotion and Disease Prevention Research and Director of the Division of Health Behavior Research at the University of Southern California. Dr. Johnson's current research is in determinants of health-related lifestyles and approaches to prevention of behavioral risks for disease. This research includes tobacco, alcohol, and other drug use, nutritional practices and physical exercise, and communication strategies for health promotion. Dr. Johnson received his B.A. and Ph.D. in Social Psychology from Duke University.

Snehendu Kar, Dr.P.H., received his M.Sc. in Psychology in 1958 from the University of Calcutta, India, and his Doctorate and Master's degrees in Public Health and Behavioral Sciences from the University of California at Berkeley. His professional and research interests include acculturation and health, health communication in multicultural communities, empowerment and health education, and health promotion indicators. Dr. Kar has been a Professor of Public Health at UCLA since 1979. He is currently the Director of the MPH Program for Health Professionals (MPHHP) in Health Promotion and Health Education, and Co-Director of Public Health Practice. Previous positions include: Associate Dean and Chair of the School and Department of Public Health (1984-1988), Head of the Behavioral Sciences and Health Education Division (1980-1984), and Chair of the Asian American Studies IDP (1994-1996) at UCLA, Associate Professor and Assistant Professor at the School of Public Health at the University of Michigan,

Ann Arbor (1967-78), and the Deputy Assistant Director General (Research) at the Ministry of Health and Family Planning, Government of India, New Delhi.

Earl Massey has been the Executive Director of Surviving in Recovery since its inception and is one of its original founders. Mr. Massey also served as a case manager for an HIV/AIDS drop in center, as a substance abuse counselor for a recovery program, a special counselor for UCLA's Drug Abuse Research Center and is a qualified Pre and Post Test Counselor for HIV/AIDS. He has worked in the fields of HIV/AIDS and chemical dependency for the past seven years. Mr. Massey has also personally experienced the substance abuse recovery process for the past eight years and considers himself to be in "recovery."

Raquel Ortiz, was born and raised in Buffalo, New York. Ms. Ortiz earned her Bachelor of Science Degree in Elementary Education. She relocated to California in 1982 and went to work for The Los Angeles Unified School District. For the past fifteen years her active experience has been in educating, assisting and empowering community members to overcome and stop cycles in their lives relating to issues of substance abuse, teen pregnancy, parenting, gangs, domestic violence, and issues with youth at risk. It has been her endeavor to make a positive difference in the communities that she serves.

Mallie J. Paschall, Ph.D., is a Health Research Analyst with the Research Triangle Institute. He received his doctorate in 1995 from the Department of Health Behavior and Health Education at the University of North Carolina at Chapel Hill. Dr. Paschall's research focuses on the epidemiology, etiology, and prevention of risk behaviors among adolescents and young adults. He has published a number of articles on the etiology and prevention of adolescent and young adult violence, and is currently involved in a study on the prevention of alcohol abuse by college students.

Mary Ann Pentz, Ph.D., is Professor of Preventive Medicine and Director of the Center for Prevention Policy Research (CPPR) at the University of Southern California, where she has been since 1983. For over a decade, Dr. Pentz has developed and tested school and community prevention interventions for adolescent drug use, stress, smoking and prosocial skill development. She has over 100 publications in the area of drug abuse prevention and has served as a Chair of the NIDA Epidemiology and Prevention study section and as a member of several national evaluation review boards for community prevention studies. Her recent work in the CPPR focuses on the potential of local community policy change as a drug abuse prevention strategy in combination with prevention programs. A new NIDA study will develop and test a four-year prevention program that focuses on both protective and risk factors for drug abuse. Dr. Pentz received her Ph.D. in School and Clinical Psychology from Syracuse University.

Christopher Ringwalt, Dr.P.H., directs Research Triangle Institute's Program in Substance Abuse and Other Risk Behavior Prevention and Epidemiology, and is Chair of the Alcohol, Tobacco, and Other Drug (ATOD) Section of the American Public Health Association. His primary research interests include adolescent risk behaviors including violence and ATOD use. He currently serves as principal investigator for a number of projects, including: a grant from CDC to investigate the relationship between the development of ethnic identity and risk behaviors among African American adolescents; a grant from NIAAA to develop the capacity of faculty in a historically Black university to conduct alcohol-related research; an assessment of ATOD prevention needs of populations within North Carolina, supported by CSAP; a study of school-based drug prevention curricula, sponsored by NIDA; and a CSAP-supported study of drug prevention strategies infused into managed care settings serving public employees.

Ruth Roemer, J.D., is Adjunct Professor Emerita at the University of California Los Angeles, School of Public Health, Department of Health Services. She received her J.D. degree from the Cornell Law School in 1939. Prof. Roemer has specialized in health law and legislation. Her research has involved studies of mental hospital admission law, education and legal regulation of health personnel, laws governing abortion and family planning, organization of health services, and legislation for tobacco control. She has served as a consultant to the World Health Organization on health legislation. In 1987, Dr. Roemer was president of the American Public Health Association (APHA), and in 1991, she was awarded APHA's highest award, its Sedgwick Memorial Medal for Distinguished Service in Public Health.

Sadina Rothspan, Ph.D., received her Ph.D. in social psychology from the University of Southern California and has spent the last ten years assisting with research projects designed to reduce risky behaviors and foster healthy lifestyles. Dr. Rothspan is formerly the Project Manager for Bright STARS, the elementary school extension to Project STAR. Project STAR has received nation-wide attention for its success at reducing marijuana, cigarette, and alcohol use among middle and high school students. Bright STARS intends to foster the effectiveness of Project STAR by increasing resiliency skills through academic and social competence. Dr. Rothspan is currently continuing her education as a post-doctoral fellow in epidemiology at the University of California, Los Angeles.

Kathy Sanders-Phillips, Ph.D., a developmental psychologist, is a faculty member in the Department of Pediatrics at the UCLA School of Medicine and is currently a Senior Researcher with the UCLA Drug Abuse Research Center. Much of her research has focused on psychosocial factors influencing health behaviors and health outcomes in low income Black and Latino women and children, particularly the impact of exposure to violence on health decisions and behaviors. She has also conducted several community-based health interventions in South Central Los Angeles. She has published several papers on the impact of community-based health interventions on health behaviors in low-income, ethnic minority residents. In 1991, Dr. Sanders-Phillips was a University of California Wellness Lecture awardee for her work on exposure to violence and health behaviors in Black and Latino populations. Dr. Sanders-Phillips serves as a member of the National Advisory Council for the National Institute on Drug Abuse (NIDA) and is currently an advisory board member of the Tobacco-Related Disease Research Program at the University of California (UC). She is the former chair of the UC AIDS Taskforce and a former member of the Extramural Science Advisory Board for NIDA.

Silvana Skara is a doctoral student in the Preventive Medicine (Health Behavior Research) Program at University of Southern California in Los Angeles, California. She received her B.A. in Psychology from California State University, Long Beach. She is currently involved in research on school-and community-based tobacco, alcohol, and other drug abuse prevention interventions being conducted at the Institute for Health Promotion and Disease Prevention Research, University of Southern California, Los Angeles, California.

Saskia Subramanian, Ph.D., is an Assistant Research Sociologist in the Department of Psychiatry and Biobehavioral Sciences at UCLA. She has participated in a variety of family and youth oriented studies, including an evaluation of child abuse prevention programs for high risk populations, an investigation of community based projects designed to reduce unplanned teen pregnancy rates, and ethnographic research on female crack addicts in residential rehabilitation facilities. Dr. Subramanian is currently part of an interdisciplinary research team examining family formation, relationship satisfaction, and well-being through a twenty-one-city survey project.

Felicia Sze, M.P.H., is currently serving as a Presidential Management Intern as the Special Assistant to the Region Manager for the U.S. Department of Health and Human Services, Office for Civil Rights, Region IX. Previously, she acted as the Special Projects Coordinator for the Office of Public Health Practice at the UCLA School of Public Health. She received a Bachelor's degree in Molecular and Cell Biology–Genetics at the University of California, Berkeley in 1996 and a Master's in Public Health at UCLA in 1998. Her research interests include minority health issues, welfare reform policy and immigrant health.

David Takeuchi, Ph.D., is currently Professor of Sociology at Indiana University at Bloomington. His research interests focus on the social and cultural factors associated with health problems and health seeking behaviors, particularly with ethnic minority populations. His current projects include large scale community studies of Chinese Americans in Los Angeles and Filipino Americans in San Francisco and Honolulu.

Gencie Turner, Ph.D., is a Research Associate in the Department of Preventive Medicine, USC School of Medicine. She earned her doctorate in Health Behavior Research at USC in 1993. Research interests include women's health, cancer prevention and control, and adolescent substance abuse prevention. The majority of her experience has been with quasi-experimental and survey research, including being a Principal Investigator on a cancer screening and early detection project funded by the NCI. Currently she is studying the effects of life transitions on substance use.

Serineh Voskanian is completing her Bachelors of Science in Health Promotions and Disease Prevention Studies at the University of Southern California with a minor in Bioethics. Her research in the University of Southern California Department of Preventive Medicine is performed under the supervision of MaryAnn Pentz and Malcolm C. Pike. Through her research, she hopes to better understand the factors influencing patient behavior in order to apply this knowledge in patient care as a physician.

Index

White Americans
  African Americans' distrust of, 175
  billboards, alcohol/tobacco, 238
  cigarette smoking and other tobacco
    uses, 249, 251
  delinquency, juvenile, 114
  disrupted families, 110
  emergency room visits, 173
  fertility rates, 20
  Head Start, 113
  health and quality of life, 19, 23
  health related information, sources of,
    29-30
  infant mortality rates, 22
  influences on drug use in youth, 221
  life expectancy, 20
  marijuana, 105
  onset of drug use, 220
  parental education, 109-110
  population statistics, 20, 21, 23
  rates of drug use/abuse, 13-15, 104-106,
    111, 172, 203
  religion, 110
  social influence programs, 115
  Surgeon General, U.S., 243
  See also Ethnicity

Women/mothers organizing to prevent
    drug abuse
  appealing power of the issue, 91
  collective concern and engagement,
    91-92
  community level, the, 93-94
  conclusions, 96-97
  family roles, 79-81
  implementing the process, 92, 93-96
  individual-level concerns, 92-93
  organizations in three culturally diverse
    communities, 86-90
  organizing multicultural communities,
    82-83
  review of issues related to substance
    abuse prevention, 283
  task performance and goal accomplish-
    ment, 92
  See also Black/Hispanic women,
    psychosocial factors influencing
    substance abuse in; Gender
World Health Organization (WHO), 233

Yunus, Muhammad, 92